T0261595

Tics and Tourette Syndrome
Key Clinical Perspectives

Tics and Tourette Syndrome
Key Clinical Perspectives

ROGER FREEMAN

Clinical Professor Emeritus, Department of Psychiatry, and Associate Member, Department of Pediatrics, University of British Columbia, Vancouver, Canada

2015
Mac Keith Press

© 2015 Mac Keith Press
6 Market Road, London N7 9PW

Editor: Hilary Hart
Managing Director: Ann-Marie Halligan
Commissioning and Production Editor: Udoka Ohuonu
Project Management: Pat Chappelle

The views and opinions expressed herein are those of the authors and do not necessarily represent those of the publisher

All rights reserved. No part of this publication may be reproduced, stored in a retrieval system, or transmitted in any form or by any means, electronic, mechanical, photocopying, recording or otherwise, without the prior permission of the publisher

First published in this edition 2015

British Library Cataloguing-in-Publication data
A catalogue record for this book is available from the British Library

ISBN: 978-1-909962-41-5

Cover design: Karl Hunt

Printed by Berforts Information Press, Eynsham, Oxford, UK

CONTENTS

AUTHOR'S APPOINTMENTS

Clinical Professor Emeritus, Department of Psychiatry, and Associate Member, Department of Pediatrics, University of British Columbia, Vancouver, Canada

Neuropsychiatry Clinic, BC Children's Hospital, Vancouver, Canada

Member and former Chair, Professional Advisory Board, Tourette Syndrome Foundation of Canada

Former Member, Medical Advisory Board, Tourette Syndrome Association (USA)

Dedication

To the memory of Dr Ronald Charles Mac Keith (1908–1977)
Mentor and Colleague

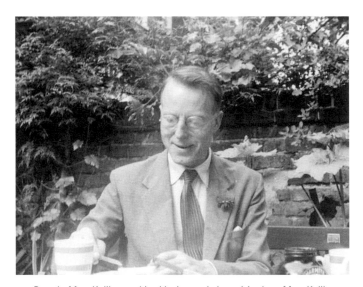

Ronnie Mac Keith, used by kind permission of Andrew Mac Keith.

FOREWORD

I first met Dr Roger Freeman in the mid-1990s when he graciously allowed me to shadow him as he diagnosed and treated children with tic disorders at the Neuropsychiatry Clinic at the Children's Hospital, Vancouver, British Columbia, Canada. At that time I was writing a book on the history of Tourette syndrome, and I quickly recognized the depth and breadth of Dr Freeman's expertise about tics and related disorders. I was most impressed, however, with how this knowledge fed into Freeman's skills as a diagnostician and clinician. His initial interviews with patients and their families were remarkable in that he listened to and engaged patients and their families rather than mechanically dispensing pharmaceuticals. Certainly, Freeman prescribes medications for the treatment of tics and eruptive vocalizations when appropriate, but his primary aim is to evoke the uniqueness of each patient in order to determine appropriate and effective intervention strategies. Freeman's search to understand Tourette syndrome led him to spearhead the worldwide '*TIC* database' that by 2013 had recorded the differing signs and symptoms of almost 7500 individuals diagnosed with Tourette syndrome. The findings of the database have reinforced Freeman's belief that his patients must be approached in the contexts in which each experiences Tourette syndrome, including at home with their families and in their schools.

Today, Roger Freeman is one of the most respected Tourette syndrome clinicians in the world. Why this is so, is evident in the pages that follow. *Tics and Tourette Syndrome: Key Clinical Perspectives* is an intellectual and clinical tour de force. It draws on Freeman's lifetime of experiences, insights and clinical research. Dr Freeman explores Tourette syndrome and tics from diagnosis and lived experience. What emerges is a nuanced examination of most assumptions about the identification, diagnosis and treatment of Tourette syndrome and tics.

Tics and Tourette Syndrome is aimed at those working in neurodisability and child development, with some extensions into adult development of those with developmental problems. It also will appeal to a wide range of clinicians including neurologists, pediatricians, physiatrists, specialist occupational therapists, physical therapists, orthopedic surgeons, audiologists, speech pathologists and psychologists. Throughout the book Freeman inserts brief but fascinating and compelling patient case studies as exemplars of the conditions and processes he is discussing. Drawn from his 50 years of practice, these cases alone are worth the price of the book.

Although this foreword is not intended to serve as a book review, it may be useful to alert readers to some of the important contributions that they will discover. *Tics and Tourette Syndrome* begins with an examination of how patients (and their families) often ask different questions and have different goals from those of the clinicians who diagnose and treat them.

Freeman notes that the progress in identifying and treating Tourette syndrome in the past four decades has sometimes been a double-edged sword. On the one hand, it has authorized the belief that childhood tics and eruptive vocalizations constitute an organic disorder rather than resulting from repressed early childhood psychological stress. On the other hand, the diagnosis has sometimes become promiscuous, resulting in 'diagnostic creep', in which children with mild tic presentations can inappropriately be labeled and treated as if they meet the criteria for Tourette syndrome.

There are more than a few other unique contributions and discussions that readers will discover in the pages that follow, including: details on stereotypies and stereotypic movement disorder; help for clinicians dealing with patients with Tourette syndrome, such as surgeons, ophthalmologists, optometrists, dentists and other medical specialists, who might not realize why their patient cannot keep still; the variability and frequency of copro-phenomena, which have been greatly misunderstood; and misleading information that may be found, especially on the internet, about the onset, course and effective treatments for Tourette syndrome.

All of these issues and many more are examined in 27 concise and accessible chapters. Drawing on his case studies, Freeman elucidates symptom patterns, including anger, rage and inappropriate sexual behavior. He also examines the occurrence of physical symptoms such as headache, pain and enuresis. While he has wisely decided not to reproduce every new claim and study related to Tourette syndrome (although he provides a citation road map of how a reader may do so), he does review important new research claims, such as the role of autoimmune antibodies in the etiology of Tourette syndrome, and the implication of new hypotheses for interventions and treatments.

Tics and Tourette Syndrome should be required reading for all clinicians and others who diagnose and treat movement disorders. Although aimed at clinicians, this volume will greatly benefit affected individuals and their parents, whether they read the book from cover to cover or simply use it as a resource to answer specific questions. Finally, it will prove incredibly useful not only for those who want to learn specifically about tics and Tourette syndrome, but also for clinicians and lay persons who seek to understand the complexity of neuropsychiatric syndromes in general.

Howard I Kushner, PhD
Nat C Robertson Distinguished Professor
Program in Neuroscience and Behavioral Biology;
and Department of Behavioral Sciences and Health Education
Rollins School of Public Health
Emory University
Atlanta, GA

ACKNOWLEDGMENTS AND CONFLICT OF INTEREST DECLARATION

Acknowledgments

I was fortunate indeed to attend Johns Hopkins School of Medicine, where the focus was on learning and broad experience rather than — as for many of my college classmates at other medical schools — competition to memorize vast amounts of factual material, much of which would be soon forgotten. In addition to an elective in child psychiatry under Leo Kanner, I spent a summer doing gout research under Harry Klinefelter, research on dogs that included translating a cardiology book from Dutch to English, and in my senior year providing Victor McKusick with translations of papers from several languages on rare syndromes when he was starting his epochal work on genetics after leaving spectral phonocardiography.

After I returned from internship and general psychiatric training at McGill University in Montreal, Philadelphia became my base for 9 years during which I started working with teams of pediatricians and therapists as well as having a small role in the early research on temperament led by Stella Chess, and at St Christopher's Hospital for Children (Temple University) where I started a child psychiatric service for children with disabilities within John Bartram and Henry Baird's team in what was then the Handicapped Children's Unit.

Fellowship in the American Academy for Cerebral Palsy and Developmental Medicine started my long association with colleagues in neurodisability and sensory impairment in many countries, and specifically the UK (Ronald Mac Keith, Martin Bax, Philip Graham and Michael Rutter, among others). At all points I benefited from mentors in fields other than my own, an influence which has shaped the remainder of my career.

During my 44 years in Vancouver my closest research colleague has been James E Jan, neurologist, and in the tic field I have had particularly close associations with Larry Burd, Jack Kerbeshian, Mary Robertson, Diane Fast, Sam Zinner and Paul Sandor, along with too many others to list here, including those in the Tourette Syndrome International Database Consortium, Donald Cohen and James Leckman at Yale University, and those I was fortunate to work with at the Tourette Syndrome Association (USA) and the Tourette Syndrome Foundation of Canada. When Howard Kushner spent a year in Vancouver teaching 'The History of the Brain' at Simon Fraser University I was privileged to sit in on his course and to benefit from his encyclopedic knowledge of the history of Tourette syndrome as well as his observing some of our clinical work.

Recognition is due to the US Centers for Disease Control and Prevention, whose collaborative support for the Tourette Syndrome Association has made the rapid development of behavioral treatment possible. I would be remiss if I did not highlight the excellent work of the German researchers Kirsten Müller-Vahl, Aribert Rothenberger, Veit Roessner, and Tobias Banaschewski and the German Tourette Syndrome Association. Anyone with a reasonable knowledge of German can profit from reading Müller-Vahl's 2010 book.

The many members of the *TIC* database consortium and their patient data made it possible to generate illustrative points throughout the book. Daniel Picchietti helped bring my knowledge of sleep disorders and particularly restless legs syndrome up to date.

Udoka Ohuonu (Commissioning and Production Editor) and Ann-Marie Halligan (Managing Director) have been stalwart supporters of the high standards of medical writing for which Mac Keith Press is known. Finally, Pat Chappelle has done the most thorough and inspired copy editing I have ever encountered. Seeing the many errors in recent books and papers I had thought that this skill had atrophied to the point of extinction, but my faith has been restored.

Conflict of interest declaration

In 1972–73 I acted as one of three consultants to the US Food & Drug Administration's Bureau of Drugs in reviewing stimulant medications for childhood ADHD. In that capacity I eventually became highly critical of a pharmaceutical company's submission, and later wrote (in general) about problems in the drug approval process (Freeman 1973: Drug research: out of sight, out of mind. *J Spec Educ* 7: 223–8) and twice testified before the Kennedy Senate Subcommittee. That testimony has been published (Freeman 1974: Statement for Senate Health Subcommittee Hearings. In: *Examination of the Pharmaceutical Industry 1973–74, US Senate Hearings.* Washington, DC: US Government Printing Office, pp. 2866–74; and testimony before Senator Edward Kennedy, pp. 2861–5). I testified twice for plaintiffs in actions against the specific company alluded to above. I later declined to accept the opportunity to join in a multisite trial on a drug I considered to be too risky for Tourette syndrome.

However, this personal history of sometimes critical or adversarial actions does not indicate that I have never cooperated with, or at times appreciated, contacts with pharmaceutical companies. I have received small honoraria for advisory board meetings where there was no restriction upon my expression of opinion. I have served as a consultant on tetrabenazine for Shire Pharmaceuticals when they owned the rights to that drug and Valeant Canada for the same drug later. Some end-of-year surplus funding from Roche Canada for an open study that was never undertaken was allowed to be added to my Tourette Syndrome and Tic Research Endowment Fund without any conditions attached. In one desperate case a company acted with amazing rapidity (within a day) to provide a drug not then available in Canada (and requiring a special exemption because Tourette syndrome was not an approved indication in the USA) for one of my most severely affected patients. In that case the drug made (and continues to make) all the difference in that young man's life after more than 17 different medications had proven unsuccessful.

LIST OF ABBREVIATIONS

ADHD attention-deficit/hyperactivity disorder
ASD autism spectrum disorder
BFRB(D) body-focused repetitive behavior (disorder)
CBIT Comprehensive Behavioral Intervention for Tics
CBT cognitive–behavioral therapy
CMT chronic motor tic disorder
CTD chronic tic disorder (TS+CMT+CVT)
CVT chronic vocal tic disorder
C-YBOCS Children's Yale–Brown Obsessive–Compulsive Scale
DCD developmental coordination disorder
DCDQ Developmental Coordination Disorder Questionnaire
DMDD disruptive mood dysregulation disorder
DSM *Diagnostic & Statistical Manual of Mental Disorders*
DSM-III-R *Diagnostic & Statistical Manual of Mental Disorders, Version 3, Revised* (1987)
DSM-IV-TR *Diagnostic & Statistical Manual of Mental Disorders, Version 4, Text Revision*
    (2000)
FAS fetal alcohol syndrome
FGA first-generation antipsychotic
GAD generalized anxiety disorder
ICD International Classification of Diseases
MDD major depressive disorder
OCB obsessive–compulsive behaviors that are significant but do not reach OCD level
OCD obsessive–compulsive disorder
ODD oppositional–defiant disorder
PANDAS pediatric autoimmune neuropsychiatric disorders associated with streptococcal
    infections
PKD paroxysmal kinesigenic dyskinesia
PLMS periodic limb movements in sleep
PMTD persistent motor tic disorder (same as chronic motor tic disorder in DSM-IV-TR)
PTSD post-traumatic stress disorder
PVTD persistent vocal tic disorder (same as chronic vocal tic disorder in DSM-IV-TR)
PTD provisional tic disorder (same as transient tic disorder in DSM-IV-TR)
RLS restless legs syndrome (Willis–Ekbom disease)
RMB repetitive motor behavior
SGA second-generation antipsychotic
SIB self-injurious behavior

SLD specific learning disability
SMD stereotypic movement disorder
SSRI selective serotonin reuptake inhibitor
TBI traumatic brain injury
TS-only Tourette syndrome without comorbidity
TS+ Tourette syndrome with comorbidity
TSA Tourette Syndrome Association (USA)
URI upper respiratory infection
WED Willis–Ekbom disease (restless legs syndrome)
YBOCS Yale–Brown Obsessive–Compulsive Scale
YGTSS Yale Global Tic Severity Scale

1
INTRODUCTION

If everybody is thinking alike, then somebody isn't thinking.

George S Patton, Jr

I have a confession to make. When I gave talks about children's developmental problems over 40 years ago, I poked fun at the development of a plethora of service organizations for unusual or rare disorders, and used the example of the Tourette Syndrome Association, which almost always got a laugh from the audience. Fast forward to more modern times…

- As I was leaving the Emergency Room I heard the 34-year-old accident victim with a head injury in the next cubicle being interviewed. Asked how he felt, he replied "Like I'm going to do a Tourette's!" "What?" he was asked. "You know, start cursing big-time!"
- Discussing politically incorrect or racist statements, a *Time* magazine article commented "It's as if the U.S. were experiencing collective Tourette's, regurgitating decades of dutifully sublimated hate" (James Poniewozik, Dec. 4, 2006, vol. 168, no. 23, p. 52).
- On October 26, 2011, Diane Sawyer, a well-known TV interviewer, reported on her exclusive interview with Bernie Madoff who was in prison for his all-time record defrauding of American investors (he was not permitted to be on TV). She stated that he showed a "nervous tic", with the implication that this was an indication of his discomfort, that her questions were 'getting' to him.

The first incident is an indication of how coprolalia (the blurting out of inappropriate words) has entered public consciousness as the hallmark of Tourette syndrome. In the second, the writer expects the general reader to understand the allusion to impulsive coprolalia. The third is an instance of the confidence that people have about the signal function of tics, because it required no explanation.

How times change! Forty years ago I could say anything about Tourette syndrome without fear of contradiction — no longer! How could I have known that I would later consider it an honor to serve the Tourette Syndrome Association's Medical Advisory Committee and other committees for nine years, as well as the Tourette Syndrome Foundation of Canada, when I had made fun of the very idea of an organization for this 'rare' condition previously? From a 'disease' confidently asserted to be rare and exotic to a common problem that is the subject of jokes in the popular media, the increasing information about Tourette syndrome now represents both a success and, sometimes, a problem for those with tics and their families.

Many textbooks in medical specialties, home medical 'encyclopedias' and internet-based information contain authoritative-sounding but often wrong, conflicting, or confusing information, and paint an overly bleak picture of life's typical course with tics and Tourette syndrome (some examples are given in Appendix 1). Since parents searching for help often go to these sources (especially when there is a long wait to see a specialist), it is important to be aware of the major errors that they are likely to encounter. Among these are: the prevalence is 'rare'; the cause is psychological stress of some kind; tics will go away if you ignore them, but get worse if you pay attention; it is always 'life-long' and 'serious'; it requires treatment with medication (often life-long); coprolalia is common, or rare, or a necessary characteristic; comorbidity, if mentioned at all, is not given an adequate perspective.

One can easily see why a parent would be confused and maybe horrified to receive such a diagnosis and physicians might be reluctant to impart it. When parents do receive a diagnosis, the meanings derived from it may amplify their fears, invade their hopes and expectations, and cause serious problems in their family life. It is absolutely essential for the clinician to recognize what makes Tourette syndrome unusual (if not unique) among childhood chronic recurrent illnesses or disorders, because it is these characteristics that drive the initial sufferings of parents and open an opportunity for relief.

Since the course of most persistent tic disorders in childhood is typically unstable, as experienced by parents it has many of the characteristics of a seemingly progressive neurological disease that has befallen their child. Subsequent diagnoses of comorbid (apparently new) disorders may compound this sense of catastrophe. Other conditions in childhood such as eczema and asthma are typically recurrent, but the manifestations are usually the same or similar with each exacerbation. Not so usually with Tourette syndrome! "It's always changing", many parents spontaneously lament, and the majority of children have — or develop — comorbid disorders.

It is said that a person's tics may be referred to as "just his/her fashion". And for many with mild tics this may be entirely appropriate and non-stigmatizing.

But consider this. In Franz Kafka's famous novella *The Metamorphosis*, Gregor Samsa, a seemingly ordinary traveling salesman, awakens to find himself turned into a sort of giant beetle or verminous insect. He continues at first to think of himself as late for work, and his family's reactions of disbelief, horror, shame and progressive alienation make up much of the bizarre tale. But can this be an allegory for what happens with the sudden onset of multiple tics? Can the child's taken-for-granted identity become transformed? Is the child still who he or she was, imbued with the same hopes and expectations, or not? Can this be expressed, shared within the family, later articulated for the busy clinician? If not, how important is what is missed?

Case example

'Dominic', a bright 11-year-old, had had tics and anxiety for two years. When his psychiatrist, becoming more aware of his vocal tic, mentioned that he now met the criteria for Tourette syndrome, he became upset and started to withdraw from his friends. He

> explained that he was "*no longer the same person*". He didn't want anyone to rein-
> force the perceived change by commenting about his tics.
>
> **Comment:** *In this instance the severity of the reaction seems to have been contin-
> gent upon the rigidity of his thinking and emotional sensitivity, already evident for
> years. This reaction was not relieved, at least in the short term, by discussion of the
> relationship of Tourette syndrome to other tic disorders and the arbitrariness of the cri-
> teria. For other children, applying the diagnosis might result in relief that the symptoms
> had a name.*

In reality, then, one of the most serious problems plaguing clinical practice with patients who have tics is the vast variability in symptoms, severity, interference, associations and complications, all accorded meanings by the experiencing person, their family and social group. Many patients have only minor tics with minimal to no comorbidity that never constitute serious or obvious problems or threats to self-esteem. For them the question is: *Is the Tourette syndrome or other tic diagnosis important? A benefit or harm? If so, how?* Other patients have upsurges in symptoms — old or new — several times a year that challenge accommodation by parents, teachers and peers. Some (fortunately relatively few) render James Leckman's evocative phrase "the self under siege" (Leckman et al. 2006) highly appropriate: dreadful, constantly changing tics, comorbid torturing symptoms, and a greatly impaired existence. These are the cases where the medieval 'demonic possession' concept becomes comprehensible, even to those for whom religion holds no interest or commitment. Yet even in such situations the personal meanings will differ.

It is typically stated that the history of Tourette syndrome starts with Itard in 1825, who described the noblewoman Marquise de Dampierre in Paris, well known for her swearing uncontrollably in public. However, there is a much earlier description of what may have been Tourette syndrome (perhaps combined with obsessive–compulsive disorder [OCD]), published in 1486. Two Dominican monks, Sprenger and Kramer, were appointed inquisitors by Pope Innocent VIII and are reputed to be the authors of the manual of the Inquisition (the *Malleus Maleficarum*), whose task it was to root out heretics and cases of demonic possession. It became the basis for witch trials and in 200 years went through 20 editions (Mackay 2009). The pertinent selection reads as follows.

In the time of Pope Pius II the following was the experience of one of us... A certain Bohemian brought his only son, a priest, to Rome to be delivered because he was possessed ... When he passed any church and genuflected ... the devil made him thrust out his tongue; and when asked whether he could not restrain himself from doing this, he replied: 'I cannot help myself at all, for so he uses all my limbs and organs, my neck, my tongue, and my lungs, whenever he pleases, causing me to speak or to cry out; and when I try to engage in prayer he attacks me more violently, thrusting out my tongue.' A venerable bishop ... who had been driven from his see by the Turks, piously took compassion on him, and by fasting on bread and water for forty days, and by prayers and exorcisms, at last through the grace of God delivered him, and sent him back to his home rejoicing.

Another variation on a similar 'case' in the *Malleus* is given (in German) by Müller-Vahl (2010).

3

Practice point

Even with the best available scientific information, aspects of the individual's experience and the relationships among his or her symptoms will remain opaque. A wise clinician does not take for granted that he or she fully knows what a patient is experiencing or how a symptom is affecting him or her, and will inquire, and listen.

Public health importance

The public health aspects of Tourette syndrome have recently become a focus of attention by the US Government (Centers for Disease Control and Prevention [CDC] National Center on Birth Defects and Developmental Disabilities) in partnership with the Tourette Syndrome Association USA (TSA-USA). In 2009 the CDC published the first American national survey of Tourette syndrome prevalence.

Case studies and examples

Throughout the book there are examples representing actual persons or combinations of features (with names and other identifying information altered to protect privacy: the names given are in quotation marks to indicate this). These are not full stories, nor do many tell of an outcome; they are snapshots or parts of a life course to illustrate a specific point or confusion. Many of them are excerpted from clinical encounters of up to 47 years ago, in more than one country. Briefer points are termed 'case examples', a few with more in-depth information are termed 'case studies'.

Case examples

'Eli' was a 12-year-old Chinese immigrant boy, doing well in school and exceptionally bright, who developed fairly severe tics including some coprolalia despite having no other comorbidity. After the diagnosis was imparted by a specialist, the parents went to the internet. They developed a worry that for a time seriously skewed family life: putting limits on his computer usage (which had been recommended) led to angry opposition from him; they feared this reaction would cause his tics to worsen and stay worse, maybe even cause brain deterioration, so they allowed unlimited usage. When this got completely out of control, the police were called on more than one occasion to deal with the violence triggered by separating him from his computer.

'Zachary', age 12, was referred because of a 5-year history of significant tics: eye-blinking, head-turning, throat-clearing, spitting, touching things to his tongue, skipping, and having to even up sensations felt to be on only one side of his body. He would get a feeling where the tic was going to emerge, and it was very hard to resist. His parents described a clear waxing–waning pattern, worse with stress. He had not encountered much teasing, had friends, was doing well in school and displayed a sense of humor.
    Comment: *This is a typical, straightforward, relatively uncomplicated case.*

Why are tics important in neurodisability?

First, there is an increased likelihood of the occurrence of tics in neurodisability due to differences in brain structure and function. Second, there is a decreased likelihood of their identification because other matters concerning the disability may seem much more important, or the tics may be misidentified as something else (e.g. stereotypy or other repetitive behaviors). Third, even after the establishment of the importance of the role of tics in the totality of the person's symptoms and functioning, this may change and require reassessment because of upsurges of new or old tics, responses of the tics to changes in environmental factors, reactions to medications to treat other non-tic issues, or misunderstandings.

Scope

The focus of this book is clinical and the basis for material being included is clinical utility. It would be fruitless to try to summarize the cutting edge of scientific publishing. By its very nature much will be pruned back or modified; what remains may have little clinical utility at present, and will in any event be modified by the time of publication. For the reader who wishes to try to keep up-to-date with the voluminous literature, a regular PubMed or Google Scholar search is recommended.

What seems most practical and, it is hoped, of some lasting value is to portray realistically the many issues represented by the diagnosis and clinical management of tics and their sometimes co-occurring problems. The wide range of variation along several dimensions poses a special challenge. Also given consideration are the common reasons for misdiagnosis or delayed diagnosis, the benefits and harms of a diagnosis, common myths or misunderstandings, self-injurious tics, adult-onset tics, medication-refractory Tourette syndrome, tics that present problems when co-occurring with some other neurodevelopmental disorder, conditions that may be confused with tics (such as stereotypies and autistm spectrum disorder), the family and school context, and associations with sensory peculiarities. Omitted are some categories from the *Diagnostic and Statistical Manual of Mental Disorders, 5th Edition* (DSM-5) that pose excessive complexity or are deemed relatively unrelated to tic disorders (such as personality disorders and schizophrenia), although that is not to say that the combination of any condition with a tic disorder might not pose special problems.

'Simple' or single tics

Although the boundaries of tic disorders are arbitrary, we need to realize that there is a difference between persons with persistent single tics and those with a complex changing picture, whether they meet Tourette syndrome criteria or not. Most of what is discussed in this book will apply to the latter, but not necessarily to the former. There is actually little research on the former group.

Limitations

With the DSM-5, released in May 2013, there were changes in the diagnostic criteria for tic disorders. How these may affect the continued relevance of information and opinion in this book and previous works that are still available is unknown. Despite unprecedented years of preparation involving participants from countries other than the USA and disciplines other than psychiatry, as well as rounds of public input, controversy has been stirred about many aspects (including the addition of new disorders, the broadening of some diagnostic criteria, and the potential for increasing opportunities for pharmaceutical companies) and has reached the media (Gornall 2013). Publication of proceedings, revisions of textbooks and a blizzard of articles will follow for several years. Unless a new, significant and replicated etiologic finding and links to possible new treatments are forthcoming, this book's focus on tic disorders, not just Tourette syndrome, is not dependent upon every detail of the arbitrary diagnostic criteria. Although some changes of direct relevance will be mentioned, this book is not intended as a comprehensive handbook for super-specialists in the field (for this, see Martino and Leckman 2013, though published before the DSM-5), nor as a treatment manual for exceptionally complex cases.

If some of the statements or recommendations seem arguable or idiosyncratic, the reader will do well to keep in mind that there are few aspects of tics and Tourette syndrome that are not contested or contestable, and that is one way in which progress occurs. "The critical discussion of even our best theories always reveals new problems" (Karl Popper 1994, p. 159).

Several good recent resources include books by Woods et al. (2007), Robertson and Cavanna (2008), Brown (2009), Pliszka (2009), Singer (2010), Fahn et al. (2011), Walkup et al. (2012), Burn (2013), and Martino and Leckman (2013).

Conventions and abbreviations in this book

Persons with tics or Tourette syndrome will be referred to, when in a clinical context, by using the traditional appellation 'patients', not 'clients'.

Tourette syndrome itself has been referred to in a number of ways: Gilles de la Tourette disease, disorder, or syndrome; Tourette's disorder or syndrome, and Tourette disorder or syndrome, with related abbreviations. Of course there are other referents for some of the acronyms, such as TD = tardive dyskinesia, TS = tuberous sclerosis, etc. In this book, TS-only refers to non-comorbid or 'pure' Tourette syndrome, and TS+ to those with comorbidity.

TIC database

Throughout this book findings are reported from the *TIC* database. The *TIC* project (*T*ourette Syndrome *I*nternational Database *C*onsortium) was established in 1996 with the aim of finding out more about the large differences characterizing clinical cases of Tourette syndrome among sites, each of which had different selection criteria resulting in variable published results. At that time the prevalence of Tourette syndrome was thought to be about 1 in 10,000 so that epidemiologic research on representative community samples was felt to be impracticable. Possible, however, would be the compiling of clinical information on a large sample of the world's clinics and the identification of common trends in the data.

A collaboration was initially set up among sites in Vancouver, BC; Grand Forks, North Dakota; and Winnipeg, Manitoba. The Tourette Syndrome Foundation of Canada sponsored a meeting in Montreal at which a short and simple data entry form was designed, to enable use in standard clinical practice without requiring much time per patient or specific research funding.

Introduction

Over the next several years, 67 sites in 27 countries joined and started submitting data to the registry. Medical specialists involved varied at each site and included psychiatrists, neurologists, pediatricians and medical geneticists. Results from the first 3500 cases were published in 2000 (Freeman et al. 2000) and by 2007 there were 6805 cases (Freeman 2007). This number was more than enough to meet the original goals, and the total dataset is now fixed at 7481 (24% of whom are adults). The dataset was made available in anonymized form to any Consortium member for research projects and publications. A list of publications may be found in Appendix 4.

REFERENCES

American Psychiatric Association (2013) *Diagnostic and Statistical Manual of Mental Disorders, 5th edn.* Arlington, VA: American Psychiatric Association.

Brown TE, ed. (2009) *ADHD Comorbidities: Handbook for ADHD Complications in Children and Adults.* Washington, DC: American Psychiatric Publishing.

Burn DJ, ed. (2013) *Oxford Textbook of Movement Disorders, 2nd edn.* Oxford: Oxford University Press.

Centers for Disease Control and Prevention (2009) Prevalence of diagnosed Tourette syndrome in persons aged 6–17 years – United States, 2007. *MMWR Morb Mortal Wkly Rep* 58: 581–5.

Fahn S, Jankovic J, Hallett M (2011) *Principles and Practice of Movement Disorders, 2nd edn.* Edinburgh/ New York: Elsevier/Saunders.

Freeman RD (2007) Tic disorders and ADHD: answers from a world-wide clinical dataset on Tourette syndrome. Tourette Syndrome International Database Consortium. *Eur Child Adolesc Psychiatry* 16 (Suppl 1): 15 23.

Freeman RD, Fast DK, Burd L, et al. (2000) An international perspective on Tourette syndrome: selected findings from 3500 individuals in 22 countries. *Dev Med Child Neurol* 42: 436–47.

Gornall J (2013) DSM-5: a fatal diagnosis? *BMJ* 346: f3256. doi: 10.1136/bmj.f3256.

Leckman JF, Bloch MH, Scahill L, King R (2006) Tourette syndrome: the self under siege. *J Child Neurol* 21: 642–9. doi: 10.1177/08830738060210081001.

Mackay C (2009) *The Hammer of Witches: A Complete Translation of the Malleus Maleficarum.* Cambridge, UK: Cambridge University Press.

Martino D, Leckman JF, eds (2013) *Tourette Syndrome.* New York: Oxford University Press.

Müller-Vahl K (2010) *Tourette-Syndrom und andere Tic-Erkrankungen in Kindes- und Erwachsenenalter.* Berlin: Medizinisch Wissenschaftliche Verlagsgesellschaft.

Pliszka SR (2009) *Treating ADHD and Comorbid Disorders: Psychosocial and Psychopharmacological Interventions.* New York and London: Guilford Press.

Popper KR (1994) *The Myth of the Framework: In Defense of Science and Rationality.* London: Routledge.

Robertson MM, Cavanna A (2008) *Tourette Syndrome, 2nd edn.* Oxford: Oxford University Press.

Singer HS, Mink JW, Gilbert DL, Jankovic J (2010) *Movement Disorders in Childhood.* Philadelphia: Saunders/Elsevier.

Walkup JT, Mink JW, McNaught KStP, eds (2012) *A Family's Guide to Tourette Syndrome.* Bloomington, IN: iUniverse/Bayside, NY: Tourette Syndrome Association.

Woods DW, Piacentini JC, Walkup JT, eds (2007) *Treating Tourette Syndrome and Tic Disorders: a Guide for Practitioners.* New York: Guilford Press.

2
DIAGNOSIS AND DEFINITIONS

Although all definitions are imperfect, the description of Tourette syndrome is of a pattern of tics varying over time, often starting with a single tic and progressing to greater number and complexity, in upsurges or 'bouts' of old and/or new patterns that can come to the attention of almost any kind of specialist as well as primary care clinicians. Typical tics are repetitive, randomly occurring, rapid contractions of muscles or muscle groups. There are three general categories: Tourette syndrome requiring at least one vocal tic and two or more motor tics present for at least a year; persistent motor or vocal tic disorder (not both); and provisional tic disorder. Distress or impairment are not required. Tic onset is often unclear because the first tic wasn't identified as a tic but as something else. Some repetitive movements may be wrongly assumed to be tics or simply co-occur. Because tics can be temporarily affected by excitement, stress, or talking about them, it may be wrongly concluded that these factors are causative and should be strictly avoided. A major factor in clinicians missing the diagnosis is non-simultaneity; another is confusion with stereotypies. Tics may rarely occur in various neurologic conditions, but usually accompanied by other neurologic signs or symptoms. When the clinical picture or subsequent course seems atypical or puzzling, further consideration and consultation are in order. No tests are usually necessary for the tic diagnosis. Comorbidity is the rule, rather than the exception, and its presence always requires careful consideration, especially since it often results in more impairment than do the tics themselves. Information on the internet is typically perused by patients and parents, but contains much that is misleading.

What is a tic?

A tic is described as a stereotyped (but not by everyone), repeated (but not rhythmic), usually rapid and brief movement or vocalization. The diagnosis of the typical case of Tourette syndrome is relatively straightforward. The description is of a pattern of waxing and waning tics over time, with the comment to the effect that "something new always replaces them" or "it's changing". As we shall see in further detail in Chapter 7, a tic can take many forms, some quite surprising, and therefore can come to the attention of almost any kind of specialist.

The official DSM-5 criteria (American Psychiatric Association 2013) are a substantial change from those in the former *DSM Version 4, Text Revision* (DSM-IV-TR) (American

Psychiatric Association 2000). Essentially there are three categories that cover most tic disorders:

(1) *Tourette's disorder* requires multiple motor and one or more vocal tics both present at some time (not necessarily simultaneously) for at least one year, a waxing and waning course, onset before age 18, and not attributable to effects of a substance or other medical condition.
(2) *Persistent motor or vocal tic disorder* is defined by having single or multiple motor or vocal tics but not both, with the specification "with motor tics only" or "with vocal tics only".
(3) *Provisional tic disorder* requires one or more tics present for less than one year, when the criteria for the other two categories have never been met. This is a replacement for the older category of 'transient tic disorder' in DSM-IV-TR.

Rarely the category 'other specified tic disorder' may be used when there is a specific reason given to not make one of the three diagnoses above, and 'unspecified tic disorder' when there is insufficient information or no specification of the reasons. (Note that the general term 'disorder' is used, whereas this book and many others use 'syndrome' for Tourette syndrome, instead.)

Problems with the diagnoses
There is a problem with lists of kinds of tics, often portrayed along two dimensions: simple versus complex and motor versus 'vocal'. Some repetitive patterns are almost certain to be tics, others may be something else, and the dividing line between simple and complex is often less clear than the lists imply.

Another problem is that while 'vocal' is in the definition, it is not clearly defined as 'noises made with the vocal cords and surrounding structures', and therefore has gradually spread far beyond that meaning. (Why are whistling and sniffing on some lists as 'vocal'?) How does this become accepted? Because 'phonic' is often substituted for 'vocal' further confusion is introduced. Why is clicking your teeth, drumming on a table, or noisily knocking your knees together not 'phonic'? Strictly speaking, if you need at least one vocal tic for part of the diagnosis, and you say sniffing is the only 'vocal' tic present, then you may be considered by some (but not others) to meet the diagnostic criteria for Tourette syndrome. This is not always a trivial matter.

Practice point
"Tourette syndrome is the most severe tic disorder" is a common statement of purported and unquestioned fact, but is *wrong*. Why? By imposing arbitrary criteria on the tic spectrum we construct the category Tourette syndrome at one end (more complex by definition, and therefore deceptively assumed to be identical to 'severe'), but that is not the same as a continuum of impairment or social impact; those can be considered as two continua that are not simply congruent with each other. Furthermore, individual

---

impact and social impact are not congruent either because of individual differences in symptom tolerance and many other factors. This little-considered point is the source of much misunderstanding and is rarely made clear. Distress or impairment are not required for a tic disorder diagnosis.

What do parents want from an assessment?

Parents want information about causes, cures, the future, and treatment possibilities (usually excluding medications, at first).

The history

It is a fundamental observation that many parents cannot initially identify when tics began, because the identity of the first tic *as a tic* was not clear. With additional contact, observation and experience, the parent's dating of tic onset may move backwards (rarely forwards) in time. Children whose tics have apparently not lasted the arbitrary 12 months are often in this category: seen again and with a revised history, they then *do* qualify for the diagnosis of Tourette syndrome. The arbitrary 12-month time criterion is thus not very useful, and we find that if there are multiple and especially complex tics, it will almost certainly turn out to be a persistent tic disorder, not a 'provisional tic disorder'. The DSM-IV-TR 3-month rule (if there was ever a 3-month or greater period with no tics, then you didn't have Tourette syndrome) was always unworkable, since the threshold for tic recognition, tic recall, and the murky definition of tics were all problematic; it was thankfully abandoned in DSM-5.

Practice point

First, because many of the issues to discuss with parents involve speculation about whether the child's course will be average or otherwise, and because many children are prone to hear only part of what is said or to take qualified statements as concrete, it is always good practice to talk with the parents separately. Second, there are likely to be discrepancies between what the patient or parents have read on the internet and what you will tell them; these merit explanation [for example, no tests for the Tourette syndrome diagnosis, status of Tourette syndrome in the continuum of tic disorders, and evidence for the current validity of PANDAS (*p*ediatric *a*utoimmune *n*europsychiatric *d*isorders *a*ssociated with *s*treptococcal infections — see Chapter 19)]. Third, patients or parents with limited English require special consideration. Finally, there is usually a tendency for mothers to become the experts on their children, the fathers less so. If the latter aren't included, differences in understanding may be exacerbated. See the fathers also! Do not depend upon mothers to adequately interpret to their partners what you say to them.

Practice point

'Diagnostic creep': Some repetitive movements may not be tics (though most people don't know how to distinguish them), and much swearing is not coprolalia. If you do have a tic, there is often a tendency to identify every other repetitive motor behavior as a tic, too ('diagnostic overshadowing': Jopp and Keys 2001, Jones et al. 2008). Thus, nail-biting, nose-picking, joint-cracking, lip-licking and bruxism may be awarded honorary status as tics, and may even be used to make up the required number of tics for the diagnosis of Tourette syndrome.

Perceived role of stress and anxiety, temporary and permanent

As pattern-seekers, we may exaggerate the role of 'stress' and anxiety. While it is true that for many individuals excitement (positive or negative), stress and anxiety may temporarily be associated with a behavior such as increased tics, this is nonspecific and not causative. Many reactions and motor patterns may be increased under similar circumstances (e.g. anorexia, fidgetiness, urinary frequency and tremor). Reactions to stress-related situations may be invoked as the sufficient cause of tics and they may therefore be seen as 'psycho-somatic' or 'somatizing' and to be treated by 'reducing stress'.

Another important factor in causing parental fear of 'stress' is that they observe that talking about tics or other ways of 'paying attention' to them seems to increase the tics. Since they don't distinguish momentary or temporary increases from permanently resetting the tics at a higher level, they may feel that their reactions to some activity (e.g. video games) are *creating* (not just temporarily exacerbating) the problem.

The irregular waxing and waning of childhood tics is the source of many misunder-standings.

Case example

'Susan' went through a difficult period around age 11 when she had a loud barking tic. It bothered a child living next door who was sensitive to noise. To her mother's relief the tic diminished and was almost gone a few months later. Other less bothersome tics started soon afterwards. She noticed that when Susan played computer games she became very excited and the tics increased, including occasional barking. She engaged in a struggle to control her daughter's computer time, because she feared the activity would bring back the barking and it would continue indefinitely.

> **Practice point**
> Parents need to be helped to understand the fundamental difference between temporary aggravations of tics by various factors (including what they do with the child) and factors that will permanently exacerbate the condition. In this instance it might be good to limit computer time for a variety of reasons, but not to expect it to change the course of the tics.

Automatic suppression

Automatic suppression may deprive the clinician of the advantage of direct observation. (This refers to suppression that seems to not be effortful.) It thus isn't always easy to make the diagnosis. Non-simultaneity is a major problem: seeing one tic (if any) in the office, and only *hearing about* a few other tics in the past that were isolated in time lacks an immediate impact, so that the diagnosis may be missed or delayed. Parents may have a sense that they are not believed or that the basis for their anxiety is not fully appreciated (a major example is presented in the case example of 'Joshua' in Chapters 7 and 17).

> **Practice point**
> A major reason for failing to make the diagnosis of Tourette syndrome is in the definition, which seems clear but leads to confusion. The definition actually is clear: *tics in Tourette syndrome do not have to occur simultaneously*, but if they are not experienced together, their impact may seem too unimpressive for the clinician to make the diagnosis. Further, single isolated tics are often attributed by the parent or the clinician to some other symptom or cause, whereas if they occur simultaneously the diagnosis is much less likely to be missed.

What can happen before they reach you?

A further problem from the parental side is that the path leading to you as the competent clinician can be tedious and tortuous, and along the way much conflicting information and opinion may be picked up that must eventually be sorted out, consuming precious time. Timing is an issue too, because the first contact (usually with a primary care physician) may be at (or near) the height of a tic upsurge, but the referral to a specialist or clinic imposes a delay, and at that point the tic level is likely to have diminished. The clinician may then not be very impressed with the symptoms and the additional problem of non-simultaneity may result in no diagnosis.

Premonitory sensations or urges

Tics are sensorimotor — not just motor — phenomena, a fundamental concept established by Joseph Bliss (1980) from his own experience. They are reported by the great majority of adults, most young people, but not all young children. Their strength can be assessed and tracked by the Premonitory Urge for Tics Scale or PUTS (Woods et al. 2005), confirmed by Crossley and Cavanna (2013) and Crossley et al. (2014) for adults. These sensations may be more troublesome than the motor or vocal output, may adversely affect quality of life, and may remain when tics disappear. They are a fundamental focus of behavioral treatment.

[As will be seen later, the claim that premonitory sensations are unique to tics and a dependable distinction from other movement disorders, such as stereotypic movement disorder (SMD) and stereotypic behavior in autism spectrum disorder (ASD), is disputed in this book.]

What else could it be?

There are a large number of possibilities, many rare or with atypical presentations (Jankovic 2001, Jankovic and Mejia 2006). Although tics are most common in the head, neck and shoulder areas, they can start anywhere. If in an unusual location without other obvious tics, other types of movement disorder may be suspected. Atypical tics without a family history and occurring close to the onset of a neurologic disorder or brain trauma suggests a cause-and-effect relationship and can be termed 'tourettism'.

• *Coughs* can have many causes (Irwin et al. 2006). A respiratory tic should be suspected when each cough is stereotyped (e.g. always being done twice or some other number of times) and when it is absent in sleep and is not a cause of nocturnal awakening. As is true with many other tics, there is an urge to get it 'just right', so it may become ritualized. One may be tempted to call it a tic when a long-lasting symptom has no objective findings, but the diagnosis by exclusion may be incorrect. They may be confused with atypical asthma. The rule is: look for other tics (present now or in the past), and because patterns may not be identified as tics, take a history of other repetitive behaviors.

Practice point

When unsure if a particular movement is a tic, look for another tic or tics in the history or present, and take a history of other repetitive behaviors.

A difficulty can arise when there is a combination of factors, such as a previous upper respiratory infection (URI) with subsequent airway sensitization persisting for weeks or months and aggravated by allergy, and can trigger tics. The history may be difficult to elicit. The following case example illustrates this complexity.

Case example

'Dean' was 10 when he was examined in an emergency department because of very frequent, loud coughing for a month that kept him home from school most days. Reportedly his school found the 'cough' disruptive. His friends became reluctant to

play with him. During an influenza outbreak there was much publicity about contagion and Dean was regarded as suspiciously contagious. History revealed that he had had prolonged 'coughing' after each bout of a URI. After several visits the previous other minor tics were described and appreciated for the first time.

  Comment: *The URI was probably a trigger for a symptom that had both airway sensitization and a tic disorder as factors.*

The evidence-based clinical practice guidelines of the American College of Chest Physicians (Irwin et al. 2006) try to distinguish 'habit cough,' 'tic cough' and 'psychogenic cough' in both adult and child populations. Such coughs may have persisted since childhood. They recommend that the diagnosis of 'habit cough' be made only after ruling out tic disorders (and some uncommon disorders) and when cough improves after behavior modification or psychological/psychiatric treatment. Misdiagnosis is not uncommon. A problem with these guidelines is that automatic suppression is not mentioned and that patients or their parents often forget much earlier tics. It is not clear how tics can be so successfully ruled out.

• *Dystonias* are involuntary, sustained, patterned movements caused by opposing muscle contractions and twisting abnormal postures. They can be local or more general, and can interfere with swallowing, chewing or speech (Nambu et al. 2011, Albanese et al. 2013, Frucht 2013) and can occur in any muscles.

• *Chorea* is involuntary, abrupt, irregular, continuous and dance-like; the movements randomly migrate.

• *Akathisia* is an unpleasant inner restlessness that may make it impossible to sit still; it often leads to pacing and agitation.

• *Wilson disease* (treatable autosomal recessive inborn error of copper metabolism on 13q14.3 with basal ganglia damage, hepatic cirrhosis, and highly variable neurological signs): see Chapter 13.

• *Stereotypies and stereotypic movement disorder* are discussed in detail later, in Chapter 11. Some of those occurring in ASD may be confused with tics.

• *Benign ocular myokymia* (eyelid twitches, unilateral upper or lower, not usually both). At one time or another most people have eyelid twitches. These are *felt* but only visible on close inspection, and thus not readily observed by others. They may last minutes to days, and usually subside spontaneously. They may occur in muscles elsewhere. They are not tics, rather contractions of a bundle of muscle fibers, not whole muscles or groups of muscles. Their cause is unknown, despite common assertions in the ophthalmologic literature to treat them by reducing stress and fatigue and avoiding alcohol, caffeine, smoking and eyestrain.

In a Tourette syndrome support group meeting with parents the question was asked: "How many of you also have — or have had — any tics?" The majority raised hands, but most of them were referring to myokymia and didn't know the differences.

Rarer possibilities include the following.

• *Rett syndrome* can present with tic-like repetitive stereotypies before regression occurs (Temudo et al. 2007).

• *Neuroacanthocytosis* is a group of at least four heterogeneous disorders with genetic variability. One type is autosomal recessive, with abnormally spiculated red blood cells and a movement disorder that has Tourette-like features (mostly chorea-like, often with vocalizations, orofacial dyskinesia, parkinsonism, stereotypy, self-injurious behavior [SIB], cognitive changes, and motor and vocal tics in up to 40% of patients) (Saiki et al. 2004; Walker et al. 2006, 2010).

• *Huntington disease* (autosomal dominant) in rare cases in childhood may present with a non-choreic movement disorder involving tics, with impulsive and/or compulsive behavior and OCD features (Kerbeshian et al. 1991, Jankovic and Ashizawa 1995, Angelini et al. 1998, Becker et al. 2007).

• *Neurodegeneration with brain iron accumulation* (NBIA1, formerly Hallervorden–Spatz disease) is a rare progressive genetic disorder with onset usually in the second or third decade with dystonia, increasing dementia, rigidity, spasticity, stereotypy and OCD features, and rarely tics (Nardocci et al. 1994, Scarano et al. 2002).

• *Hyperekplexia* is a sudden gross-motor involuntary response to a sensory provocation, as in the 'Jumping Frenchmen of Maine' (Howard and Ford 1992).

• *Infections* (apart from PANDAS: see Chapter 19) that may affect brain structure or function can be the precursor of tic onset. For example, Dale et al. (2003) described a boy who, after encephalitis caused by varicella zoster, developed ADHD and multiple tics associated with basal ganglia imaging abnormalities.

Although tics are most common in the head, neck and shoulder areas, they can start anywhere. If in an unusual location without other obvious tics, other types of movement disorder may be suspected.

• *Stroke and various brain lesions* (Kwak and Jankovic 2002).

• *Pseudo-tics, 'psychogenic' tics, conversion or functional neurological movement disorders* are other kinds of movements that can be confused with tics (Kurlan et al. 1992,

Dooley et al. 1994, Jankovic 2001, Tan 2004, Ferrara and Jankovic 2008, Schwingenschuh et al. 2008) (see Chapter 9). Tics may be 'hidden' within the performance of complex stereotypies.

• *Psychogenic nonepileptic seizures* are another form of 'pseudo-tics', thoroughly discussed in Plioplys et al. (2007) and Schachter and LaFrance (2010). The latter define them as "events that resemble epileptic seizures but without epileptiform activity and with psychological underpinnings" (p. 3). These are to be distinguished from physiologic nonepileptic seizures that are cardiogenic, migrainous or sleep-induced.

• *Psychosis* (can be accompanied by movement disorders).

Case examples

'Paul', age 22, came in because he thought he might have Tourette syndrome. He had a history of eye-blinking, throat-clearing, and moving his legs up and down, as well as clenching his fists. He had been on thioridazine; a trial of haloperidol led to akathisia. Further history revealed that 4 years previously he saw satanist grafitti on a washroom wall, which seized his awareness and in response he made movements to prevent the robbing of his soul. He added: "I have to clench my fists or the comfort will leak away through my left foot." He had undergone two unsuccessful exorcisms in the previous year. He had other concerns "too secret to reveal". He was referred to a psychiatrist for exploration of his psychotic preoccupations.

    Comment: *It is possible that he had tics as well as motor responses to delusions.*

'Manuel', age 20, was a university student referred for possible Tourette syndrome. He had a clear history of motor tics (eye-blinking, platysma contractions, shoulder-shrugging, facial grimacing, head-shaking and mouth-opening). However, he had no obvious vocal tics. Instead, he showed extreme fear of vomiting, which was manifested since childhood as hyperawareness of food in his mouth, of nausea, and of eating and losing weight. He gulped and made clicking sounds when focused on not vomiting. But he also had odd ideas connected with some of his tics: if he made a lot of clicks, he'd have less anxiety later; he opened his mouth wide "to feel that it's still there", and shook his head "to feel my brain move". He was extremely bothered by his brother looking into his room because once his eyes had been in there, they would seem to stay there.

    Comment: *Although he had tics, he also seemed to have somatic preoccupations verging on the hypochondriacal or even psychotic. If his gulping and clicking were not classified as tics, then by definition he did not qualify for Tourette syndrome, rather for persistent motor tic disorder.*

• *Paroxysmal movements.* There are an increasing number of channelopathies that present with unusual patterns of abnormal movements. One of these is paroxysmal kinesigenic dyskinesia (PKD) (Kato et al. 2006, Méneret et al. 2013, Silveira-Moriyama et al. 2013). This is usually an autosomal dominant (occasionally sporadic) genetic disorder with onset in childhood or adolescence involving a rare (1/150,000) mutation in the *PRRT2* gene that is treatable with low dosages of anticonvulsants like carbamazepine or phenytoin. It may remit spontaneously in adulthood, and treatment radically improves the patient's life. For this reason three cases are briefly presented here that were referred as possible Tourette syndrome.

Case examples

Fifteen-year-old 'Eric' was referred for abnormal movements suspected of being tics. However, a written description of his symptoms by his father explained that he tended to fall over when he started to move after a long period of inactivity. There were periods of remission, but the symptoms could occur more than once a day. This led to him being teased and some avoidance of activities. His electroencephalogram was normal and he had no tics. The clinical picture was consistent with PKD and this was confirmed by a neurogeneticist. A low dose of phenytoin completely controlled his abnormal movements. Several years' follow-up showed good symptom relief and generally successful young adult functioning.

A 12-year-old boy from a remote rural area was referred for possible tics, but his abnormal movements had never been observed by a clinician until the specialist interview, in which he was asked to move after a period of sitting still. He fell over. He also was found to have classic obsessive–compulsive symptoms and a periodic perceptual alteration termed visual fragmentation. Once the diagnosis was made by an astute neurologist he was given a low dose of carbamazepine and responded with relief of all his symptoms. The story continues, however: this experience led to his decision to become a physician and many years later he was reached by the initial team and found to be a successful practicing physician (Jan and Freeman 1994). His PKD symptoms as well as the others had recurred when for brief periods he stopped taking his medication as a child, but as an adult he did not need to continue it and had complete cessation of his dyskinesia.

A mother of a patient worked in a library, filing books in the stacks. She became very anxious when she learned that she would be promoted to working at a desk to help library visitors. On inquiry the problem, despite an increased salary, was that she would be embarrassed by people being able to observe a symptom she tried to hide: sometimes when she got up or started to move she would briefly fall over but would not feel faint. She had been told years before by a neurologist that this was a 'neurotic' anxiety-related problem. A current neurological consultation identified PKD. Her daughter, who had tics, was then found to have the same disorder.

• *Gratification disorder* or infantile masturbation is another repetitive pattern that can be confused with dystonia or epilepsy (Nechay et al. 2004). This may start as early as 2 months of age (10.4 months in the recent study by Rödöö and Hellberg 2013) and is especially likely to be misdiagnosed when there is no direct manual-genital stimulation. There is even one documented case occurring in utero (Meizner 1987). For diagnosis, a video clip of the behavior in question is helpful.

The diagnosis of comorbid disorders will be discussed in Chapter 10.

What do physicians tend to get wrong in their referrals?
In a small local study referral letters to a neuropsychiatry clinic were analyzed for accuracy of information. These letters were received from pediatricians in 44% of cases, family physicians in 38%, neurologists in 12%, and psychiatrists in 6%. The most important factor in the *missed diagnosis* of Tourette syndrome was *non-simultaneity*. Unless this point is grasped, when a parent provides a history of a repetitive motor pattern that was assumed to be a habit, an allergy, imitation of others, etc., it may be uncritically accepted as such, because it is not linked with the presenting tic(s) due to separation in time. Even experienced specialists who have attended lectures on tics and Tourette syndrome may sometimes make this mistake.

A secondary factor is the lack of awareness of the differences between tics and other stereotypies. As will be seen in Chapter 11, these two patterns may usually be distinguished by age at onset, duration of episodes, and variability of the pattern over time, as well as (often) the child's attitude toward their pattern.

The worldwide web: a mixed blessing
Parents are almost certain to use the internet as a source of information, either before you see them, or thereafter, no matter what you advise. It is therefore important to have a general idea of how dependable the information there is, and a more detailed knowledge of the common misunderstandings or confusions that are likely to have their origin there. For these reasons a brief discussion is appropriate at this early point. Information on the internet regarding tics and Tourette syndrome can be very confusing for the following reasons.

• Anyone can put something on the internet and make it look impressive.
• Many sites have a mixture of well-explained and accurate information, as well as inaccurate or even bizarre information.
• Some sites are woefully out of date and though not revised for years, remain accessible.
• Information is not usually peer-reviewed, and even when reviewers' names are appended, they may not be responsible for all recent errors.
• Sites originating from medical schools and professional organizations are not necessarily more accurate than some created by individuals.
• Sources of genuine disagreement are often not indicated; only one opinion is present.
• The diagnostic subcategories and their criteria are arbitrary and temporary, but this is

usually not explained (things presentated as 'facts' are more appropriately considered 'factoids').

A recent survey (Reichow et al. 2013) of the results of a Google search on 'tics' turned up 19,500,000 items, and for 'Tourette' 1,340,000! A table of the findings and associated errors is in Appendix 1. The implications of these errors, which many parents may believe, will be taken up at other places in this book. Suffice it to say here that questions with implications for parental anxiety may be answered in unhelpful ways, and the most important to be aware of, right from the start, are (1) the common injunction to rigorously ignore tics or they will worsen; (2) types of tic disorders and the diagnostic criteria; (3) the symptoms that are often listed as tics, but need not be tics; (4) the genetic/familial implications; (5) causes of tics; (6) frequency and impact of coprophenomena; (7) the worst-ever age for tics (in terms of frequency, complexity, severity and interference with activities); (8) adverse effect on tics of stimulant treatment for ADHD; and (9) the role of diet and stress.

Some of the most common or disturbing misinformation on the internet is summarized below.

• *Ignore tics or else!* This is the most common and perhaps the most harmful error. "Reminders [to the child] imply the tics are bothering you" (what a surprise!). "If the child knows you're worried, he may worry, producing tension rather than acceptance" (and consequently more tics). "Don't allow teasing by siblings." "Stop all family conversation about tics" (as if you have the power to achieve this). "Get relatives and teachers to ignore the tics" (and if you can't and the tics worsen — and they will! — you can feel guilty...). On the other hand, "if ignored, usually tics disappear in 2–12 months." One might well wonder how these injunctions, if taken seriously, would work out in a typical family.

• *Vocal or phonic?* As pointed out previously, but meriting repetition here: the DSM definition, for better or worse, is of at least one vocal — not phonic — tic (and more than one motor tic). Dictionary definitions of 'vocal' signify involvement of the vocal chords, whereas many sites (and articles) refer to 'phonic' or 'phonic/vocal' as if they are synonymous with vocal, e.g. "A simple phonic tic can be almost any sound or noise." One site tries to be helpful by reporting that "most prefer phonic because vocal cords are not involved in all tics that produce sound." That is true, but would imply that tapping and hitting objects, or clicking teeth to make a sound, are 'phonic' tics, and there is no survey of 'most' clinicians' opinions on this topic. One may wonder how 'vocal' in the diagnostic criteria changed to 'phonic' in the best-known rating scale, the Yale Global Tic Severity Scale or YGTSS (Leckman et al. 1989). Some researchers highly respected in the field have indicated that they do not distinguish between the two words. That is evident in the most recent textbook (Martino and Leckman 2013).

Whether 'vocal' or 'phonic' is better, the definition calls for 'vocal', and continues to do so in DSM-5 after ample opportunity for discussion and revision, but they are not the same (all vocal tics are phonic, but not the reverse). The compelling reason to recognize this is as follows: the current definition of Tourette syndrome is not only descriptive, but depends upon arbitrary criteria for the description of tics, the number of two kinds of tics, and the duration of tics. Thus although the condition referred to is *real*, the category is *socially constructed* and is meant to be for purposes of communication, especially for research, and not final. To continuously refine the methodology of research studies is appropriate, but allowing sloppiness in the definition is not — it is a serious flaw. To ignore this is to allow unknown degrees of heterogeneity into the groups studied, and in some instances to affect whether an individual receives services or has a helpful understanding of his or her diagnosis. Although the importance of this point may be arguable, in this book it is regarded as significant.

• *Prevalence and nature of coprolalia.* Most sites report that it is 'rare', of the order of 10%, or any figure down to as low as 2% of patients. None indicates the fact that it may sometimes be transient or not impairing, though one mentions that it may be truncated so as to not be clear. Many sites are specific that it involves 'shouting'.

• *Comorbidity* is now commonly mentioned, but most often there is confusion because it is not tied into the presentation of associated disorders or problems such as 'rages', sleep disorder or specific learning disability. One site describes children with Tourette syndrome as "usually normal, bright and sensitive", right after listing the high rates of comorbid disorders!

• *Stimulant drugs for ADHD.* Only a minority of websites specify that stimulants can usually be used for ADHD in the presence of tics, and that recommendations against it have changed. One site recommends avoiding decongestants. Another states specifically that stimulants precipitate tics and that the drug may set the tic level permanently at a higher level.

• *Questionable behaviors as tics.* Several sites list bruxism, torticollis, lip-licking or sniffing as tics (which often is incorrect or doubtful).

• *Causes of tics* list hypothyroidism, drugs, and contributory factors such as 'any form of mental or physical stress'.

• *Prognosis.* Most state that tics may abate or disappear, but they disagree on when this occurs, and how often. One states confusingly "TS almost always persists throughout life. Fortunately, by age 18, approximately 50% of patients are essentially free of tics…"

• *Tics in sleep: do they disappear, or not?* This is completely inconsistent.

• *All that twitches is not a tic.* Only one site explains that eyelid twitches (benign ocular myokymia) are not tics, but it fails to mention that such benign twitches may occur elsewhere than in the eyelids.

• *PANDAS.* A few sites indicate there is still controversy over the validity of the concept (see Chapter 19), but others discuss it as settled fact.

• *Differential diagnosis.* Some sites make an effort to distinguish tics from stereotypies, but the most complete discussion adds that the latter are "rare in normal children", that those children do not have urges to perform their movements, and that they are not able to suppress them. These declarations are incorrect and lead to misdiagnoses.

• *Genetics.* The present best agreement on the pattern is erroneously reported on some sites: "Tics and TS should be considered as a possible cause if a child with a family member who has TS has a learning or behavior problem" (this without any tics!). And from a medical school site: the inheritance is "usually from both maternal or paternal sides of the family".

• *Meaning for individuals of studies on groups.* Findings on groups cannot definitively prove, disprove or predict something for an individual within that group. This fundamental principle was not expressed or explained on any site examined.

• *What 'worse' and 'better' mean.* This is rarely elaborated.

• *Specific and nonspecific treatments.* Exercise, a healthy diet and adequate sleep are good in general, but are not specific treatments for tics. This distinction is rarely made.

Finally, three other caveats:

(1) Although misdiagnosis is uncommon, the changing pattern of tics and the patient's sensitivity to new or uncomfortable sensations creates a risk that an unrecognized new or co-occurring condition may be missed because its effects appear as new tics, and the distinction can be difficult.

(2) Can there be harm from diagnosis? It is often assumed that early diagnosis (the earlier, the better) is a good thing, but this assumption has its limits and overdiagnosis can be harmful (Moynihan et al. 2012, Coon et al. 2014). A diagnosis of Tourette syndrome (specifically) can have mostly unpredictable harms unless it is part of a more comprehensive process. Here's how. The family members may have, or acquire, a stereotypically negative view of the diagnosis. The teacher if told the diagnosis may modify expectations and misinterpret symptoms. Sensitive children may come to feel they are pariahs, freaks of nature, and overreact to any new or obvious tics; it may affect their educational placement, admission to a private school, job placement, or the granting of insurance. In short, feelings, expectations, and the reactions of others may be — or seem to be — changed for the worse, especially when ongoing support is not available. Medication is unlikely to solve such problems.

(3) Can we talk about tics adequately? Silly question – or is it? The fair reply is *yes* and *no*

and *maybe*… Language in use inevitably contains short-cuts and ambiguities. When we talk about 'tics' how much precision do we need? How much is possible or practical in every-day life? There is no laboratory test and descriptions are only approximations. And those descriptions used in the definition apply only to movements and sounds, not to the 'urges' that we now (since 1980) believe are a fundamental part of the experience of a *sensori*motor disorder. (You can 'have' and be troubled by the sensory part alone, residual from your ear-lier tics, or perhaps even arising de novo.) When we decide that a continuum of tic char-acteristics can be specified and is useful, we have to provide cut-off points to refer to the 'categories' on that continuum, cut-off points that are not natural. Tourette syndrome is such a part of the continuum. We omit the sensory part entirely. Then we may say that I — or my son — has Tourette syndrome. Now I and my readers or listeners may assume that we share some degree of meaning.

When it seems important to inform my son's teacher — or a police officer if he gets into trouble — that he has some unwanted movements or sounds that meet a committee's crite-ria and is given a name for communication convenience, will we say something like that, or simply "he has Tourette syndrome and doesn't have control over it…"? Not likely the former!

But of course it is much more complicated than this. Since the majority of persons meeting criteria for Tourette syndrome also 'have' comorbid disorders whose characteris-tics also vary and have likewise been constructed by a committee, we are unlikely to bring that subject up at all in our everyday communications. If legal issues arise, will we be able to avoid simplistic and uncertain assumptions about 'urges', 'needs', and their pleasurable or unpleasant character?

This is a problem we have, whether we realize it, or think about it, or not. But be assured that it is lurking there anyway.

REFERENCES

Albanese A, Bhatia K, Bressman SB, et al. (2013) Phenomenology and classification of dystonia: a consen-sus update. *Mov Disord* 28: 863–73. doi: 10.1002/mds.25475.

American Psychiatric Association (2000) *Diagnostic and Statistical Manual of Mental Disorders, 4th edn, Text Revision.* Arlington, VA: American Psychiatric Association.

American Psychiatric Association (2013) *Diagnostic and Statistical Manual of Mental Disorders, 5th edn.* Arlington, VA: American Psychiatric Association.

Angelini L, Sgrò V, Erba A, et al. (1998) Tourettism as clinical presentation of Huntington's disease with onset in childhood. *Ital J Neurol Sci* 19: 383–5.

Becker N, Munhoz RP, Raskin S, et al. (2007) Non-choreic movement disorders as initial manifestations of Huntington's disease. *Arq Neuropsiquiatr* 65: 402–5.

Bliss J (1980) Sensory experiences of Gilles de la Tourette syndrome. *Arch Gen Psychiatry* 37: 1343–7.

Coon ER, Quinonez RA, Moyer VA, et al. (2014) Overdiagnosis: how our compulsion for diagnosis may be harming our children. *Pediatrics* 134: 1013–23. doi: 10.1542/peds.2014-1778.

Crossley E, Cavanna AE (2013) Sensory phenomena: clinical correlates and impact on quality of life in adult patients with Tourette syndrome. *Psychiatry Res* 209: 705–10. doi: 10.1016/j.psychres.2013.04.019.

Crossley E, Seri S, Stern JS, et al. (2014) Premonitory urges for tics in adult patients with Tourette syndrome. *Brain Dev* 36: 45–50. doi: 10.1016/j.braindev.2012.12.010.

Dale RC, Church AJ, Heyman I (2003) Striatal encephalitis after varicella zoster infection complicated by Tourettism. *Mov Disord* 18: 1554–6. doi: 10.1002/mds.10610.

Dooley J, Stokes A, Gordson KE (1994) Pseudo-tics in Tourette syndrome. *J Child Neurol* 9: 50–1. doi:

10.1177/088307389400900112.

Ferrara J, Jankovic J (2008) Psychogenic movement disorders in children. *Mov Disord* 23: 1875–81. doi: 10.1002/mds.22220.

Frucht SJ (2013) The definition of dystonia: current concepts and controversies. *Mov Disord* 28: 884–8. doi: 10.1002/mds.25529.

Howard R, Ford RR (1992) From the Jumping Frenchmen of Maine to posttraumatic stress disorder: the startle response in neuropsychiatry. *Psychol Med* 22: 695–707. doi: 10.1017/S0033291700038137.

Irwin RS, Glomb WB, Chang AB (2006) Habit cough, tic cough, and psychogenic cough in adult and pediatric populations: ACCP evidence-based clinical practice guidelines. *Chest* 129: 174S–179S.

Jan JE, Freeman RD (1994) Familial paroxysmal kinesigenic choreoathetosis in a child with visual hallucinations and obsessive–compulsive behaviour. *Dev Med Child Neurol* 37: 366–9. doi: 10.1111/j.1469-8749.1995.tb12015.x.

Jankovic J (2001) Differential diagnosis and etiology of tics. *Adv Neurol* 85: 15–29.

Jankovic J, Ashizawa T (1995) Tourettism associated with Huntington's disease. *Mov Disord* 10: 103–5.

Jankovic J, Mejia NI (2006) Tics associated with other disorders. *Adv Neurol* 99: 61–8.

Kato N, Sadamatsu M, Kikuchi T, et al. (2006) Paroxysmal kinesigenic choreoathetosis: From first discovery in 1892 to genetic linkage with benign familial infantile convulsions. *Epilepsy Res* 70 (Suppl 1): 174–84.

Kerbeshian J, Burd L, Leech C, Rorabaugh A (1991) Huntington disease and childhood onset Tourette syndrome. *Am J Med Genet* 39: 1–3.

Kurlan R, Deeley C, Como P (1992) Psychogenic movement disorder (pseudo-tics) in a patient with Tourette syndrome. *J Neuropsychiatr Clin Neurosci* 4: 347–8.

Kwak C, Jankovic J (2002) Tourettism and dystonia after subcortical stroke. *Mov Disord* 17: 821–5. doi: 10.1002/mds.10207.

Leckman JF, Riddle MA, Hardin MT, et al. (1989) The Yale Global Tic Severity Scale: initial testing of a clinician-rated scale of tic severity. *J Am Acad Child Adolesc Psychiatry* 28: 566–73. doi: 10.1097/00004583-198907000-00015.

Martino D, Leckman JF, eds (2013) *Tourette Syndrome.* New York: Oxford University Press.

Meizner I (1987) Sonographic observation of in utero 'masturbation'. *J Ultrasound Med* 6: 111.

Méneret A, Gaudebout C, Riant F, et al. (2013) *PPRT2* mutations and paroxysmal disorders. *Eur J Neurol* 20: 872–8. doi: 10.1111/ene.12104.

Moynihan R, Doust J, Henry D (2012) Preventing overdiagnosis: how to stop harming the healthy. *BMJ* e3502: 1–6.

Nambu A, Chiken S, Shashidharan P, et al. (2011) Reduced pallidal output causes dystonia. *Front Syst Neurosci* 5: 89. doi: 10.3389/fnsys.2011.00089.

Nardocci N, Rumi V, Combi ML, et al. (1994) Complex tics, stereotypies, and compulsive behavior as clinical presentation of a juvenile progressive dystonia suggestive of Hallervorden Spatz disease. *Mov Disord* 9: 369–71. doi: 10.1002/mds.870090322.

Nechay A, Ross LM, Stephenson JBP, O'Regan M (2004) Gratification disorder ('infantile masturbation'): a review. *Arch Dis Child* 89: 225–6.

Plioplys S, Asato MR, Bursch B, et al. (2007) Multidisciplinary management of pediatric nonepileptic seizures. *J Am Acad Child Adolesc Psychiatry* 46: 1491–5. doi: 10.1097/chi.0b013e31814dab98.

Reichow B, Shefcyk A, Bruder MB (2013) Quality comparison of websites related to developmental disabilities. *Res Dev Disabil* 34: 3077–83. doi: 10.1016/j.ridd.2013.06.013.

Rödöö P, Hellberg D (2013) Girls who masturbate in early infancy: diagnostics, natural course and a long-term follow-up. *Acta Paediatr* 102: 762–6. doi: 10.1111/apa.12231.

Saiki S, Hirose G, Sakai K, et al. (2004) Chorea–acanthocytosis associated with tourettism. *Mov Disord* 19: 833–6. doi: 10.1002/mds.20050.

Scarano V, Pellecchia MT, Filla A, Barone P (2002) Hallervorden–Spatz syndrome resembling a typical Tourette syndrome. *Mov Disord* 17: 618–20. doi: 10.1017/S.

Schachter SC, LaFrance WC, Jr, eds (2010) *Gates and Rowan's Nonepileptic Seizures, 3rd edn.* Cambridge/New York: Cambridge University Press.

Schwingenschuh P, Pont-Sunyer C, Surtees R, et al. (2008) Psychogenic movement disorders in children: a report of 15 cases and a review of the literature. *Mov Disord* 23: 1882–8. doi: 10.1002/mds.22280.

Silveira-Moriyama L, Gardiner AR, Meyer E, et al. (2013) Clinical features of childhood-onset paroxysmal kinesigenic dyskinesia with *PRRT2* gene mutations. *Dev Med Child Neurol* 55: 327–34. doi: 10.1111/dmcn.12056.

Tan E-K (2004) Psychogenic tics: diagnostic value of the placebo test. *J Child Neurol* 19: 976–7.

Temudo T, Levy A, Barbot C, et al. (2007) Stereotypies in Rett syndrome: analysis of 83 patients with and without detected *MECP2* mutations. *Neurology* 68: 1183–7.

Walker RH, Danek A, Dobson-Stone C, et al. (2006) Developments in neuroacanthocytosis: expanding the spectrum of choreatic syndromes. *Mov Disord* 21: 1794–805. doi: 10.1002/mds.21108.

Walker RH, Saiki S, Danek A, eds (2010) *Neuroacanthocytosis Syndromes II.* Berlin: Springer.

Welch HG, Schwartz LM, Woloshin S (2011) *Overdiagnosed: Making People Sick in the Pursuit of Health.* Boston, MA: Beacon Press.

Woods DW, Piacentini JC, Himle MB, Chang S (2005) Premonitory Urge for Tics Scale (PUTS): initial psychometric results and examination of the premonitory urge phenomenon in youths with tic disorders. *J Devel Behav Pediatr* 26: 397–403.

3
PRESENTATION TO CLINICIANS

Tics can present to primary care or specialist physicians, psychologists, or other clinicians, shortly after initial onset or at any later point. Diagnostic delay is common, because simple tics are often attributed at first to other possible causes. Tics that remain single and simple occur but are usually not presented as problems; it is new ones or more complex ones that eventually come to attention. If earlier tics were not identified as such the history may be unclear. This may be the case with rare instances of adult onset. Except with simple tics or those in young children, most tics are preceded by premonitory urges or unpleasant sensations. Active efforts to suppress tics are often made when in school or public places, with differing degrees of success. There is a common belief that suppression leads to later rebound, but strong evidence of this is lacking. Active or automatic suppression can lead to no display or minimal occurrence of tics in the clinician's office, especially when time is short, making appreciation of tic impact difficult. Contrariwise, talk about tics may cause them to appear, even ones not currently in the patient's repertoire. Tics can consist of any movement or sound, so are easy to attribute to some other cause or to have social meanings attributed to them, including as apparent indicators of sexual abuse. Comorbidity is the rule, rather than the exception, so that assessment is complex. Because of the confusion of tics with 'nerves' it is important to explain that emotional factors may influence tic severity but are not sufficient causes.

Typically a child develops one or more tics (that may not be recognized as such) at around age 5–7 years. Excessive eye-blinking (with brief blepharospasm), eye-rolling, facial grimacing, head-shaking, sniffing and throat-clearing are very common. The history is often that new tics tend to progress in a rostral–caudal direction, head, neck and upper limbs before lower limbs. At that point the child may be seen by a primary care physician or referred to a specialist, but often the delay is several years, and misdiagnosis and missed diagnosis are common.

The first or second simple tic may be attributed to some other common condition, such as allergies, eye problems, infections, nervousness, stress, or bad habits from imitating another person. There are also many misidentifications that clinicians make, discussed below. Much confusion and sometimes suffering by the patient and family may be the result of this delay. The child may be disciplined, interrogated, and brought to many clinicians who fail to recognize symptoms as tics, provide unhelpful advice, perform useless tests or treatments, or attribute the tics to attention-seeking behavior or to stresses in the family situation that are at most aggravating factors, and thereby inadvertently worsen the situation. The child may develop a sense of futility about understanding him- or herself, or about the helpfulness of clinicians.

All clinicians would benefit from reading the experience of a boy in England growing up with Tourette syndrome (Van Bloss 2006). His book also contains some of the most useful descriptions of what Tourette syndrome is like for the patient.

Blepharospasm itself is of interest. This is the brief forced closing of the eyes that occurs after some eye-blinking tics, but not with normal eye-blinking unless there is some associated itch or irritation. It is definitely not the prolonged spasm that may constitute a serious progressive disorder in adult life. It is almost never spontaneously reported by parents or patients, yet it is a fairly reliable marker for tics. Insufficient attention has been paid to this in the medical literature. Close attention to patients doing this, or even to excessive eye-blinking seen by strangers on television, will indicate that this is not just a matter of more frequent blinking, but an additional component. It may be combined with other facial muscles into a complex grimace.

Meanings are necessarily created by parents (and patients) and help to fill a void. They may determine subsequent attitudes and reactions to the tics. The waxing–waning pattern permits almost any theory to seem plausible.

Premonitory sensations or urges are quite typical, but not all tics are preceded by them or described by very young children, especially very frequent simple tics. The latter may occur out of awareness (Goetz et al. 2002). They may occur in the same location as the tic that follows, or elsewhere, and they may be more disturbing than the tics, as well as ineffable (Turtle and Robertson 2008). *Note:* because urges may be disturbing even when tics are not apparent (i.e. are suppressed), it is always important to ask about them and how they feel, and to do so again later, not only initially (because they may change over time and with further development).

> **Practice point**
> Premonitory urges may be as disturbing as tics, sometimes more so, and should always be asked about.

Some older adolescent and adult patients have no tics left to see or hear, but are still aware of the urges. It may be assumed that their tics have 'gone' so that their tic disorder has also gone, but their fundamental sensory difference has not.

Consequences of tic suppression

An important recent paper (Specht et al. 2013) has tested the assumption that suppressing the tics will increase the urge and therefore a more severe tic may eventually have to follow. Children and parents may say that if the child concentrates in school on tic suppression it will cause distraction and exhaustion so that at the end of the day the tics rebound to a worse level. From this conclusion, advice follows not to try to suppress tics. But the study found that this did not happen. So why do people believe this? Dr Douglas Woods (personal communication

2013) suggested that tics occurring at the end of the day, if worse, may be assumed to be due to rebound from tic suppression at school, but there are other potential explanations: (1) we don't know if the child was actually suppressing all day; (2) something unidentified in the home environment might be making the tics worse; (3) parents may be away at work and then be impressed by the tic level they experience after coming home; (4) fatigue after school may be responsible, and may make suppression less effective.

> **Practice point**
> Despite widespread belief in the 'fact' that 'rebound' results from tic suppression, it is not well supported by present evidence.

Goetz et al. (2002) in a paper aptly entitled 'Home alone' showed that adult tics were least likely to occur in the presence of a clinician in the office, and that patients with long-standing tics did not recognize many of their own tics on home videotapes made by themselves. This observation seemed to fit with automatic suppression. However, Piacentini et al. (2006) in a study with children found much greater tic stability across different situations.

Effects of tic-related conversation

Persons with tics may say that their urges to tic are increased when they hear 'tic talk'. Some evidence for this has been provided by Woods et al. (2001) and a study of tics in two siblings (Dufrene et al. 2013). A puzzle is that if tic-related talk increases urges and tics, why are tics often reduced in an initial meeting with a clinician in which much tic talk inevitably occurs?

Unusual presentations

Unusual presentations can cause considerable confusion. Because the history is sometimes unclear (earlier, more common types of tics weren't identified as such, and may not be recalled) the dramatic tic or other unusual movement that presents to a specialist may point in another direction, or convince someone that it isn't Tourette syndrome.

> **Case example**
> *A 7-year-old boy whose family spoke limited English presented to the emergency depart-ment with recent onset of gluteal contractions. This was initially diagnosed as myoclonus epilepsy and he was admitted. Subsequently a perceptive pediatric neurologist talked with the parents more thoroughly and learned that there had been a previous bout of excessive eye-blinking and throat-clearing. He was then re-diagnosed with Tourette syndrome.*

Tics with apparent sexual significance

Since a tic can be almost any movement, sound or combination, tics that appear as fragments or even fairly full enactments of sexual activity can be shocking, or in young people danger-ously misunderstood. You cannot always be sure whether this represents a complex copro-praxic act, a replay of a sexual encounter that could signal a report of sexual abuse, or the imi-tation of an observed, talked-about or read-about action. Although one cannot always be sure of the causative factors even after investigation, the authorities who may become involved often know nothing about Tourette syndrome and may therefore too readily jump to another more familiar explanation without due consideration. The emergence of an action with obvi-ous sexual meaning to the observers in a young child can precipitate a crisis, especially in jurisdictions where reporting to child welfare authorities is mandatory. The possibilities for traumatizing a child and family by a less than comprehensive investigation is a serious one. So is missing child sexual abuse.

Practice point

Tics can mimic sexual acts and trigger mistaken (but understandable) assumptions and reporting to child welfare authorities. Clinicians should be aware of this and be prepared to collaborate with the authorities so that there is no harmful outcome.

Cough

Persistent 'cough' (already mentioned in Chapter 2) may have many causes, but tic is one of them (Irwin et al. 2006). The typical picture is that it has a stereotyped pattern (e.g. always a specific number of coughs with each bout) unlike other coughs, may have a different quality, and usually disappears in sleep, whereas coughs of other origin usually are worse at night and may disrupt sleep. If these differences are not recognized and the presence (past or present) of other tics not questioned, the diagnosis may be missed. When seen initially, a persistent, apparently solitary cough may be suspected to be caused by gastroesophageal reflux and a treatment trial (usually a proton-pump inhibitor) instituted. Although extra-esophageal symp-toms such as cough may be entertained, this is difficult to link to reflux and is probably over-diagnosed (Richter 2004). Many publications in the otolaryngology and respirology literature completely omit mention of cough as a possible respiratory tic.

Practice point

Respiratory tics usually differ from cough or similar symptoms by their unusually stereo-typed nature and absence in sleep. The presence or history of more typical tics is impor-tant to obtain. Invasive and unnecessary procedures or treatment are desirable to avoid. Collaboration with colleagues in pediatrics, respirology, otolaryngology and allergy may be required.

It is not rare for children who have some tics to develop severe, prolonged or bizarre movement episodes that are suspected of being epileptic in origin (Plioplys et al. 2007).

One case history described an adolescent boy whose reduction in medication eventually led to a return of very frequent vocal tics when he was under unusual stress. He had two episodes in hospital before it was recognized that his air swallowing had produced ileus (Frye and Hait 2006). We had an unpublished instance of pneumomediastinum from severe vocal tics, described here.

Case examples

'Alex' was a 15-year-old boy who had had multiple tics since age 7, but he underwent a very severe exacerbation that led to hospitalization when he was unresponsive to neuroleptic medication. His forced expirations (with Valsalva maneuvers) were loud and very frequent. By the time he was admitted he had some swelling in his neck, and several days after entering the hospital he was found on chest radiograph to have air in his mediastinum. He finally responded to aripiprazole, and 5 years later was attending university with only periodic upsurges of severe symptoms.

   Comment: *The mediastinal air is a very unusual complication.*

An 8-year-old girl presented with tics, but also 'encopresis'. It turned out that her incontinence was due to her vocal tics, which included a Valsalva maneuver.

A 12-year-old boy had periodic diurnal urinary incontinence. This was due to his abdominal contractions combined with a full bladder when he played long sessions of computer games.

Misinterpretations of common tics

Tics can be almost any movement or sound, often ones that seem inimitable. But they can also mimic other sources of sound or movement.

Case examples

A 6-year-old boy developed a new loud barking tic. His parents were renting an apartment that had a restriction: no pets were allowed. A neighbor complained to the landlord that someone was violating this restriction: the 'pet' was the patient! Because of automatic tic suppression, the tic was not performed in the landlord's presence. The clinician had to write a letter to the landlord and it helped that a recording had been made.

Some jurisdictions have child abuse reporting laws that require anyone to report a suspicion that a child is being abused. A 10-year-old girl with Tourette syndrome developed a screaming tic during springtime; in summer when it was hot and windows were left open her screams led to a report to the abuse hot-line that fortunately was cleared when the Tourette syndrome was explained to the investigator.

Tics can also have *social meanings attributed to them by others*. Two common examples are that an eye-wink can be received as negating what was just said, or as a sexual come-on; lateral eye-rolling when being talked to by a superior may be interpreted as an unspoken negation.

Other unusual presentations or associated behaviors

Vomiting, retching and aerophagia can sometimes be considered a tic, or at least tic-like. Rickards and Robertson (1997) presented 10 cases with many associated symptoms. Four of the 10 had 'forced touching' such as of hot objects; two, 'coughing'; three, tongue protrusion; one, eye-poking; one evolved into spitting; and two put fingers down their throats. An OCD-like state might have been involved in some, but "their setting in the context of other tics and abnormal behaviors led to these being called tics" (p. 534). For one patient retching was the presenting symptom. Pathological laughter has been described by Cavanna et al. (2010). The wide variety of associated behavior patterns is striking. (No matter how many instances of Tourette syndrome are seen, surprises and confusions are always a possibility.)

The initial examination

Having discussed how tics may appear, we need to briefly consider how one assesses the total picture since comorbidity is the usual situation. Tics themselves, if not observed directly (especially with suppression or at a low point in tic severity) should be supplemented by viewing a video recording. This can be difficult when a child is very sensitive about being recorded, but determined parents can usually succeed. Most parents, if they do not have or cannot afford a video recorder know someone who has one or who can simply use the camera in a modern 'smart' phone for this purpose.

> **Practice point**
> If you cannot observe the tics or related behaviors, and their range, video samples are essential for a proper diagnosis and an appreciation of the impact of the tics, especially complex tics which are not seen in the office.

Coexisting disorders or symptoms are very important, often crucial. One must beware the tendency to attribute all symptoms to the tic diagnosis itself ('diagnostic overshadowing'). A high index of suspicion of comorbid disorders is a fundamental part of every evaluation.

> **Practice point**
> It cannot be overemphasized that an evaluation of comorbid disorders and other symptoms must be part of every assessment of tic disorders.

Although misdiagnosis of a tic disorder when it is actually a different rare disorder is very uncommon, it is always good to perform or obtain a comprehensive physical examination.

If the patient is being seen by a psychiatrist or in a 'mental health' facility, rather than by a neurologist, pediatrician or other specialist, it is of the utmost practical importance to explain that no assumption is being made about emotional causes of the patient's tics or other symptoms. Seeing a psychiatrist still has a significant stigma attached to it, and many assume that that is an automatic indication that tics are *caused* by emotional disturbance. After the diagnostic session is completed it may be appropriate to re-emphasize that tics are not caused by emotions and that emotional *influences* do not signify necessary and sufficient *causation*.

Practice point

Stigma associated with 'mental' or psychiatric disorders remains and can have important negative effects. Never forget that for better or worse tic disorders are in the Diagnostic and Statistical Manual of *Mental* Disorders and many patients are seen and treated by psychiatrists. To patients or their families the meaning may be clear but wrong: tics are signs of something wrong with you mentally and associated with presumed 'mental' causes. That this is incorrect needs to be explained and sometimes reinforced. *It is a myth that conditions seen by psychiatrists are the same as those seen by other clinicians.*

Another question important for the child, parent or adult patient is: "How have tic upsurges affected you (or been handled)? How do you feel when one is starting?" A related question for parents is "How do you feel when you take your child out in public? How do your other children feel or react?"

WHAT SHOULD YOU (OR CAN YOU) TELL THE PATIENT OR FAMILY AT THE FIRST VISIT OF A CHILD OR ADOLESCENT?

- If you can make the tic disorder diagnosis with confidence, then you should ask what they already think they know (such as from the internet, relatives or others), then explain how the diagnosis is made without physical tests.
- Say more (depending upon the child's age and course so far) about the usual fluctuating course, the likelihood of upsurges with some new tics, the frequent rising baseline experienced as overall worsening of the condition, but the usually benign course into adolescence.
- Discuss possibilities for treatment and when to consider medication or behavioral treatment.
- Explain what to do about follow-up, referral (if any) to ongoing services elsewhere, and how to access oneself or responsible others if and when needed.
- Discuss other needs such as explanations to school or other activity, and to important relatives (including siblings, grandparents, and the other parent, if not present).

If you cannot satisfy yourself as to comorbidity, other arrangements must be made and what you can tell should explain the current limitations and further steps needed. An inquiry should also be made about caregiver or partner strain.

Adult-onset tics or 'tourettism'

Oliver Sacks (1982) discussed postencephalitic states involving parkinsonism, myoclonus and tics after the epidemic of encephalitis lethargica following World War I. Many of those patients developed parkinsonism or catatonia later, until in the late 1960s levodopa made it possible to 'awaken' those patients, often followed by complex Tourette-like states in those who had never had tics or whose tics developed from other movement disorders. Other neurological conditions in which Tourette-like states can emerge are tardive tourettism associated with chronic psychoactive drug treatment, 'senile chorea', Huntington chorea, strokes, brain damage, tumors and degenerative diseases.

An *adult form of Tourette syndrome* apparently with onset in adulthood also can be seen occasionally (Klawans and Barr 1985, Goetz et al. 1992, Chouinard and Ford 2000, Pappert et al. 2003, Agrawal and Shrestha 2009, Jankovic et al. 2010). In many cases these persons have had earlier tics that were forgotten or misdiagnosed. Truly adult onset should be considered an indication for further medical investigation.

Practice point

Although tics reported to be of adult initial onset are likely to be an exacerbation of earlier tics that were not diagnosed or were forgotten, this cannot be safely assumed and may warrant further medical investigation.

Problems with tic diagnoses: what's in a name?

Sometimes the accuracy of the tic diagnosis is important, and not necessarily for the most obvious reasons. Adhering closely to the diagnostic criteria, some people given the Tourette syndrome label don't belong there [they may have 'honorary tics' that are actually better classified as repetitive motor behaviors (RMBs) or stereotypies, or one or more of the required motor or vocal tics is accepted by history only, or a 'phonic' tic is assumed to be 'vocal']. From the practical individual standpoint these fine points may not matter, but for research, for developing guidelines, and sometimes for qualifying for benefits such as special-needs school supports, it may. For example, if a school system is set up so that Tourette syndrome specifically qualifies for support but 'lesser' tic disorders don't, this can make a difference. If a clinician or bureaucrat believes what is often incorrectly stated as a fact, namely that Tourette syndrome is 'the most serious of the tic disorders', then any 'lesser' disorder may be accorded less importance and fall short of credibility for help. (This is a misunderstanding: remember that the label 'Tourette' may seem more impressive than 'persistent motor or vocal tic disorder'.)

Practice point

Tic disorders are defined differently from others: no impairment or distress are necessary for the diagnosis, leaving room for many other factors to influence their significance, including personal and social tolerance for the tics.

REFERENCES

Agrawal A, Shrestha R (2009) New onset of idiopathic bilateral ear tics in an adult. *Clin Neurol Neurosurg* 111: 307–8. doi: 10.1016/j.clineuro.2008.11.014.

Cavanna AE, Ali F, Leckman JF, Robertson MM (2010) Pathological laughter in Gilles de la Tourette syndrome: an unusual phonic tic. *Mov Disord* 25: 2233–8. doi: 10.1002/mds.23216.

Chouinard S, Ford B (2000) Adult onset tic disorders. *J Neurol Neurosurg Psychiatry* 68: 738–43. doi: 10.1136/jnnp.68.6.738.

Dufrene BA, Watson TS, Echeverria DJ, Weaver AD (2013) Effects of tic-related conversation on rate of tics in two siblings. *J Obsess-Comp Relat Disord* 2: 281–5. doi: 10.1016/j.jocrd.2013.05.004.

Frye RE, Hait EJ (2006) Air swallowing caused recurrent ileus in Tourette's syndrome. *Pediatrics* 117: e1249–52. doi: 10.1542/peds.2005-2914.

Goetz CG, Tanner CM, Stebbins GT, et al. (1992) Adult tics in Gilles de la Tourette's syndrome. *Neurology* 42: 784–8.

Goetz CG, Leurgans S, Chmura TA (2002) Home alone: methods to maximize tic expression for objective videotape assessments in Gilles de la Tourette syndrome. *Mov Disord* 16: 693–7. doi: 10.1002/mds.1159.

Irwin RS, Glomb WB, Chang AB (2006) Habit cough, tic cough, and psychogenic cough in adult and pediatric populations: ACCP evidence-based clinical practice guidelines. *Chest* 129: 174S–179S.

Jankovic J, Gelineau-Kattner R, Davidson A (2010) Tourette's syndrome in adults. *Mov Disord* 25: 2171–5. doi: 10.1002/mds.23199.

Klawans HL, Barr A (1985) Recurrence of childhood multiple tics in late adult life. *Arch Neurol* 42: 1979–80.

Pappert EJ, Goetz CG, Louis ED, et al. (2003) Objective assessments of longitudinal outcome in Gilles de la Tourette's syndrome. *Neurology* 61: 936–40.

Piacentini J, Himle MB, Chang S, et al. (2006) Reactivity of tic observation procedures to situation and setting. *J Abnorm Child Psychol* 34: 647–56. doi: 10.1007/s10802-006-9048-5.

Plioplys S, Asato MR, Bursch B, et al. (2007) Multidisciplinary management of pediatric nonepileptic seizures. *J Am Acad Child Adolesc Psychiatry* 46: 1491–5. doi: 10.1097/chi.0b013e31814dab98.

Richter JE (2004) Ear, nose and throat and respiratory manifestations of gastro-esophageal reflux disease: an increasing conundrum. *Eur J Gastroenterol Hepatol* 16: 837–45.

Rickards H, Robertson MM (1997) Vomiting and retching in Gilles de la Tourette syndrome: a report of ten cases and a review of the literature. *Mov Disord* 12: 531–5. doi: 10.1002/mds.870120409.

Sacks OW (1982) Acquired tourettism in adult life. *Adv Neurol* 35: 89–92.

Specht MW, Woods DW, Nicotra CM, et al. (2013) Effects of tic suppression: suppressibility, rebound, negative reinforcement, and habituation to the urge versus extinction learning. *Behav Res Ther* 51: 24–30. doi: 10.1016/j.brat.2012.09.009.

Turtle L, Robertson MM (2008) Tics, twitches, tales: the experiences of Gilles de la Tourette's syndrome. *Am J Orthopsychiatry* 78: 449–55.

Van Bloss N (2006) *Busy Body: My Life with Tourette's Syndrome.* London: Fusion Press.

Woods DW, Watson TS, Wolfe E, et al. (2001) Analyzing the influence of tic-related talk on vocal and motor tics in children with Tourette's syndrome. *J Appl Behav Anal* 34: 353–6. doi: 10.1901/jaba.2001.34-353.

4
PREVALENCE AND EPIDEMIOLOGY

The definition and boundaries of the tic disorders have changed over time and have made a significant difference in how these categories are viewed, by both clinicians and the general public. We still don't have solid agreement on what is a tic, and what is not (there are exceptions to all definitions); whether a tic is solely an abnormal movement pattern or necessarily includes a sensory component; or on the relationships with associated disorders and symptoms. Both 'tic' and 'Tourette' have been hijacked by the larger culture, like many of the associated named disorders, leading to further confusion. Many commendable efforts have been made to characterize tic disorders and to educate clinicians and the public, and ultimately to help those who really suffer, but one should not lose sight of the complex and enduring confusions that this category represents. Prevalence figures (numbers) are not adequate to represent the clinical importance of tic disorders.

For many decades, perhaps until around 1975, Tourette syndrome was thought to be rare and exotic. If it's believed to be rare, then the clinician may not make the diagnosis. The currently accepted population prevalence is between 0.5% and 1.0%, and between three and four times as frequent in males as in females. Several studies in special education classes and in special populations have reported much higher figures (Baron-Cohen et al. 1999a,b; Kurlan et al. 2001). The figures obtained depend upon the definition, the age of ascertainment, and the methods employed. Be aware that many current textbooks give wildly varying prevalence rates. A review book (Shiau and Toren 2006) for medical students prior to licensing examinations cites 3–5/100,000, 100 times less than the currently accepted rate, while Harrison's well-known text (Kasper et al. 2005) cited the recent 0.5%, even two editions previous to the most recent one.

The Avon Longitudinal Study of Parents and Children (Scharf et al. 2012) found that 0.7% of 13-year-olds had Tourette syndrome. Co-occurring OCD and ADHD were much lower than in clinical studies, as might be expected. Chronic motor tics occurred in 0.3% and chronic vocal tic disorder in 0.2%. The male:female ratio was 3.6 to 1. Of those with tic disorders, the combination of OCD and ADHD occurred in 8.2%, OCD in 22% (9% of chronic tic disorder) and ADHD in 17% (14% of chronic tic disorder). Since the study was based upon parent ratings, not direct assessment of the children, the authors caution that the ADHD rate of co-occurrence may be a minimum.

Consider this. Increases in the purported incidence of ASD have been widely reported in both scientific and popular media, leading to controversial beliefs in various environmental causes such as the measles–mumps–rubella vaccine, *but the increase in the reported prevalence of Tourette syndrome is much more substantial*, and has so far occasioned very little notice. This is not the place to thoroughly explore the ramifications of this specific group of categories [see Bowker and Star (1999) for a fascinating study of classification and its consequences], but it would be wrong to forget that the medical diagnosis as such is socially constructed and that its meanings cannot be permanently frozen. We will see later that there are paradoxes in how the categories are used and how research is carried out that suggest caution in accepting current 'facts' as final.

Scahill et al. (2005) have provided an in-depth review of the public health significance of tic disorders, and the US Government has conducted its own prevalence study (Centers for Disease Control and Prevention 2009).

A fundamental question germane to the role of comorbidity is: now that there is much evidence that psychopathology and disruptive behavior in Tourette syndrome is closely associated with co-occurrence of other disorders, especially ADHD (Freeman et al. 2000), are tics themselves ('TS-only') associated with an increased risk of such problems? The conclusion is 'yes': in cases of persistent tics (not provisional tics) without comorbidity there is a somewhat (but not greatly) increased risk of learning problems and disruptive behavior. More research is needed to clarify the extent and nature of these problems (but is unlikely to settle them).

The high rate of reported comorbidity has occasioned some debate about what is the 'real' Tourette syndrome, and phrases like 'full-blown Tourette syndrome'. One different way to look at it is that Tourette syndrome with highly complex comorbidity (TS+) may be the 'forme pleine' of 'full-blown Tourette syndrome', while TS-only can be considered a 'forme fruste' or a partial manifestation of TS+, which is the 'real' status. It seems highly unlikely that this confusion can be settled to general satisfaction, and just as there were problems when Tourette syndrome was assumed to be rare, now there are problems when it is thought to be common (not only overdiagnosis but much more diagnostic overshadowing).

Yet another consideration is that TS+ can be conceptualized as in the story of the blind men and the elephant, who each correctly perceive a part of the beast, but no one the totality. Whatever the model, the complexity is such that we are likely to continue to see explanations and descriptions that neglect the varying whole, and some research that does the same (Freeman 2014). This may be one of the hindrances to research advance.

In the *TIC* database (Freeman et al. 2000) a quite regular positive association was found between comorbidity score (number of comorbid disorders) and rates of non-diagnostic behavior patterns. This is easy to observe in Table 4.1, where rates of the behavior problems rise with increasing comorbidity. Children with complex diagnoses are thus very likely to have developmental/behavioral problems that are not directly part of diagnostic categories, but represent management challenges.

TABLE 4.1
Comorbidity and non-diagnostic problems in children in the *TIC* database (n=4238)

	Comorbidity score							
	1 (n=1474)		*2 (n=1477)*		*3 (n=950)*		*4 (n=337)*	
	n	*%*	*n*	*%*	*n*	*%*	*n*	*%*
Anger (now)	274	18.6	452	30.6	40	41.6	156	46.3
Sleep (now)	224	15.2	306	20.7	216	22.7	98	29.1
SIB	138	9.4	174	11.8	166	17.5	87	25.8
Social skills problems	142	9.6	236	16.0	253	26.6	120	35.6
Coprophenomena	127	8.6	167	11.3	165	17.4	62	18.4

Excluded: intellectual disability, autism spectrum disorder and psychosis.
SIB, self-injurious behavior.
All $p<0.001$.

REFERENCES

Baron-Cohen S, Mortimore C, Moriarty J, et al. (1999a) The prevalence of Gilles de la Tourette's syndrome in children and adolescents with autism. *J Child Psychol Psychiatry* 40: 213–8. doi: 10.1111/j.1469-7610.00434.

Baron-Cohen S, Scahill VL, Izaguirre J, et al. (1999b) The prevalence of Gilles de la Tourette syndrome in children and adolescents with autism: a large-scale study. *Psychol Med* 29: 1151–9.

Bowker GC, Star SL (1999) *Sorting Things Out: Classification and Its Consequences.* Cambridge, MA: MIT Press.

Centers for Disease Control and Prevention (2009) Prevalence of diagnosed Tourette syndrome in persons aged 6–17 years – United States, 2007. *MMWR Morb Mortal Wkly Rep* 58: 581–5.

Freeman RD (2014) Blame the disorder. *Can J Neurol Sci* 41: 233 (editorial).

Freeman RD, Fast DK, Burd L, et al. (2000) An international perspective on Tourette syndrome: selected findings from 3500 individuals in 22 countries. *Dev Med Child Neurol* 42: 436–7. doi: 10.1111/j.1469-8749.2000.tb00346.x.

Kasper DL, Braunwald E, Fauci AS, et al., eds (2005) *Harrison's Principles of Internal Medicine, 16th edn.* New York: McGraw-Hill.

Kurlan R, McDermott MP, Deeley C, et al. (2001) Prevalence of tics in schoolchildren and association with placement in special education. *Neurology* 57: 1383–8.

Scahill L, Sukhodolsky DG, Williams SK, Leckman JF (2005) Public health significance of tic disorders in children and adolescents. *Adv Neurol* 96: 240–8.

Scharf JM, Miller LL, Mathews CA, Ben-Shlomo Y (2012) Prevalence of Tourette syndrome and chronic tics in the population-based Avon Longitudinal Study of Parents and Children cohort. *J Am Acad Child Adolesc Psychiatry* 51: 192–201. doi: 10.1016/j.jaac.2011.11.004.

Shiau CJ, Toren AJ, eds (2006) *Toronto Notes 2006, 22nd edn.* Toronto: Toronto Notes for Medical Students.

5
ETIOLOGY

The cause(s) of tic disorders are of great interest to patients and their families, but there are not many facts to impart, rather perhaps more 'factoids' to remove. It is of great importance to clarify that tic disorders (and specifically including Tourette syndrome) are not mental disorders as lay people understand them, nor is it believed that tics have emotional factors or parenting errors as necessary and sufficient causes. Nor would it be correct (as we now understand) to say that sufficient cause is to be found in a difference in a single brain structure. From this point what can be said will differ depending upon the educational level of the recipient, what they have already read or been told, and also most importantly why causation is important to them.

From the standpoint of the clinician, at this time there are few important facts on this topic (reviewed by Bloch et al. 2011, Felling and Singer 2011, McNaught and Mink 2011). However, patients and parents typically ask about it: they may have read about 'chemical imbalances', dopamine or genetics, or be concerned that they or some environmental factor may have caused it in some way. The frequent observation that 'stress' aggravates tics may lend this credence, especially when something stressful has occurred prior to tic onset (such as a parental separation or a head injury). Some tics can be interpreted as deliberate or a 'bad habit', and the child repeatedly admonished or punished.

The following are other possibilities observed as explanations: (1) imitation of others' repetitive behavior (most common when younger siblings develop tics); (2) change in living situation (e.g. from one parent to another); (3) change of school; (4) allergies; (5) infections (even if they have never heard of 'PANDAS'); (6) excessive engagement in computer or video games (Kühn et al. 2011); (7) traumatic experiences.

There is general agreement among researchers that there is not one major causative factor contributing in all cases. A cortico-striatal thalamo-cortical circuit is thought to be involved (Rubenstein 2011). One mechanistic explanation, based largely on an animal model of tics, posits that tics occur when basal ganglia disinhibition affects the thalamic/cortical neurons as well as associative and limbic domains, perhaps thereby accounting for some of the comorbid symptoms of Tourette syndrome (Bronfeld and Bar-Gad 2013).

Genetics
The genetics are still obscure and poorly understood (O'Rourke et al. 2009, Paschou 2013).

That most people with tics have relatives with tics and/or obsessive–compulsive patterns has been shown in many studies, but it is highly likely that there are multiple genetic and environmental factors (and there may be different contributing genes in different families) interacting during development. Originally it was thought that there must be a dominant gene fully penetrant in males, but not in females. This concept gave way to that of a complex disorder with multiple genes, multiple mechanisms and combinations with environmental factors (Leckman and March 2011, Roth and Sweatt 2011, Deng et al. 2012). Genetic heterogeneity is likely. There have been occasional announcements of candidate genes, but none has been replicated (Plomin 2005). In spite of this, there are still websites implicating a dominant gene for tics, Tourette syndrome and even OCD. Most recently histidine decarboxylase deficiency in the basal ganglia has been identified as a rare cause in humans and in a mouse model of tics (Baldan et al. 2014).

Having said this, it is important to realize that the interplay of genes and environment that contributes to the causation of neurodevelopmental disorders (not just tic disorders) is much more complex and dynamic than most clinicians have been taught; these interactions are not necessarily additive (i.e. static) nor necessarily the same combinations in different individuals. The current status of research in this rapidly moving field is wonderfully elaborated in the book edited by Kendler et al. (2011). Nevertheless, the results are not yet significant for treatment interventions for tic disorders (and are therefore beyond the scope of this book). Evidence that stress early in life and even in adolescence can have epigenetic and other effects on an individual (see, for example, van der Knaap et al. 2014) indicates that the old dualism between genetics and environment, nature versus nurture, should really be discarded.

Conceptually there is a question as to whether tics really represent a separate entity, or rather that there is a fundamental core in neurodevelopmental disorders from which various symptoms may emerge and be given different names, this being a brief statement of the proposal by Gillberg (2010) in his papers on what he has termed ESSENCE (*e*arly *s*ymptomatic *s*yndromes *e*liciting *n*eurodevelopmental *c*linical *e*xaminations). In line with this concept, he has pointed out that major problems in more than one domain before age 5 years often signal major problems in the same or overlapping domains later. Such children therefore merit comprehensive work-ups.

Interpreting genetic theories about Tourette syndrome for patients and their family members may be problematic. Many people are not conversant with basic genetic ideas, and it is possible that the familial aspect may increase stigma attached to Tourette syndrome or make it seem less likely to change, as has been suggested for schizophrenia (Bennett et al. 2008).

Obtaining genetic information on the internet is fraught with difficulties because sorting through the information and understanding it may be difficult and confusing (Roche and Skinner 2009). Emotional factors may override well-presented genetic information (Klitzman 2010). Having access to genetic information is not always comforting, nor can it always be shared or discussed by a family.

A major misunderstanding
It is essential to understand that *Tourette syndrome cannot be inherited!* It is a descriptive

category with criteria and cut-off points defined by a committee (and revised now in DSM-5). It is not a 'thing' with a natural boundary. A committee description cannot be biologically inherited. If any literature on Tourette syndrome has made this fundamental point, it must be rare since it has not trickled down to information available on the internet, nor in many papers. *This is not trivial.* It is important because patients and families may make decisions to have children on the basis of the assumption that a child has a specific and known risk to inherit Tourette syndrome as such, because the parent has been diagnosed with Tourette syndrome (especially if impairing). They do not understand that it is *a tendency to manifest tics* (of any severity or complexity on a spectrum) or perhaps OCD that may be one of many factors. The reification of the name is so powerful that explanations often are not understood: "Things perceived as real are real in their consequences" (Thomas and Thomas 1928, p. 572).

Practice point

The assumption that familiality means a pattern of genetic inheritance producing a condition with the specific criteria in DSM-5 is widespread and not even challenged in most publications about tic disorders.

Case example

'Sharie' was first seen at age 48 years after she saw a story in her local newspaper. She complained of tics, anxiety and depression. "I hate it, knowing that it's always there and I have to do it. I'm afraid that some day it'll come back like it was when I was a child." Back then she had had squealing, snorting, touching and coprolalia. She described being very aware of a feeling of tightness around her mouth and shoulders and inside her head. She was teased and her mother hated the faces and noises she made; they were attributed to her attention seeking. She had been taken to many physicians, none of whom made the diagnosis, except for a suggestion of 'St Vitus dance'. Three of her children had tics but didn't know about hers, she said; they had not themselves been diagnosed. One grandchild had tics. If she told them, she felt they would blame her for their tics. Her self-esteem problems created difficulty making friends, and her moods seemed closely related to her attitude toward her tics. Many years later two of her teenage grandchildren were referred. One had Tourette syndrome with coprolalia and trichotillomania, the other Tourette syndrome with coprolalia, OCD, ADHD and dyslexia. Others in that generation were reported to have tics as well.

Comment: This family had a dense tic pattern with a high rate of coprolalia along with a variety of co-occurring disorders, but had not been able to openly share information about the patterns that had been present over at least three generations.

> **Practice point**
>
> Patients and family members need to understand that the working definitions of tic disorders are arbitrary, not "nature carved at its joints" (Campbell et al. 2011). Otherwise they may make incorrect assumptions that can affect their feelings, the meanings given to categories, and even decisions in relation to the category of Tourette syndrome.

Limitations of psychoeducation about etiology and genetics

The power of education is limited (Freeman 2014). Consider a not uncommon situation: an individual has grown up with a severe and impairing tic disorder known to other family members. Now a young child in the family is diagnosed with a chronic tic disorder, let us say Tourette syndrome. Assumptions are made and expectations affected by the emotionally laden image of the tic disorder in that family's history. Now the wise and experienced clinician provides the best information about the range of symptoms and outcomes in tic disorders, including that one person's condition is not predictive of another's. Nevertheless, that clarification may not have the major reassuring effect desired. For some family members accurate information may need repeating and even require ongoing counseling, but it is doubtful that the baleful image of Tourette syndrome will be neutralized. (One tries anyway.)

Video and computer gaming

Parents often bring up video and computer gaming as possible causes of tics. There is some evidence that extensive participation may be harmful (Chan and Rabinowitz 2006), but it could not be a sufficient cause of tic disorders. However, that there may be a neural basis for addiction to video games comes from a study of frequent gamers, who were found to have higher volume in their left ventral striatum that could reflect altered reward processing (Kühn et al. 2011). Extensive gaming may worsen tics, at least temporarily.

Causal factors in comorbid disorders

In many individuals with comorbidity their symptoms may be increased by environmental factors, just as may be true for tics. One will not immediately know that this is so without trying to modify factors whose effect is plausible. A relationship between stress and tic onset and severity has been proposed by Buse et al. (2014) because of the stress activation of the hypothalamic–pituitary–adrenal axis. The case study of 'Brendan' in Chapter 16 (pp. 244–5) illustrates this point clearly. However, we need to be mindful of very important advice regarding both causation and prognosis, as follows.

Practice point

There is reason for optimism:

"… no causal influences in multifactorial disorders are fully determinative. Even when the dice seem loaded against the individual, successful coping may still be attainable and the onus is on the clinician to identify and foster the processes that might lead to success." (Rutter 2013, p. 484)

Role of non-genetic environmental factors

Recent studies have shown that unrecognized and not always obvious environmental factors can influence tic frequency and severity (but are not necessary causes). However, "almost all variables that describe environments include a complex mixture of genetic and environmental mediation" (Rutter 2013, p. 475). Patients and parents can be encouraged to identify these.

Practice point

Before launching into a lecture on genetic and environmental factors in replying to a question about the cause of tics, find out what the person has already learned and why the question is important.

REFERENCES

Baldan LC, Williams KA, Gallezot J-D, et al. (2014) Histidine decarboxylase deficiency causes Tourette syndrome: parallel findings in humans and mice. *Neuron* 81: 77–90. doi: 10.1016/j.neuron.2013.10.052.

Bennett L, Thirlaway K, Murray AJ (2008) The stigmatizing implications of presenting schizophrenia as a genetic disease. *J Genet Counsel* 17: 550–9.

Bloch M, State M, Pittenger C (2011) Recent advances in Tourette syndrome. *Curr Opin Neurol* 24: 119–25. doi: 10.1097/WCO.0b013e328344648c.

Bronfeld M, Bar-Gad I (2013) Tic disorders: what happens in the basal ganglia? *Neuroscientist* 12: 101–8. doi: 10.1177/1073858412444466.

Buse J, Kirschbaum C, Leckman JF, et al. (2014) The modulating role of stress in the onset and course of Tourette's syndrome: a review. *Behav Modif* 38: 184–216. doi: 10.1177/0145445514522056.

Campbell JK, O'Rourke M, Slater MH, eds (2011) *Carving Nature at Its Joints: Natural Kinds in Metaphysics and Science.* Cambridge, MA: MIT Press.

Chan PA, Rabinowitz T (2006) Cross-sectional analysis of video games and attention deficit hyperactivity disorder symptoms in adolescents. *Ann Gen Psychiatry* 5: 16.

Deng H, Gao K, Jankovic J (2012) The genetics of Tourette syndrome. *Nat Rev Neurol* 8: 203–13. doi: 10.1038/nrneurol.2012.26.

Felling RJ, Singer HS (2011) Neurobiology of Tourette syndrome: current status and need for further investigation. *J Neurosci* 31: 12387–95.

Freeman RD (2014) Blame the disorder. *Can J Neurol Sci* 41: 233 (editorial).

Gillberg C (2010) The ESSENCE in child psychiatry: early symptomatic syndromes eliciting neurodevelopmental clinical examinations. *Res Devel Disabil* 31: 1543–51. doi: 10.1016/j.ridd.2010.06.002.

Kendler KS, Jaffee SR, Romer D, eds (2011) *The Dynamic Genome and Mental Health: the Role of Genes and Environments in Youth Development.* New York: Oxford University Press.

Klitzman RL (2010) Misunderstandings concerning genetics among patients confronting genetic disease. *J Genet Counsel* 19: 430–46.

Kühn S, Romanowski A, Schilling C, et al. (2011) The neural basis of video gaming. *Transl Psychiatry* 1: e53. doi: 10.1038/tp.2011.53.

Leckman JF, March JS (2011) Developmental neuroscience comes of age. *J Child Psychol Psychiatry* 52: 333–8. doi: 10.1111/j.1469-7610.2011.02378.x.

McNaught KSP, Mink JW (2011) Advances in understanding and treatment of Tourette syndrome. *Nature Rev Neurol* 7: 667–76. doi: 10.1038/nrneurol.2011.167.

O'Rourke JA, Scharf JM, Yu D, Pauls DL (2009) The genetics of Tourette syndrome: a review. *J Psychosom Res* 67: 533–45. doi: 10.1016/j.jpsychores.2009.06.006.

Paschou P (2013) The genetic basis of Gilles de la Tourette syndrome. *Neurosci Biobehav Rev* 37: 1026–39. doi: 10.1016/j.neubiorev.2013.01.016.

Plomin R (2005) Finding genes in child psychology and psychiatry: when are we going to be there? *J Child Psychol Psychiatry* 46: 1030–8. doi: 10.1111/j.1469-7610.2005.01524.x.

Roche MI, Skinner D (2009) How parents search, interpret and evaluate genetic information obtained from the Internet. *J Genet Counsel* 18: 119–29.

Roth TL, Sweatt JD (2011) Epigenetic mechanisms and environmental shaping of the brain during sensitive periods of development. *J Child Psychol Psychiatry* 52: 398–408. doi: 10.1111/j.1469-7610.2010.02282.x.

Rubenstein JLR (2011) Development of the cerebral cortex: implications for neurodevelopmental disorders. *J Child Psychol Psychiatry* 52: 339–55. doi: 10.1111/j.1469-7610.2010.02307.x.

Rutter M (2013) Resilience – clinical implications. *J Child Psychol Psychiatry* 54: 474–87. doi: 10.1111/j.1469-7610.2012.02615.x.

Thomas WI, Thomas DS (1928) *The Child in America: Behavior Problems and Programs.* New York: Knopf.

van der Knaap LJ, Riese H, Hudziak JJ, et al. (2014) Glucocorticoid receptor gene (*NR3C1*) methylation following stressful events between birth and adolescence. The TRAILS study. *Transl Psychiatry* 4: e381. doi: 10.1038/tp.2014.22.

6
CLINICAL COURSE AND PROGNOSIS

Tics are usually rapid, randomly occurring movements or vocalizations that are of varying complexity, variably suppressible, and subject to changes under stress or excitement. For most patients the onset, whether or not identified as such, occurs in early childhood, often motor tics before vocal ones. The tics are unstable and change their form, complexity, number, frequency of upsurges and degree of impairment, with a 'worst-ever' period around the ages of 10–12 years. During adolescence instability diminishes so that the majority experience improvement, often to the point that their tics are no longer noticed (whether or not they still experience the sensory urges). Most tics, and certainly complex tics, are preceded or accompanied by 'premonitory urges' to tic, with brief relief following the performance of the tic. Little is known about the evolution of tics into old age.

It used to be accepted that tics in Tourette syndrome became worse in adolescence, as our society tends to assume is true of much else. However, the groundbreaking report of Leckman et al. (1998) changed this. It is now generally believed that it is in the preadolescent period at roughly ages 10–12 years that tics are usually at their worst (most unstable), and this has been recently confirmed in another follow-up study (Spencer et al. 1999, Bloch et al. 2006a, Bloch and Leckman 2009). Of 46 children who were followed, 39 reported improvement during adolescence; 19 experienced OCD symptoms and among these, the worst-ever period was 2 years later than the peak of Tourette syndrome symptoms.

Before this point, a single tic may appear around age 5–6 years and be attributed to something other than a tic, then disappear or diminish for a variable period, then another perhaps different one or two appear, and so on, until at some point there are several tics, some of them complex. Between tic exacerbations (termed 'upsurges' here) the baseline of zero often rises so that some tics are always present. Previous explanations no longer suffice, and referral to specialists may result in a correct diagnosis.

It is also said that motor tic onset usually precedes vocal tic onset and coprolalia (if it occurs) (Freeman et al. 2009).

Another important clinical observation is that during an upsurge of tics other brain functions may be affected, such that there may be increased irritability and emotional lability, not ascribable totally to the distractions caused by greater tic awareness.

However, an interesting quality of life study by Bernard et al. (2009) showed that tic severity was not predictive: it was the presence of ADHD (specifically inattentive type) and OCD that was. Other studies have generally confirmed that tic severity is less salient than comorbidity (and specifically ADHD) in the impact on quality of life of the patient and family (Bawden et al. 1998, Woods et al. 2005, Wilkinson et al. 2008).

One serious reservation about the use of the studies cited in counseling parents and patients is the uncertainty as to whether Tourette syndrome that is imbedded in comorbid or co-occurring combinations of diagnoses that have not themselves been included in studies may have a different course. We simply do not know. However, some light has been thrown on this question by Rizzo et al. (2012b). Their conclusions on a 10-year clinical follow-up were that 'pure Tourette syndrome' has a good long-term clinical course; those with comorbidity at onset had a less positive prognosis.

Practice point

In general, it can be said that for most children with persistent tic disorders the tics will get worse (severe and/or unstable) around ages 10–12 years before they get better (stabilize, diminish or disappear) in late adolescence or early adult life.

Various predictors of later adult status have been proposed (one being maternal smoking, with a small effect). Fine-motor coordination difficulties were assessed on a group of young people with Tourette syndrome and followed up at an average of 7.5 years later (Bloch et al. 2006b). Those children with fine-motor weaknesses had worse tic severity and overall psychosocial functioning, but the neuropsychological test results were not predictive of severity of future OCD.

Tracking tics and prognosis

Tics in individuals can be tracked over time with the Yale Global Tic Severity Scale (YGTSS) or the Parent Tic Questionnaire (Chang et al. 2009). Several follow-up studies have shown substantial improvement of tics in adult life, for example Burd et al. (2001) at approximately 15 years later reported that 44% of their original 54 patients were virtually tic-free, 59% improved in overall severity, and there was a 42% reduction in the number of comorbidities. It has been suggested that compensatory neural reorganization may underlie adolescent improvement in tics (Jackson et al. 2011).

Sensory tricks: a provocative possibility

Here we have a fascinating case to consider (Gilbert 2013): a 19-year-old male with severe persistent tics from age 10 was refractory to many different and concurrent medications. He discovered that he could abolish the urge and his severe tics by means of gentle pressure to his head, so would wear a bandana or hat and rest his chin on his hand. A video shows that when his hat or bandana is removed, the tics immediately return. (Some mild tics were not changed thereby.) Sensory tricks like this are typical of dystonia, not tics, but have been reported before, in one-third of a group of 45 tic patients (Wojcieszek and Lang 1995).

Perhaps the reputed limitation mostly to dystonia is due to clinicians not asking tic patients about sensory tricks, and that the phenomenon represents an influence of the sensory cortex. If so, transcranial magnetic stimulation might be effective but so far it has been applied to the motor rather than the sensory cortex. It may be that the belief that such practices are typical of one but not another movement disorder, like the assumption about premonitory sensations absent in stereotypy, has inhibited a broader possibility that could have therapeutic value.

Malignant tics

A subset of patients was given this identifier by Cheung et al. (2007). They reviewed 333 patients who had had two or more emergency department visits or one or more hospitalizations on account of their tics (injuries, SIB, violence, suicidality) in a 3-year period, and compared their history and characteristics with those not meeting these criteria; 5.1% were identified, that group having an increase in OCD, tic complexity, coprophenomena, mood disorder and poor response to medication.

Tics in old age

There is no long-term longitudinal follow-up study of a community sample of tic disorders into old age. Therefore any general statements about a lifetime course of tics are based upon clinicians' stories of referred cases, an obviously biased group, and should be taken with appropriate reservations. There is a case report (Hartman and Yuvarajan 1994) with onset at 72 after possible encephalitis (perhaps representing better what can be termed 'tourettism'). Sutula and Hobbs (1983) reported tic onset in an 81-year-old with no neurological etiology identified. Klawans and Barr (1985) reported four cases of remission of childhood simple tics between the ages of 14 and 20 years, with recurrence at ages 62–71 years. They argued that late-onset tics may be on a continuum with childhood tics, not a new neurological disorder.

Because this is such a difficult and relatively neglected area, more should be said about it. It would seem that prior to the more modern view of Tourette syndrome as sensorimotor rather than purely motor (Bliss 1980) and the understanding of the neurodevelopmental origins of tics, comorbidities and higher prevalence, very few individuals were properly diagnosed and most were never seen by specialists. Their tics were likely to be seen as psychogenic or an indicator of psychological dysfunction (as they still commonly are) and thus could have negative repercussions on self-image and family relationships. These putative outcomes may still be actively affecting the quality of life of countless older persons. Since there is no adequate case series available, a few examples may be instructive.

Case examples

A 55-year-old woman was seen only because a friend saw an article in a women's magazine that seemed to describe her symptoms and when she contacted the TSA the author's name was provided. In short, she had a typical early history of multiple motor and vocal tics, regarded as a psychiatric disorder that led to mental hospitalization for a time, electroconvulsive therapy (ECT), and the breakdown of her marriage. After diagnosis she responded to low-dosage (4mg/d) pimozide maintenance. What was a sad commentary about the lack of early diagnosis was an awkward relationship with a brother. The diagnosis having been made, a suggestion was accepted to meet separately with him. During the explanation about her Tourette syndrome he started crying and confessed that he had always believed that he had been the cause of her movement disorder; this was the first time he had considered that it might be otherwise. He revealed that because her tics began after an episode of sexual touching about which he had felt guilty, he had assumed that that was the cause.

A 67-year-old man had had obvious multiple tics as a child, misdiagnosed as a psychiatric ('neurotic') disorder. When local psychotherapy failed to improve his symptoms he was admitted to a residential treatment center in another city. It is thought that this may have affected his later nagging sense of inferiority and his insecure relationships with others.

Aside from the negative effects of persistently misunderstood symptoms, there is a possibility that when elderly persons encounter health problems their unfortunate Tourette-related experiences with physicians may adversely influence their help-seeking and compliance with medical recommendations. Increasing health problems with age often result in using more medications, some of which may interact with medications for tics. Pain and discomfort from tics may be less tolerable in old age. Some tics might aggravate the social isolation that is all too common among elderly people.

A survey might assist in validating or invalidating these suggestions. There may be no way to recruit a representative sample of elderly persons with tics, but a start can be made through contact with their children or other relatives who may be attending support groups. If indeed elderly persons with tics are suffering in the community because of their lack of diagnosis and counseling, outreach through online blogs, social media, magazine articles and service organizations might well be of significant help to at least some.

Simple or single tics

Most studies and most referrals to specialists are for persistent tics or Tourette syndrome. Very little is known about single tics that are mostly simple and therefore unlikely to be diagnosed. Do they have associated comorbid disorders? How often are they impairing, and in what way? We do not know.

REFERENCES

Bawden HN, Stokes A, Camfield CS, et al. (1998) Peer relationship problems in children with Tourette's disorder or diabetes mellitus. *J Child Psychol Psychiatry* 39: 663–8.
Bernard BA, Stebbins GT, Siegel S, et al. (2009) Determinants of quality of life in children with Gilles de la Tourette syndrome. *Mov Disord* 24: 1070–3. doi: 10.1002/mds.22487.
Bliss J (1980) Sensory experiences of Gilles de la Tourette syndrome. *Arch Gen Psychiatry* 37: 1343–7.
Bloch MH, Leckman JF (2009) Clinical course of Tourette syndrome. *J Psychosom Res* 67: 497–501. doi: 10.1016/j.jpsychores.2009.09.002.

Bloch MH, Peterson BS, Scahill L, et al. (2006a) Adulthood outcome of tic and obsessive–compulsive symptom severity in children with Tourette syndrome. *Arch Pediatr Adolesc Med* 160: 65–9. doi: 10.1001/archpedi.160.1.103

Bloch MH, Sukhodolsky DG, Leckman JF, Schultz RT (2006b) Fine-motor skill deficits in childhood predict adult tic severity and global psychosocial functioning in Tourette's syndrome. *J Child Psychol Psychiatry* 47: 551–9. doi: 10.1111/j.1469-7610.2005.01561.x.

Burd L, Kerbeshian J, Barth A, et al. (2001) Long-term follow-up of an epidemiologically defined cohort of patients with Tourette's syndrome. *J Child Neurol* 16: 431–7. doi: 10.1177/088307380101600609.

Chang S, Himle MB, Tucker BTP, et al. (2009) Initial psychometric properties of a brief parent-report instrument for assessing tic severity in children with chronic tic disorders. *Child Fam Behav Ther* 31: 181–91. doi: 10.1080/07317100903099100.

Cheung M-YC, Shahed J, Jankovic J (2007) Malignant Tourette syndrome. *Mov Disord* 22: 1743–50. doi: 10.1002/mds.21599.

Freeman RD, Zinner SH, Müller-Vahl KR, et al. (2009) Coprophenomena in Tourette syndrome. *Dev Med Child Neurol* 51: 218–27. doi: 10.1111/j.1469-8749.2008.03135.x.

Gilbert RW (2013) Tic modulation using sensory tricks. *Tremor Other Hyperkinet Mov* 3: tre-03-115-3129-1 (case report). Published online Mar 26, 2013 (http://tremorjournal.org/article/view/115).

Hartman JA, Yuvarajan R (1994) Case report: Tourette syndrome in the elderly. *Int J Geriatr Psychiatry* 9: 157–9.

Jackson SR, Parkinson A, Jung J, et al. (2011) Compensatory neural reorganization in Tourette syndrome. *Curr Biol* 21: 580–5. doi: 10.1016/j.cub.2011.02.047.

Klawans HL, Barr A (1985) Recurrence of childhood multiple tics in late adult life. *Arch Neurol* 42: 1979–80.

Leckman JF, Zhang H, Vitale A, et al. (1998) Course of tic severity in Tourette syndrome: the first two decades. *Pediatrics* 102: 14–9.

Rizzo R, Gulisano M, Calì PV, Curatolo P (2012) Long term clinical course of Tourette syndrome. *Brain Dev* 34: 667–73. doi: 10.1016/j.braindev.2011.11.006.

Spencer T, Biederman J, Coffey B, et al. (1999) The 4-year course of tic disorders in boys with attention-deficit/hyperactivity disorder. *Arch Gen Psychiatry* 56: 842–7. doi: 10.1001/archpsyc.56.9.842.

Sutula T, Hobbs WR (1983) Senile onset of vocal and motor tics. *Arch Neurol* 40: 693–4.

Wilkinson BJ, Marshall RM, Curtwright B (2008) Impact of Tourette's disorder on parent reported stress. *J Child Fam Stud* 17: 582–98. doi: 10.1007/s10826-007-9176-8.

Wojcieszek JM, Lang AE (1995) Gestes antagonistes in the suppression of tics: 'tricks for tics.' *Mov Disord* 10: 226–8. doi: 10.1002/mds.870100219.

Woods DW, Himle MB, Osmon DC (2005) Use of the impact on family scale in children with tic disorders: descriptive data, validity, and tic severity impact. *Child Fam Behav Ther* 27: 11–21. doi: 10.1300/J019v27n02_02.

7
PHENOMENOLOGY AND SOCIAL CONSEQUENCES

Tics can be of any movement or sound, an astounding range of possibilities. Stress or anxiety can trigger an increase in tics. Suppressibility varies from person to person and from time and situation to others. Suggestibility may be a factor in temporarily increased severity of tics from tic-talk and observation of others' tics. Tics inhabit a conceptual space between voluntary and involuntary, despite assertions made that they are generally beyond control. There is some evidence for increased sensitivity to inner and outer stimuli. Echophenomena are common. Exploring meanings is important. Even when done well, though, meanings may remain relatively unchanged and continue to cause difficulty. Unless the patient's course is relatively mild and stable you can expect to see your patient again for a problem that may seem to have been adequately explained. This may not occur at a convenient time, either.

The 'strange range' of tic characteristics

Tics can take on almost any movement or noise that a human can make, and some that may seem beyond the range of human capability (Leckman et al. 2006). Movements of the ears were described by Keshavan (1988) and Cardoso and Faleiro (1999). In several local cases known to the author (one described in Chapter 3) a family lived in rental housing where the rental contract specified 'no pets'. Neighbors complained that the family was violating the contract, so the landlord sent a warning: get rid of the pet or be evicted. The author had to send a letter explaining that the 'pet' was the patient! Another patient who had never lived in the area developed a Brooklyn-like accent. Another male patient with constant impairing speech dysfluency and severe tics only minimally responsive to medication reported that his tics (and speech) were substantially improved when he cross-dressed as a female. Even harder to believe was that the degree of improvement depended upon whether he dressed completely as a woman or only with external clothing. Faced with skepticism, he presented video recordings made by his friends, which fully validated his description.

Effects of 'stress' and life events

Stress is experienced by everyone, with many variations, but is a rather nebulous concept that can be overused to explain almost anything. Stress and excitement seem to increase the frequency and/or intensity of tics for many persons; this is probably the origin of the notion that tics are *caused* by stress or emotional factors. It is very important that parents and patients understand the difference. Anxiety disorders are a fairly frequent accompaniment of Tourette syndrome, and may be the predominant symptom because of effects on family and school. Special attention may need to be paid to environmental changes that can impact on sensitive, anxious children. Common examples are a more frightening or demanding teacher, teasing, bullying, and an increase in task level or complexity.

Situational variability

An interesting study (Woods et al. 2008) has found that differential reinforcement in various contexts may play a role in explaining the often-observed variability in tic expression. The factors involved were not always obvious. This important finding needs replication and extension.

Suppressibility

Suppressibility, that is, the conscious control of tics, is usually partial and brief. In a study of the developmental aspects of both premonitory sensations and suppressibility of tics in 254 patients, Banaschewski et al. (2003) found 64% able to partially suppress their tics although only 37% reported premonitory sensations. They concluded that awareness of the sensations is not necessary for suppression. Blanket statements that tics are 'involuntary' may be convenient, but are misleading and may have unintended and unfortunate consequences. Schools trying to decide whether or not a child's disruptive behavior is to be treated as a disciplinary matter are not pleased to learn from the clinician that "it depends... sometimes more, sometimes less". Persons with tics know that the extent of suppressibility is variable. If tics are simply described as 'involuntary' then any behavior may have an automatic excuse. Suppressibility can sometimes interfere with capturing a video clip to show to the clinician, and lead to the clinician not taking the tics seriously.

Case study

'Joshua' is an extreme example with an unfortunate outcome. He had an underappreciated history of past episodic SIB. When he developed violent 'whiplash-like' twisting of his neck, the physicians who saw him observed no tics and the parents were unable to capture a sample video because "He won't do it" when aware of an attempt to capture his pattern, which the parents blamed on his exciting computer games. The physicians told the parents that his tics could not be the cause; they attributed his muscle-wasting and bilaterally asymmetric neurologic signs as due to a sports injury and did not refer to neurology. A sports medicine referral resulted in an opinion that the referral was inappropriate. Referral back to a pediatrician (each step involving a wait) also resulted in no belief that his described tic could be the cause. When finally seen in the emergency department his neurologic signs had progressed and an MRI showed damage to his spinal cord and some changes in his cervical vertebrae. A hard collar was supplied to limit the effects of his tic, but complete recovery was not to be expected. Joshua refused

---

to accept this prognosis and family conflict developed (elaborated further in Chapter 17).

> **Comment:** *There are four other reports in the English-language literature (Krauss and Jankovic 1996, Dobbs and Berger 2003, Lin et al. 2007, Isaacs et al. 2010). Joshua now has an impaired gait, permanent deltoid wasting, and numbness and paresthesias in his arms and legs. This very unusual situation seems to be attributable to several factors: extreme tic suppression making it hard for consulting physicians to believe the parents' description, lack of appreciation of the predictive importance of past SIB in the case history, and stubborn rejection of the possibility of such severe tic SIB. We do not expect non-experts to be familiar with literature on rare symptoms or outcomes, but persistence in a negative belief as occurred here seems unjustifiable.*

AUTOMATIC SUPPRESSION

Automatic suppression is a common but perhaps not universal aspect of tics: few tics may be displayed in an interview, sometimes none at all, but on the way out, or in the car, or at home, out they come. This presents at least two clinical problems: first, patient or family description may not be believed, or not fully appreciated; second, it contributes to the impression that the tics are voluntary. Sometimes automatic suppression (as well as deliberate suppression) interferes with capturing a video clip to show to the clinician. A theoretical puzzle is how to reconcile exacerbation by 'stress' with reduction of tics in the physician's office (not a place generally associated with lack of stress). It seems that no study has dealt with this seeming paradox.

> **Practice point and key concept**
>
> It is not possible to estimate the relative proportions of conscious and automatic control of tics in any particular individual in different situations and at different times, nor may control apply equally to all a person's tics. For this reason tics cannot be said to be generally either 'voluntary' or 'involuntary'.

Suggestibility

Suggestibility may have a complex relationship with suppressibility. Many persons with tics feel an increased urge to perform a tic when they observe it in another, or even read about it or are asked about it (Woods et al. 2001). (See also the effects of tic talk, in Chapter 2.) But that does not mean that they will keep that urge-related tic. The following illustration shows how important this misunderstanding may sometimes be.

> **Case example**
>
> *'Ayden' was 12 when seen for assessment. He had some obvious but not severe or disruptive tics. His schoolwork and motivation had deteriorated and there were problems that had developed in his family. It seemed that he was clinically depressed. Seen alone,*

though, he was surprised to learn that the new tic urges he had developed after seeing different tics in other persons would not become permanent and lead to a greatly impaired future.

   Comment: *It was an initial clinical puzzle why, after learning about tics, he continued to assert that his tics were the preeminent problem. That seemed to be because suggestibility had not been addressed in the educational part of the assessment. The provisional diagnosis of a depressive disorder was revised. This is also a good illustration of the importance of uncovering a meaning that may be central to the nature of the experience of the disorder.*

Suggestibility needs to be addressed in the interview with the patient, but also with the parents, who out of anxiety and frustration often keep asking their child why he or she is doing it, or may confuse other movements with tics. It is good to explain that this can sometimes complicate the child's efforts to develop more self-control. The power of talking about tics to influence them seems to vary among individuals and is sometimes explored in behavioral treatment.

Timing

When are tics most or least likely to occur? Although there is some variation, the usual pattern is: (1) less in school than at home; (2) more towards the end of the day; (3) within those periods, more at times between actions, when bored, or when excited. Tics may not be noticed at all when the child is engaged in gross motor activities, such as swimming or running. Consequences can be illustrated as follows: mother anticipates a call from the teacher about the tics, but it does not come; she goes to a parent–teacher conference and tics are not mentioned. One could, as was common in the past, begin to interpret the tics as a marker for a deep-seated psychological conflict or relationship problem. In school, tics may be much more noticeable in one class than another, leading to the erroneous conclusion that they are simply deliberate or attention seeking.

Premonitory sensations

Leckman et al. (2006) have provided a very good review of this subject, starting with the historic breakthrough occasioned by the subjective experiences of Joseph Bliss (1980). In an important study, Kwak et al. (2003) reported that 92% of 50 persons with Tourette syndrome reported premonitory sensations (e.g. urges, aches, pressures, itches); if prevented from performing the tic, 74% reported intensification of the sensation, 72% reported relief after doing it, and 68% described a motor tic as "a voluntary motor response to an involuntary sensation" (p. 1530). Awareness of premonitory sensations increases with a child's age.

   Although premonitory sensations are usually thought of as arising de novo (without known physical cause) from the same area as the tic or nearby, it is very important to realize that bodily sensations whose origin is physical can also trigger new tics or aggravate existing ones. Common examples are allergies, infections, and local injuries such as bruises, scrapes, insect bites, sprained ligaments, or dental or orthodontic work.

A need to reach a 'just right' feeling with one's tics (to stifle a premonitory sensation) is said to be associated with comorbid OCD, but a recent study suggests otherwise (Himle and Woods 2005).

Complicated considerations arise when there are combinations of sensory hypersensitivity, symptom prolongation for poorly understood reasons (e.g. prolonged airway sensitization after viral infections), existing tics, and psychosocial factors (school or parental worry, attributed meanings, or social disruption by symptoms). Sensations that involve dramatic complaints such as "A plate stuck in the back of my throat", "I can't get enough air" or "A hair stuck behind my eyeball" evoke great anxiety to get to the bottom of the symptom, assuming that some physical 'thing' will be found to correspond to the description.

Case example

'Mason', an 8-year-old boy with a strong history of hypersensitivities (tactile, olfactory, and a hyperactive gag reflex), ADHD combined type, some anxiety, mild obsessive–compulsive symptoms, aggression and high-functioning autism, developed an upper respiratory infection with bronchitis, and impetigo in the facial area, including his nostrils. The presenting problems were snorting and persistent nose-blowing in school that were loud enough to bother his teacher and classmates.

__Comment:__ Important here were (1) he had distressing local irritation of his nostrils and did not use tissues to blow his nose, instead blowing into the air in front of him while holding the tissue close, or using his shirt; (2) the need to understand what might be happening, and that it was not deliberate; (3) his need to understand why the noise was bothersome to others (not apparent to him); (4) the school had to be creative in allowing him time to settle in the mornings with some individual activity first, because his symptoms were worse when he felt anxious about having to immediately enter the group situation. On follow-up, the symptoms had diminished.

It appears that persons with Tourette syndrome tend to be more sensitive than average to external stimuli (Belluscio et al. 2011). This important study suggested that altered central processing rather than enhanced peripheral detection is responsible.

Symmetry

Symmetry patterns and increased awareness are common in chronic tic disorders, but we have no prevalence figures to report. Characteristic of some Tourette syndrome and OCD patients is a very strong need to even up sensations on both sides of the body, probably related to a need to arrange and order objects. Many persons without Tourette syndrome or OCD report some awareness of symmetry or lack of it, but their urge to even up is resistable. One can access this by asking, "Do you ever feel the need to even up what you do on one side of your body what you have done on the other?" Parents may respond with a "No", while the child says "Yes" and gives examples.

Case example

A 9-year-old boy was brought to our emergency department because he was leaning to one side, "like the Leaning Tower of Pisa", someone remarked. This turned out to be his way to compensate for a disturbing awareness that he had been sitting in an uneven, asymmetric pattern for a prolonged time.

Variability in tic awareness

It may be surprising to clinicians and others who are aware of a patient's tics that the perception of one's own tics can vary from acute to absent. Lang (1991) studied 170 patients with various kinds of movements, of whom 60 had tic disorders. Almost all of the 110 patients with non-tic movement disorders stated that all their abnormal movements were completely involuntary. Forty-one of the 60 with tic disorders stated that all of their tics were performed 'voluntarily' but the definitions of voluntariness were complex. The conclusion was that the tics were voluntary, but irresistible. In compulsions, the actions were also voluntary but irresistible. For an act to be voluntary one must have "the volitional ability to will to perform the act… but this requires that one can also will not to do the act" (p. 226). This description of the tic experience agrees with the description by Bliss (1980). Children and some adults often deny that they still perform a particular tic, probably partly because of the lack of awareness. (Persons are often unaware of their mannerisms and repetitive behaviors, too.)

Echophenomena

Persons with Tourette syndrome are reported to have frequent echophenomena (echolalia, echopraxia), which are considered normal in young children but are usually suppressed or controlled in adults. Clinically one may see imitation of another's tics or other movements. An experimental study by Finis et al. (2012) established that persons with Tourette syndrome are more likely to display this phenomenon than those without Tourette syndrome. The suggestion is that the mirror neuron system may be affected and that echopraxia is "a hallmark of Tourette syndrome" (Finis et al. 2012, p. 562).

Pain

Significant pain is not a frequent complaint due to tics, but it can occur in a number of ways as elaborated by Riley and Lang (1989): direct effects of sudden and repeated muscular exertion; pain from hitting a body part; deliberate self-injury; pain or discomfort from suppressive efforts; and in those who experience relief from tics by having or causing pain.

In rare cases, severe injury can result from violent tics. Isaacs et al. (2010) described a 20-year-old man with 3 years of progressive gait unsteadiness, foot deformity and numbness in his feet, thought to be due to noncompressive myelopathy from hyperextension of the cervical spine and lateral flexion tics. Other authors have also described compressive myelopathy (Krauss and Jankovic 1996, Dobbs and Berger 2003, Ko et al. 2013) and cervical disc herniation (Lin et al. 2007). This topic is discussed further in Chapter 12.

A dramatic description, presumably of Tourette syndrome (though without mention of vocalizations), is in the German poet Rainer Maria Rilke's *Das Tagebuch des Malte Laurids Brigge* (in English: *The Diary of Malte Laurids Brigge*). It describes the course down the street of a man who fits the clinical description, and the cruel reaction of others to his 'performance', as well as his reactions to being observed in a public place (Cavanna et al. 2010).

These passages complement the excellent description of the effects of obvious tics in creating a sense of 'disorder' in public spaces by Davis et al. (2004). Wilensky (1999) has poignantly shown, in her autobiographical account, how she was not fully aware of her tics, and the shock when she became more aware. The recent accounts by van Bloss (2006) and Turtle and Robertson (2008) add to the first-person descriptions of the experiences, which include the important point that patterns of upsurges are not always identifiable and predictable, and that the sensory component of tics may be impossible to adequately describe.

Tic variations can have major social effects

A tic (or indeed a non-tic repetitive motor behavior) can be tolerated until a variation is introduced, at which 'tipping point' major problems can arise. Six examples illustrate this point.

Case examples

A 3-year-old boy had typical stereotypic movement disorder which caused no difficulty until he started to make the rapid lifting of his hands show his middle finger extended. Suddenly everyone noticed. How could such a small child be 'giving the finger'? (This pattern is — in North America and other places — well known as a vulgar insult.) It appeared that this was only a mild modification of his previous pattern, probably reinforced by the attention given it by some of those around him. It soon subsided.

An 8-year-old boy frequently put his hands down his pants. His class became accustomed to it after a while. But for reasons unknown he started to smell his fingers each time he withdrew his hands, and this brought him instant and unwelcome attention as 'gross' (disgusting).

A 13-year-old girl had had tic-related gait peculiarities for a long time. She would suddenly partially squat down or make a knee-bend. Although this looked odd her friends weren't troubled by it. When she added pelvic thrusting, however, and shortly thereafter added a grunting sound, the teenagers in her class as well as strangers reacted with amusement or embarrassment.

Her classmates were quite aware of nose-picking by a 6-year-old girl. After her parents and others were unsuccessful in asking her to not do it, it was reluctantly tolerated. Soon, however, the pattern extended. After removing something from her nostril she would smell it and then eat it. This was too much to ignore.

One of the many tics that a 12-year-old boy displayed was hitting his elbows (adducting

---

his arms) against his chest, which occasionally caused soreness. Under the increased stress of school examinations a new movement was added to the pattern: abducting his arms and hitting those next to him.

Hitting himself on his thighs, especially when sitting, was a familiar tic for an 11-year-old boy. When this migrated to hitting his crotch area the tic brought much more unwelcome attention to his disorder.

Tic variations as a feature of Tourette syndrome are unusual among disorders in that they frequently pose problems of readjusting to social situations that may have been previously mastered by the patient or the family. This is often seen with the development of copro-phenomena.

Case example
Ten-year-old 'Teresa' had frequent vocal tics which required judgment as to whether to go to a movie or concert where her noises might be disruptive. This usually succeeded when the performance was loud and masked most of the tics, because she and her parents had become skilled enough to negotiate many awkward situations. These skills were inadequate, however, when coprolalia developed. When the sound level in the theater was low her tics were too obvious and their imputed meaning seemed to be of criticism of the film or performance. Explanations could not be addressed to an entire theater.

Physical interference by tics
With accelerating complexity of tics in an upsurge, one may see some interference with activities of daily living — like eating effortlessly, holding a cup, walking, running, reading smoothly like before — that can make parents wonder how far it could go, and will surely prompt a push to get to the expert or to find some apparently effective treatment.

Bullying and teasing
This important topic is discussed in detail in Chapter 18.

The fuzzy diagnostic boundary
There is sometimes a tendency to expand the concept of tics/Tourette syndrome to include other symptoms such as non-tic repetitive motor behaviors (Chapter 12), stereotypies of various sorts (including stereotypic movement disorder, Chapter 11), 'rage', and even non-epileptic spells ('freezing' tics, especially with rhythmic shaking). The boundaries are not sharp anyway. The result may be that the tic condition is seen as worse than it is; this can lead to distortion of activities and family functioning. Once confidently classified by — or for — the patient or family, it can become reified into 'my Tourette syndrome', and seem to explain too much.

Case example

Fourteen-year-old 'Peter' had tics, but also prolonged episodes that were not tics and that served to excuse him from many physical activities and from going to school, keeping him home and close to his mother. They served also to maintain dysfunctional patterns within the family. The function this behavior played was not apparent to the family until considerable therapeutic effort was expended.

Practice point

This point needs to be stressed: arriving at the most accurate categorization of the symptoms (tic and non-tic) may be essential, and to that must be added an exploration of the personal meanings of that categorization, which may be very different from the clinician's. Just as a parent may misinterpret the meanings of a seizure and what one must do about it and its risk, there is a similar need with tics. Respiratory tics and the child's explanation of them are particularly likely to cause anxious concern.

What does 'worse' mean?

When parents or patients describe a condition as 'worse', the conventional meaning is usually taken to be an increase in frequency, intensity, kind of symptom, pain or discomfort, and interference with activities. But specifically with tics, there may be other characteristics to be alert to including the following.

- *'Rising baseline phenomenon'.* Early in the course of Tourette syndrome (in the first few months or even the first few years after onset) tics may decline to zero or almost zero between upsurges; this is part of the well-known 'waxing–waning' pattern. Often the zero baseline rises with time: then some tics are always present. This is one important factor that brings a family to the clinician and demolishes the false hope that it isn't really Tourette syndrome.
- *Social impact of new tics.* Each tic has a different potential to be noticeable to others in a particular culture or activity and to bother them and the self-conscious tiqueur.
- *Tics harder to suppress in school or at work.* Change in concurrent task demands (multitasking) or the attitudes and sensitivities of others may make the effort more difficult.
- *Interference with sleep onset.* Some tics are more distracting (or worrying for the patient) than others.
- *Intrusion of new obsessions or ruminations.* A new persistent worry or a sense of being 'stuck' may make tics feel worse.
- *Demoralization with negative thinking.* New tics or other symptoms and less tic-free time can seem your destiny: "things will only get worse".
- *Increase in 'just right' urges.* Tics may take up more time and concentration when they must be re-performed perfectly.

- *Complaints by others.* New persons in one's daily life or new problems reducing the tolerance of others may become stressful, especially when it seems difficult or impossible to alter one's tics. Each new person you have to deal with (e.g. new teacher, coach, bully) raises issues of the effect of tics on their sensitivities and expectations.
- *Changes in activities* (e.g. sport or job promotion) with new demands or exposure to the public.
- *Response to increased workload or task complexity* in school or at work. It may not be an absolute increase in the tics that makes the adaptation to life 'worse'.
- *Start of new symptoms of other disorders, not attributable to tics.*
- *Expectable tic upsurges* aren't necessarily taken in stride by parents just because you as a clinician have diligently described the course of Tourette syndrome to them. Early in the family's adapting to the presence of Tourette syndrome, a tic upsurge may present as a crisis, and require reinforcement of what was previously explained. If you the clinician are not available, your patient may end up in a hospital emergency department.
- *Unexpected tic upsurges* can be those that occur with the patient on medication for tics. It is essential to explain (and perhaps re-explain later) that medication that successfully lessens the level of tics does not eliminate tic fluctuations or the appearance of new tics. If this happens it need not mean that the person's condition is 'worse', or that treatment is useless.

What does 'better' mean?

In addition to a reduction in bothersome tics, 'better' could be brought about by improved understanding (or changed meanings) by the patient, family or important others, helpful accommodations to the symptoms by the school, a valued new activity, or a troublesome teacher or schoolmate moving away.

What does 'cure' mean?

Parents may ask about the chances for a 'cure', but never have thought about the meaning of the concept. The commonly mentioned '5-year cures' for cancer don't help. It sounds odd to say that you only know when someone is cured when he or she is dead, but that is technically correct. A symptom (tics) can return after years of absence, under specific circumstances, as could occur with asthma, for example. In a sense the best one can get is an indefinite remission, but this point needs to be explained (Petrie et al. 2007).

Patients' beliefs are associated with increasing public awareness of risk factors and health outcomes in a broadening range of illnesses (Carel 2012).

The problem of our ignorance about 'simple' or single tics

Most of what has been considered concerns persistent tic disorders, not necessarily 'simple' relatively stable tics. Most of these probably do not come to specialist attention. We know relatively little about them, whether they are associated with premonitory urges, how aware persons are of their tics, how they explain them (if at all) to themselves or others, and the varying social consequences and related symptoms or comorbidities. If they subside, how often and under what conditions may they reappear? And in sum, are they really as simple as they are termed? These and other questions could be fruitful areas for investigation.

REFERENCES

Banaschewski T, Woerner W, Rothenberger A (2003) Premonitory sensory phenomena and suppressibility of tics in Tourette syndrome: developmental aspects in children and adolescents. *Dev Med Child Neurol* 45: 700–3. doi: 10.1111/j.1469-8749.2003.tb00873.x.

Belluscio BA, Jin L, Watters V, et al. (2011) Sensory sensitivity to external stimuli in Tourette syndrome patients. *Mov Disord* 26: 2538–43. doi: 10.1002/mds.23977.

Bliss J (1980) Sensory experiences of Gilles de la Tourette syndrome. *Arch Gen Psychiatry* 37: 1343–7.

Cardoso F, Faleiro R (1999) Tourette syndrome: another cause of movement disorder of the ear. *Mov Disord* 14: 888–9. doi: 10.1002/1531-8257(199909).

Carel H (2012) Phenomenology as a resource for patients. *J Lit Philosophy* 37: 96–113.

Cavanna AE, Pattumelli MG, Quarto T, et al. (2010) The 'imprisoned illness': motor tic disorder in Rainer Maria Rilke's Notebooks of Malte Laurids Brigge. *Mov Disord* 25: 1980–2. doi: 10.1002/mds.23203.

Davis KK, Davis JS, Dowler L (2004) In motion, out of place: the public space(s) of Tourette syndrome. *Soc Sci Med* 59: 103–12. doi: 10.1016/j.socscimed.2003.10.008.

Dobbs M, Berger JR (2003) Cervical myelopathy secondary to violent tics of Tourette's syndrome. *Neurology* 60: 1862–3. doi: 10.1212/01.WNL.0000064285.98285.CF.

Finis J, Moczydlowski A, Pollok B, et al. (2012) Echoes from childhood – imitation in Gilles de la Tourette syndrome. *Mov Disord* 27: 562–5. doi: 10.1002/mds.24913.

Himle MB, Woods DW (2005) An experimental evaluation of tic suppression and the tic rebound effect. *Behav Res Ther* 43: 1443–51. doi: 10.1016/j.brat.2004.11.002.

Isaacs JD, Adams M, Lees AJ (2010) Noncompressive myelopathy associated with violent axial tics of Tourette syndrome. *Neurology* 74: 697–8.

Keshavan MS (1988) The ear wigglers: tics of the ear in 10 patients. *Am J Psychiatry* 145: 1462–3.

Ko DY, Kim SJK, Chae JH, et al. (2013) Cervical spondylotic myelopathy caused by violent motor tics in a child with Tourette syndrome. *Childs Nerv Syst* 29: 317–21. doi: 10.1007/s00381-012-1939-x.

Krauss JK, Jankovic J (1996) Severe motor tics causing cervical myelopathy in Tourette's syndrome. *Mov Disord* 11: 563–6. doi: 10.1002/mds.870110512.

Kwak C, Dat Vuong K, Jankovic J (2003) Premonitory sensory phenomenon in Tourette's syndrome. *Mov Disord* 18: 1530–3. doi: 10.1002/mds.10618.

Lang A (1991) Patient perception of tics and other movement disorders. *Neurology* 41: 223–8.

Leckman JF, Bloch MH, King RA, Scahill L (2006) Phenomenology of tics and natural history of tic disorders. *Adv Neurol* 99: 1–16.

Lin J-J, Wang H-S, Wong M-C, et al. (2007) Tourette's syndrome with cervical disc herniation. *Brain Dev* 29: 61–3.

Petrie KJ, Jago LA, Devcich DA (2007) The role of illness perceptions in patients with medical conditions. *Curr Opin Psychiatry* 20: 163–7.

Riley DE, Lang AE (1989) Pain in Gilles de la Tourette syndrome and related tic disorders. *Can J Neurol Sci* 16: 439–41.

Turtle L, Robertson MM (2008) Tics, twitches, tales: the experiences of Gilles de la Tourette's syndrome. *Am J Orthopsychiatry* 78: 449–55.

Van Bloss N (2006) *Busy Body: My Life with Tourette's Syndrome.* London: Fusion Press.

Wilensky AS (1999) *Passing for Normal: a Memoir of Compulsion.* New York: Broadway Books.

Woods DW, Watson TS, Wolfe E, et al. (2001) Analyzing the influence of tic-related talk on vocal and motor tics in children with Tourette's syndrome. *J Appl Behav Anal* 34: 353–6. doi: 10.1901/jaba.2001.34-353.

Woods DW, Himle MB, Miltenberger RG, et al. (2008) Durability, negative impact, and neuropsychological predictors of tic suppression in children with chronic tic disorder. *J Abnorm Child Psychol* 36: 237–45. doi: 10.1007/s10802-007-9173-9.

8
THE LIVED EXPERIENCE

Countless experiences of daily life impinge upon persons with tic disorders and shape their reactions to themselves and others. Often these are difficult to articulate and disclose, but are worth encouraging and sharing. First-person descriptions are often more moving and helpful in fostering insight than journal articles or textbooks.

Tourette syndrome is more than its biology, epidemiology and treatment, with which clinicians spend most of their time. For the patient, living and contending with it has profound and often enduring effects (even when it later remits) that shape its trajectory and outcome. This topic is much less likely to be inquired into or offered up by the patient, and time may not foster its elicitation, but one should be aware of its importance (Kleinman 1988, Flood and Soricelli 1992, Monroe et al. 1992, Toombs 1993). Given that life with chronic tic disorders includes countless experiences of the feelings associated with the tics, that lead up to the tics, that may follow the tics, that involve others' reactions and judgments about the tics, and similarly with comorbid symptoms or disorders, against a unique personal background, much about each situation escapes capture or appreciation by others. The patient may be unable or unwilling to articulate his or her feelings. To have the opportunity to try will require time, a rare and restricted commodity. Since we are used to saying that the physician's role is to 'comfort always', whether we can cure or not, how can that be accomplished with tics, which we cannot cure? We could start by asking, of a child and his or her parents, or an adult, "How are you doing with this?"

We should also be suspicious that a child's feelings of disappointing the parent because of the disorder may be present but disavowed (or vice versa, the parent's feelings about his or her child).

In the following section excellent descriptions and stories from three books by persons with Tourette syndrome (Wilensky 1999, Van Bloss 2006, Cohen and Wysocky 2008) along with a medical anthropologic study of 17 adults with Tourette syndrome in Indiana by Buckser (2006, 2008, 2009) are utilized.

> … there's one thing about them [tics] that drives me to despair. I cannot escape from myself, from the me of constant activity, movement, clenching, grinding, flexing, shaking, pulling and pushing. One thing I cannot do is relax. Please don't tell me to sit still, because I simply can't. (Van Bloss 2006, p. 15)

> [Describing his 'counting thing'…] This counting lark often gets especially irritating when I'm in

conversation with people. I find myself counting the number of times they say certain words... (Van Bloss 2006, p. 67)

In addition to the barks and whoops, I developed some additional strange tics during the course of grades five and six. Off and on I had a smelling tic — a strong urge to sniff things, especially books and paper. Newspapers were the worst. Every time I saw a newspaper, I'd have to smell every section of it... I tried to stay away from newspapers, but then I started smelling the pages in my schoolbooks... I also began chomping my teeth so badly that I once chipped a tooth... After the chomping tic left, the touching tic began. Not only did I need to touch things, I needed to touch them in a certain way. Sometimes I needed to touch something with my left hand, then my right, then my left again, alternating hands until I touched the object just perfectly. That gave way to the sound tic. When turning up the volume on the TV, I needed to do it in a particular way. The volume had to be just so. The same was true with the radio in the car, and the slamming of the car door, and the hanging up of the telephone. If things didn't sound just right, I'd do whatever it was over and over again until it made that perfect sound, the one I needed to hear... So you can see why my extended family thought I was a bit odd. (Cohen and Wysocky 2008, pp. 37–8)

The difficult part of being in public was the unpredictability — not knowing what might happen or how people might treat me. Tourette syndrome continued to get in my way. It got me kicked out of restaurants and movies. (Cohen and Wysocky 2008, p. 77)

In these brief passages one can see the symmetry urges, the changing of repetitive patterns, the apparent restlessness that could be considered to be due to ADHD, the question of whether the smelling was a tic or a compulsion, and the unpredictable reaction of others to the tics.

Peter Hollenbeck, a neuroscientist at Purdue University, has Tourette syndrome. He did not know his diagnosis for many years. But in reminiscing about what was most important in his childhood, he has written:

... there was also a wonderful, ongoing surprise in my childhood and adolescence: those closest to me remained outwardly unperturbed by even my most baroque tics. If I have succeeded in life despite having Tourette, it is in large part because I had the good fortune to be a ticcing young boy who had some compassionate onlookers — a loving family and friends who simply let me tic — and a marvelous, intuitive doctor who convinced me that everything would be OK. (Hollenbeck 2003)

Some research has recently been undertaken on quality of life in young people with Tourette syndrome. Wadman et al. (2013) used structured interviews with 14- to 16-year-olds in the UK and found that they felt Tourette syndrome was a constant presence in their lives, but several of them felt proud of their coping skills and supportive friendships they had developed. Their major social problem was reported to be entering a group of new peers, and their most common future concern was getting a job if their tics did not abate. It is interesting that they had many fewer friends in elementary school when they had fewer coping strategies. Some peers did not believe that one boy with mild tics had Tourette syndrome because he did not match their stereotype of a person with uncontrollable swearing. Peer victimization was not apparent in this small group, as had been reported by Storch et al. (2007) and Cutler et al. (2009).

The residuals

Much too little is written about the experience of the return of symptoms that you or your loved ones hoped wouldn't happen. Isn't this strange, when 'waxing and waning' is characteristic of childhood persistent tic disorders? What is that like? Even for your doctor? Do you detect disappointment in his or her manner? Have you somehow failed? If you have urges with your tics, how is that experience changed now that your tics are 'gone'? You may wonder, "Am I back to my former self, like people want me to be? I'm still feeling something inside…" If therapy helps you manage your tics, and your urges to tic can be resisted, what is left and how do you experience the residual or an upsurge of tics? Prognostic percentages tell us little or nothing about this. Once you realize how your tics are experienced by others, the 'tic effect' is open to some choice: you can deny it, enhance it, even use it as a manipulation, and by so doing regain some lost personal power.

REFERENCES

Buckser A (2006) The empty gesture: Tourette syndrome and the semantic dimensions of illness. *Ethnology* 45: 255–74.

Buckser A (2008) Before your very eyes: illness, agency, and the management of Tourette syndrome. *Med Anthrop Q* 22: 167–92.

Buckser A (2009) Institutions, agency, and illness in the making of Tourette syndrome. *Hum Org* 68: 293–306.

Cohen B, Wysocky L (2008) *Front of the Class: How Tourette Syndrome Made Me the Teacher I Never Had.* New York: VanderWyk & Burnham.

Cutler D, Murphy T, Gilmour J, Heyman I (2009) The quality of life of young people with Tourette syndrome. *Child Care Health Dev* 35: 496–504. doi: 10.1111/j.1365-2214.2009.00983.x.

Flood DH, Soricelli RL (1992) Development of the physician's narrative voice in the medical case history. *Lit Med* 11: 64–83.

Hollenbeck PJ (2003) A jangling journey: life with Tourette syndrome. *Cerebrum* 5: 47–60.

Kleinman A (1988) *The Illness Narratives: Suffering, Healing, and the Human Condition.* New York: Basic Books.

Monroe WF, Holleman WL, Holleman MC (1992) Is there a person in this case? *Lit Med* 11: 45–63.

Storch EA, Murphy TK, Chase RM, et al. (2007) Peer victimization in youth with Tourette's syndrome and chronic tic disorder: relations with tic severity and internalizing symptoms. *J Psychopathol Behav Assess* 29: 211–9. doi: 10.1007/s10862-007-9050-4.

Toombs SK (1993) *The Meaning of Illness: A Phenomenological Account of the Different Perspectives of Physician and Patient.* Dordrecht/London: Kluwer Academic Publishers.

Van Bloss N (2006) *Busy Body: My Life with Tourette's Syndrome.* London: Fusion Press.

Wadman R, Tischler V, Jackson GM (2013) 'Everybody just thinks I'm weird': a qualitative exploration of the psychosocial experiences of adolescents with Tourette syndrome. *Child Care Health Dev* 39: 880–6. doi: 10.1111/cch.12033.

Wilensky AS (1999) *Passing for Normal: a Memoir of Compulsion.* New York: Broadway Books.

9
FUNCTIONAL ('CONVERSION DISORDER' OR 'PSYCHOGENIC') TICS

Although tics are not the most common of the functional movement disorders, they occur and may be mixed with more typical tics or other movements. These movement patterns have been challenging for a long time and can occur in children and adults with resultant suffering and disability, as well as attracting many different opinions and ideas for intervention. The prognosis is better for acute onset after a stressor and in children. Treatment recommendations are not standardized.

Persons with neurological disorders, including tics, are known to have a higher than usual occurrence of atypical features or symptoms that call the assumption of organic disease into question and are often given names that can easily be misunderstood (Stone et al. 2006). In DSM-5 the terminology now used is 'conversion disorder (functional neurological symptom disorder)'. These symptom patterns, along with disorders of sensation and pain, are actually rather common in neurologic practices, ranging from 2% to 10% for movement disorders (Ferrara and Jankovic 2008). There has been controversy over the name used, because of its presumed etiology ('conversion') and the fact that the absence of demonstrable neurologic disease does not equal psychogenesis and that some terms are unacceptable to patients.

This rather ambiguous and contested category of movement disorder is included here briefly because of its occurrence jointly with tics, confusion with tics, and difficulty in diagnosis.

A full discussion is available in the very helpful book edited by Hallett et al. (2011). Anyone reading this book will undoubtedly learn a great deal about these problems. The accompanying disk provides many video examples of functional movement disorders, and is really impressive in case you have any doubt that these patients are impaired, suffering, and present high levels of symptom complexity.

Sometimes 'functional' is contrasted with 'structural' as 'software' is to 'hardware'. Edwards et al. (2014) have made a strong case for using the word 'functional' as the most scientific of all the possibilities.

The proportion of functional disorders that took the form of tics ranged from 1% to 3% in one specialty neurology practice (Ferrara and Jankovic 2008). Girls outnumbered boys. In a further report from the same clinic, Baizabal-Carballo and Jankovic (2013) found a frequency of 4.9% of their 184 patients with functional disorder who presented 'tics'. Points of distinction between 'psychogenic' tics and typical tics were: higher proportion of females, lack of premonitory sensations, lack of family history of tics, and frequent co-occurrence of other functional disorders. Two-thirds of the children showed multiple movement types (tremor, dystonia and myoclonus being the most common). More than half of the children with functional movement disorders had a paroxysmal course.

The DSM-5 does not require a preceding psychological stressor (which is a specifier) or psychopathology. (Thus the definition has changed from DSM-IV-TR.) Incongruity with a neurological disorder and neurological assessment is a requirement. *La belle indifférence* is not (Stone et al. 2006). Prognosis is better in children than in adults and when the onset is sudden and associated with a stressor. There has been a strong tendency, still evident, to treat the diagnosis as one of *exclusion* (what is left after every conceivable test is negative), but now the trend is toward *inclusion*. These movements are unlike tics in that they are less stereotyped, suppressible, and may not have premonitory urges (Mink 2013). That does not mean that they are neurologically normal or are 'imaginary'. "Most important is for the examining physician to have sufficient knowledge of neuroanatomy and neurophysiology to determine when signs and symptoms are inconsistent with known disease processes" (Mink 2013, p. 41).

One concept is that although the functional changes are manifested through the same pathways/circuits as usual, there is a loss of the sense of 'personal agency', or that "I am the one doing this" (Parées et al. 2013). Individuals with these disorders often have had exposure to the movement disorder before, either by themselves or through family members or friends. There may be more than one functional movement disorder present.

Agreement on treatment (and by whom) is limited. Suggestion as part of a multifaceted approach is often recommended; employment of medication and many exclusionary physical tests are not.

Case examples

'Owen' was 8 years old when first seen for bouts of severe and prolonged movements that consisted of rhythmic head-shaking laterally, forward-and-back and in rotatory directions, with a sudden onset and offset. These were assessed as atypical for tics, and a functional disturbance was diagnosed. Over several years his tics became more typical than atypical. In his case a very anxious mother was able to influence clinicians to order more tests than usual, which added nothing to understanding. When last seen for follow-up 8 years later he was doing well with very few tics to be seen or heard, and was on no medication.

'Karl' was 12 years old when first seen. He had a history of tics around age 5 that then subsided for several years. Around age 11 he developed dramatic episodes in the evenings of hitting furniture and climbing on the arms of couches and falling flat on his face without the usual movements of arms protecting his face, claiming that he had to do these 'tics'. At other times (during the day) he was calm and cooperative. After being assessed initially he began to walk into walls, and on one occasion he claimed he could

not walk and propelled himself along the floor using his arms but apparently unable to use his legs. He also had multiple tics and later developed copropraxia and loud copro-lalia. Psychological testing showed a mathematical learning disability and indications of ADHD. Rituals and obsessions began. He attended the Emergency Department because of shaking, and although he maintained consciousness throughout he was given a nonspecific seizure diagnosis. He became unable to attend school, even on tic and ADHD medication, and was home-schooled. His dramatic symptoms often followed homework-related frustration. At times his tics were self-injurious. Most recently he has been participating in Comprehensive Behavioral Intervention for Tics (CBIT) therapy (see Chapter 15) and doing much better with his tics, OCD and ADHD-related symptoms.

Comment: His symptoms often varied substantially, depending upon reactions to frustration related to schoolwork and very high expectations of himself. The pediatric neurologist did not believe he had had any seizures.

REFERENCES

Baizabal-Carvallo JF, Jankovic J (2013) The clinical features of psychogenic movement disorders resembling tics. *J Neurol Neurosurg Psychiatry* 85: 573–5. doi: 10.1136/jnnp-2013-305594.

Edwards MJ, Stone J, Lang AE (2013) From psychogenic movement disorder to functional movement disorder: it's time to change the name. *Mov Disord* 29: 849–52. doi: 10.1002/mds.25562.

Ferrara J, Jankovic J (2008) Psychogenic movement disorders in children. *Mov Disord* 23: 1875–81. doi: 10.1002/mds.22220.

Hallett M, Lang AE, Jankovic J, et al., eds (2011) *Psychogenic Movement Disorders and Other Conversion Disorders.* Cambridge, UK: Cambridge University Press.

Mink JW (2013) Conversion disorder and mass psychogenic illness in child neurology. *Ann NY Acad Sci* 1304: 40–4. doi: 10.1111/nyas.12298.

Parées I, Saifee TA, Kojovic M, et al. (2013) Functional (psychogenic) symptoms in Parkinson's disease. *Mov Disord* 28: 1622–7. doi: 10.1002/mds.25544.

Stone J, Smyth R, Carson A, et al. (2006) La belle indifférence in conversion symptoms and hysteria. *Brit J Psychiatry* 188: 204–9. doi: 10.1192/bjp.188.3.204.

10
COMORBID DISORDERS AND SYMPTOMATOLOGY

Attention-deficit/hyperactivity disorder (ADHD)

ADHD typically imposes problems of various kinds on children or adults, but the presence of a tic disorder does not seem to routinely aggravate those problems (Freeman 2007, Lin et al. 2012), rather the influence tends to be the other way. Most people do not realize that in the long term, impairment from ADHD (symptoms of which are largely invisible compared with tics) may be more significant than from Tourette syndrome. Stimulant medications remain the most effective intervention for children above the age of 6 years, and group studies do not show tic exacerbations from such treatment, although in some instances this does occur and requires treatment modifications. The increasing usage of stimulant drugs has also led to higher rates of diversion for nonmedical use among adolescents. For children under 6 years, parent behavior training has evidence-based efficacy.

In the popular North American TV series 'The Sopranos' there is an episode where the mobster Tony Soprano and his wife are sitting with a clinician to receive his diagnosis on their son. He indicates that the boy has 'ADD' (sic), and when asked the basis for this he reads them the DSM-IV list of items, including fidgeting. "Fidgeting?" says Tony. "Yes." "What's a fidget?" he demands skeptically.

Public attitudes, even if usually not expressed so forcefully to the diagnosing clinician, may be skeptical — and no wonder! In spite of thousands of research publications over the past 50 years, there is no single pattern children with ADHD have in common, and no test, even though ADHD is commonly considered to be primarily neurobiologically based and strongly heritable. There are many controversies and theories as well as substantial but technical differences between current criteria in DSM-5 and the *International Classification of Diseases, 10th Revision* (ICD-10: WHO 2010). (Is ADHD a specific learning disability, or are ADHD and specific learning disability overlapping but different disorders?) Most experienced clinicians proceed with confidence in spite of these uncertainties, but one may forgive parents and some others who find this hard to accept. The problem of face validity will remain, as will the confusion caused by the category name and the acronym 'ADHD', which has not been altered in the DSM-5.

Nevertheless, in this book this conundrum, once stated, will be largely ignored.

Practice point

The category name in both DSM-IV-TR and DSM-5 includes a forward slash indicating that hyperactivity may or may not be present, as in the DSM-III-R, where the two types were termed 'attention deficit disorder with hyperactivity' and 'attention deficit disorder without hyperactivity'. Without the slash in the acronym ADHD (i.e. AD/HD), many parents reject the implication that the child must be hyperactive, so the obsolete 'ADD' persists, and will likely continue.

ADHD symptoms are the single most commonly reported accompaniment of Tourette syndrome, and they are much more often seen to need treatment than are tics. Descriptively, patients are able to pay attention to activities that interest them intensely or frighten them, but not to others, a "chronic discrepancy of focus" (Brown 2009b, p. 18). Most (about 70%) show one or more additional disorders at some point, typically requiring consideration and often appropriate treatment. The presence of ADHD can be considered to confer a risk of developing further disorders during the life span.

Practice point

ADHD is itself commonly comorbid with other disorders and more often requires treatment than do tics.

Very helpful summaries of assessment and treatment have been provided in the practice parameter of the American Academy of Child and Adolescent Psychiatry (2007a), by Brown (2009a) and by the Canadian ADHD Resource Alliance (CADDRA 2011). Adverse events during drug treatment of ADHD have been comprehensively reviewed by Cortese et al. (2013).

Another important review of the current knowledge from the standpoint of genetic and environmental risks is by Thapar et al. (2013). Risks identified so far are of small effect size or rare, and may increase the risk of disorders other than ADHD. Familial and genetic risks increase the probability of ADHD, but do not directly determine it. "It is not explained by any single risk factor alone and not all those who are exposed to a given risk show disorder" (p. 11).

Up to 6% of preschool children meet full DSM criteria for ADHD, and about half of these will experience continuing symptoms in later life. The complexity is indicated by studies showing significant rates of generalized anxiety disorder (GAD), conduct disorder, oppositional–defiant disorder (ODD) and depression. Earlier onset of ADHD predicts greater comorbidity. Almost 25% have speech or language impairments. A problem with inattention may not be obvious until school entry (Posner et al. 2009), so that an important point is that later recognition does not necessarily mean later onset.

DEFINITION

ADHD is not simply a behavior disorder characterized by excessive restlessness and distractibility, but may be better conceptualized as a complex developmental disorder of the self-management system of the brain (Brown 2009b). Criteria have changed in DSM-5 to take better account of the symptom patterns in adults; the age at onset was modified so that "several inattentive or hyperactive–impulsive symptoms were present prior to age 12 years"; it is now stipulated that the pattern must occur in more than one setting (i.e. not in school or work only, or at home only). Current severity must be specified. ADHD may not become apparent until challenges are encountered in school. Another way to conceptualize ADHD is as a disorder of executive functions that prioritize, integrate and regulate cognitive functions and therefore can produce chronic difficulties in self-management.

DIAGNOSIS (INCLUDING INSTRUMENTS AND FORMS)

Recent guidelines for ADHD, including screening instruments, are available without cost on the internet (Canadian ADHD Practice Guidelines: CADDRA 2011), and from the National Institute for Health and Care Excellence (Clinical Guideline 72: NICE 2008) in the UK. These do not take account of the changes in DSM-5.

A warning: because persons with frequent tics can appear overactive and distractible due to their tics alone, the diagnosis of ADHD can be too readily suspected. The clinician must adhere to the need for information from more than one source and an adequate history. Furthermore, there are reports of a substantial increase in the usage by young people without ADHD of stimulant medications to enhance their studying ('diversion'). For them, there may be a risk of addiction that is increased by limited physician time and cursory acceptance of their description of symptoms to make the diagnosis. There is also some evidence that the symptoms of OCD in children may appear ADHD-like and be conducive to misdiagnosis (Abramovitch et al. 2013).

PREVALENCE/EPIDEMIOLOGY

Prevalence rates in the general population range from 3% to 7%, with comorbid internalizing disorders at roughly 25%, and externalizing disorders at 50% in epidemiologic studies. Thus, 'pure' ADHD is distinctly uncommon (Ollendick et al. 2008). Community samples of Tourette syndrome yield ADHD rates of 38% (Kurlan et al. 2002), while clinic-based studies such as that of Freeman et al. (2000) show reported rates of about 60% in children (88% of them male) and 40% in adults with Tourette syndrome (79% male). Findings in a clinical sample of adult patients were similar (Haddad et al. 2009).

In the *TIC* database, several variables show statistically significant differences (p<0.001) between those with and those without ADHD (Table 10.1). Anxiety does not show a difference. It can be seen that the major differences are that SLD and conduct disorder/ODD are the two diagnoses that tend to be reported concurrently in children with TS+ADHD, and the behaviors most commonly associated with ADHD in Tourette syndrome are anger control problems and social skill deficits. In adults with Tourette syndrome, the most common diagnoses associated with ADHD are OCD and mood disorder (Table 10.2); associated behaviors are anger control problems and social skill deficits. Some differences between the children and adults are worth noting, in particular large increases in

TABLE 10.1

Children with and without ADHD (*TIC* data, n=5247): selected variables

	Without ADHD (n=2153)		With ADHD (n=3094)		p	Odds ratio
	n	%	n	%		
Female	495	23.0	374	12.1	<0.001	2.2
OCD	322	15.0	628	20.3	<0.001	1.4
SLD	241	11.2	987	31.9	<0.001	3.7
Mood disorder	164	7.6	424	13.7	<0.001	1.9
Anxiety	310	14.4	520	16.8	0.019	1.2
CD/ODD	87	4.0	633	20.5	<0.001	6.1
Sleep disorder (now)	308	14.3	656	21.2	<0.001	1.7
Anger problem (now)	334	15.5	1102	35.6	<0.001	3.2
SIB	215	10.0	456	14.7	<0.001	1.6
Social skill deficits	165	7.7	673	21.8	<0.001	3.3
Coprophenomena	190	8.8	409	13.2	<0.001	1.6

Excluded: intellectual disability, autism spectrum disorder and psychosis.
ADHD, attention-deficit/hyperactivity disorder; OCD, obsessive–compulsive disorder; SLD, specific learning disorder; CD/ODD, conduct disorder/oppositional–defiant disorder; SIB, self-injurious behavior.

TABLE 10.2

Adults with and without ADHD (*TIC* data, n=1628): selected variables

	Without ADHD (n=997)		With ADHD (n=631)		p	Odds ratio
	n	%	n	%		
Female	297	29.8	137	21.7	<0.001	1.5
OCD	281	28.2	230	36.5	<0.001	1.5
SLD	64	6.4	119	18.9	<0.001	3.4
Mood disorder	297	29.8	221	35.0	0.029	1.3
Anxiety	220	22.1	145	23.0	ns	—
CD/ODD	19	1.9	81	12.8	<0.001	7.6
Sleep disorder (now)	130	13.0	121	11.7	<0.001	1.6
Anger problem (now)	133	13.3	182	30.3	<0.001	2.8
SIB	191	19.2	180	28.5	<0.001	1.7
Social skill deficits	67	6.7	85	13.5	<0.001	2.2
Coprophenomena	151	15.1	147	23.3	<0.001	1.7

Excluded: intellectual disability, autism spectrum disorder and psychosis.
ADHD, attention-deficit/hyperactivity disorder; OCD, obsessive–compulsive disorder; SLD, specific learning disorder; CD/ODD, conduct disorder/oppositional–defiant disorder; SIB, self-injurious behavior; ns, non-significant.

OCD, mood disorder and coprophenomena. (Some of the other problem behaviors are often reported in groups of persons with Tourette syndrome, but may not take ADHD into account.)

PRESENTATION AND PHENOMENOLOGY

These differ in children and adults (Gibbins and Weiss 2007, Sibley et al. 2012); hyperactivity declines and may not be obvious in adults, which is one reason diagnosis in adults in often missed.

COMORBIDITY AND COMMON ASSOCIATIONS

Pure ADHD is "rare even in a general population sample" (Kadesjö and Gillberg 2001, p. 487). It appears that the TS+ADHD+OCD comorbidity triad is the most strongly heritable. Comorbidity issues have been extensively treated in the books by Brown (2009a) and Pliszka (2009). The most common other disorders were ODD and developmental coordination disorder (DCD). School adjustment, learning and behavior problems were also very common. In the study by Debes et al. (2010), comorbid ADHD in children with Tourette syndrome was associated with increased likelihood of teasing, avoiding social activities and need for educational support.

Anger control problems (sometimes termed 'rage' when episodes are severe and lengthy) are common in ADHD with or without comorbidity with Tourette syndrome. Children who have difficulty expressing their frustrations in age-appropriate ways, who are highly reactive and irritable, and who have difficulty processing social cues are very vulnerable to these explosive outbursts that are probably the most common reasons for visits to emergency rooms, for inpatient admissions and for medication (Carlson et al. 2009). Those authors analyzed 151 consecutive inpatient admissions; the most common inpatient diagnoses were ADHD with ODD/conduct disorder and/or SLD/language disorders (not one had a diagnosis of Tourette syndrome). So much for the idea that 'rage' is characteristic specifically of Tourette syndrome. It is of interest that only half the children admitted with a history of rages had a rage attack while in the hospital.

Motor problems in ADHD (i.e. DCD) occur in 30% to 50% of patients but mostly go untreated and often are unrecognized (Fliers et al. 2010). Patients should be assessed or at least screened (e.g. with the Developmental Coordination Disorder Questionnaire 2007: Wilson et al. 2007, 2009). Handwriting problems are also common and can be troublesome in ADHD (Racine et al. 2008) and therefore also in Tourette syndrome. In DSM-5 they have been moved from the DCD category in DSM-IV-TR to 'specific learning disorder with impairment in written expression', but in this chapter are discussed in the section on DCD.

Practice point
Think of motor problems (DCD) and handwriting problems in your assessment.

One of the most important questions is whether the symptoms of patients with TS+ADHD are due to the ADHD or to a special interaction between the two disorders. This is still uncertain, but the presence of ADHD may make it harder for children to inhibit tics, and ADHD-related behavior may exaggerate reactions of others to the child's tics (Taylor 2009b).

The presence of anxiety or sleep disorder may result in the appearance of overactivity in a child (Cortese et al. 2009) and should be taken into account in arriving at a diagnosis.

> **Practice point**
>
> Be sure to include assessment of anxiety and sleep problems in your assessment, since both can mimic ADHD and also complicate it when present.

Attentional difficulties are also the single most common abnormality in a wide variety of genetic syndromes, head injuries, infections, and preterm birth. Children with ADHD were more impaired than comparison children in most of the subjective and some of the objective measures of sleep, even when children were unmedicated and non-comorbid (Cortese et al. 2009), but the relationship remains unclear in evidence-based studies (Cohen-Zion and Ancoli-Israel 2004). Since ADHD is the most commonly reported Tourette syndrome comorbidity, one would expect persons with both disorders to have a high prevalence of sleep problems — and they do, at least according to parent reports.

Physical overactivity often diminishes in adolescence, but inattention and impulsivity combined with executive dysfunction usually continue. Conflict at home, high-risk behavior in the community and substance misuse tend to increase. Mounting complexity of school-work tends to cause declining grades and consequent avoidance or demoralization, even in bright students. Studies show rates of ODD of about 60%, conduct disorder in 25% to 40%, and major depressive and anxiety disorders in almost 30%. Reasons for lack of cooperation and collaboration in treatment are many. Parents find their role increasingly challenging. Medication and family- and school-based interventions are essential for most. The symptoms that indicate ADHD may be obscured by other behavioral presentations, so that a full assessment for associated or comorbid disorders is mandatory.

In adults, comorbidity persists in about 70%. Those with comorbid ODD/conduct disorder may be those with the most negative outcomes. There is a high rate of problems in the parents as well. In a follow-up study of 66 patients (Herrero et al. 1994), about 30% to 40% had a good outcome, 50% to 60% had continuing ADHD symptoms, and 20% had severe problems (half psychiatric, half with antisocial disturbance). Males were significantly more likely to exhibit antisocial behavior. It is important to note that more than 20% of children who presented with behavioral or antisocial problems at intake or early follow-up did not maintain these at later follow-up, so the outcome is not necessarily dismal. Those with early hyperactivity or aggression, higher comorbidity, lower socioeconomic status, lower IQ and parental psychiatric problems tend to have a more negative outcome. More than one-third had a history of substance misuse.

Many individuals who acquire an ADHD diagnosis in adulthood have already had a checkered career along with misunderstandings of their problems. A concise and helpful summary of this situation has been provided by Gibbins and Weiss (2007).

Comorbidity between ADHD and mood disorders varies in different studies from 0% to 50% both ways, but it is important that subthreshold symptoms in both directions are significant for impairment and merit attention. Diagnosis of children's mood disorders can be difficult because of the need for information from multiple informants and symptoms that are easy to misinterpret (see later section on mood disorders). The rates of bipolar disorder are controversial but there is agreement that the combination of mood and ADHD symptoms typically has a poorer outcome. The likelihood of mood as well as attentional symptoms in the parents must be taken into account. Adult psychiatrists often fail to adequately consider childhood psychopathology in their adult patients. Treating the symptoms of both disorders, and sometimes in both child and parent, requires considerable skill and experience and is not the province of primary care clinicians.

ADHD and anxiety disorders co-occur in 25% to 33%, much higher than would be expected by chance. (But note that this difference was not found in children with Tourette syndrome in the *TIC* database.) Clinicians need to assess for anxiety in these children, even when disruptive behavioral symptoms are prominent. They are worriers about their behavior, future events, and their academic and social performance. Also important is that anxiety is as common in the inattentive type as in the combined or hyperactive–impulsive types of ADHD. Risk factors for anxiety disorders include family history, shy and inhibited early behavior, and high frequency of early stressors. The two disorders do not co-segregate and therefore are believed to be transmitted independently. Academic tasks involving working memory and effortful processing are both vulnerable to anxiety. Low self-esteem is a significant risk. Anxiety symptoms may wax and wane through childhood and into adult life; in adolescence and adulthood they may become more intense. Treatment of ADHD by medication does not exacerbate anxiety when patients have both, neither does it improve anxiety directly. Psychosocial interventions are necessary along with medication. In the opposite direction, children referred for anxiety disorder symptoms have a likelihood of an ADHD diagnosis of 15% to 30%, often not suspected.

Among children with OCD, up to one-third may have ADHD (Geller 2006). Sometimes OCD is manifested in 'over-focusing' or 'getting stuck', unable to move on until getting something perfect. The onset of OCD is bimodal: around age 10 years and around 20 years. The symptom course is episodic in most, with periods of complete remission possible. Only about 10% have a deteriorating course.

Of those with ADHD, 25% to 40% have an SLD. Conversely, of those with SLD in the community, 15% to 40% have ADHD, and in clinical samples, up to 70% have ADHD, so that assessment requires screening for SLD. Inattention is most closely related to reading and math disability. SLD can also affect social functioning. Working memory and processing speed are the executive functions most strongly related to both disorders.

There is a bidirectional overlap with substance use disorders (SUDs), which affect 10% to 30% of adults in the USA. The highest risk age for onset of alcoholism and drug abuse is 15–17 years. Without treatment ADHD represents an additional risk. Once established, SUDs require both addiction and psychiatric treatments.

Diversion of short-acting stimulants (mostly by adolescents) is estimated at 11%. Long-acting forms and atomoxetine are not so subject to misuse as stimulants are (McCabe and West 2013). Many students who have not been diagnosed with ADHD now see the use of these stimulants for the purpose of doing better at studying for examinations as reasonable.

The diagnosis of ASD in the presence of ADHD is not always easy. ADHD itself can present with social interaction problems due to executive function weakness, and some children with ADHD have subthreshold ASD symptoms. In ASD almost 60% meet diagnostic criteria for ADHD, and even more in the high-functioning individuals. Co-occurrence with DCD is common. As for medication for ADHD, children with ASD may be more sensitive than average, but evidence shows that ADHD medications are effective.

All children with ADHD require screening for sleep disorders. 'Insomnia' isn't a diagnosis; it is a symptom requiring investigation. Causes include obstructive sleep apnea, restless legs syndrome/Willis–Ekbom disease (RLS/WED), periodic limb movement disorder, delayed sleep phase syndrome, some medications, and comorbid disorders (especially anxiety and ODD) (Owens et al. 2009, Mindell and Owens 2010). Melatonin can be helpful for children with initial insomnia who have ADHD (Weiss et al. 2006).

NATURAL HISTORY AND PROGNOSIS

Typically some ADHD symptoms (excess hyperactivity) seem to begin around the age when the child becomes mobile. This is well before the usual age for multiple tics to be brought to attention. But nothing obvious may be noticed until elementary school, when inability to sustain attention in class becomes a problem. Even then, the ADHD components in a child's overall situation may remain unclear until age 10–11 years, when the nature of schoolwork changes and becomes more abstract. Children with ADHD perform more poorly on academic achievement than their tested IQ would predict, and not due to associated conduct problems (Daley and Birchwood 2010).

The frequency of the ADHD diagnosis declines with age (Faraone et al. 2005), whether this change is real or reflects changes in diagnostic sensitivity. On the other hand, there is great imprecision in diagnosing adult ADHD from an item list of childhood descriptors (Suhr et al. 2009), and changed criteria are in the DSM-5. Even so, it should be noted that the increased attention paid recently to adult ADHD is a mixed blessing, offering a substantial marketing opportunity to pharmaceutical companies.

The course of ADHD is not affected by the presence of tics (Spencer et al. 2001), and in the absence of ADHD, children with Tourette syndrome are not more likely than other children to access mental health services: "In the absence of ADHD, a tic disorder alone does not appear to be associated with disruptive behavior and functional impairment" (Scahill et al. 2006, p. 189). Overall, a follow-up study by the Multimodal Treatment of ADHD (MTA) reported by Molina et al. (2009) indicated that children with ADHD, combined type, are not 'normalized' even by optimal treatment; it is "early ADHD symptom trajectory regardless of treatment type" that is prognostic (p. 484), and "sustained improvement (not normalization) relative to the child's initial presentation for treatment is achievable" (p. 496). An important follow-up study of social relationships over 20 years showed that those with ADHD as adults were the ones who showed impairment; those whose symptoms did not persist into adult life tended to have normal social relationships (Moyá et al. 2014).

TREATMENT

The MTA Study (Molina et al. 2009) has shown that stimulant medications are the most effective treatments for ADHD symptoms, but there is still some controversy over whether there is robust evidence that psychosocial methods significantly add to the outcome; they do not seem to be as demonstrably effective on their own. It is important to realize, however, that even in a study as elaborate as the MTA, medication adherence was problematic (Pappadopulos et al. 2009).

A review by Charach et al. (2013) revealed that for children with disruptive behavior under age 6, many of whom will later be diagnosed with ADHD, stimulant medication is fraught with more side-effects, and that parent behavior training programs are effective and to be preferred. (In the USA, the regulatory Food and Drug Administration [FDA] has not approved stimulant treatment of such young children anyway.)

Specific approaches to the executive function problems in ADHD with or without Tourette syndrome or OCD are covered in great and practical detail by Dornbush and Pruitt (2008), and another very useful book is that by Packer and Pruitt (2010).

A meta-analysis of studies on restriction diets and synthetic food color additives (Nigg et al. 2012) indicates that a restriction diet benefits a few children with ADHD if maintained long-term, but that research results on food coloring are equivocal because of methodological problems.

Pharmacotherapy (see also Chapter 15)

Comprehensive reviews are available of medications for ADHD (Daughton and Kratochvil 2009) and of the management of their side-effects (Graham et al. 2011). Stimulants have the strongest evidence base for short-term benefit, but not for the long term. Atomoxetine was found to be efficacious in a study by Spencer et al. (2008), but is considered by many experts to be a second-line treatment, as confirmed in a study by Newcorn et al. (2008).

Stimulants and tics

It appears that the use of stimulants is generally not contraindicated in children with tics or with a family history of tics, though occasional instances are seen where repeated challenges with such medications seem to cause temporary or sustained tic increases (Gadow et al. 1999, 2002, 2007, 2008; Gadow and Sverd 2006). The results may still be beneficial overall, and in some cases tic-suppressing medication may need to be added (Bloch et al. 2009b, Cortese et al. 2013).

Effects of stimulants and atomoxetine on the cardiovascular system are small, but monitoring during treatment (symptom history, heart rate and blood pressure) is recommended (Arcieri et al. 2012). Occasional changes in the electrocardiogram (ECG arrhythmias) can occur. Standards for baseline ECG vary by country. A pharmacosurveillance monitoring study in Italy (Ruggiero et al. 2012) found that the drugs were quite safe, but there were several uncommon adverse reactions (hepatomegaly, suicidal ideation, weight gain and drug interactions). Cardiac risk assessment before using stimulant drugs in children and adolescents has been explored and an official position taken by three Canadian organizations (Hamilton et al. 2009). This is an important contribution, including recommendations for treating children and adolescents with known or suspected cardiac abnormalities.

Psychosocial interventions

Behavioral parent training and behavioral interventions in the classroom have been effective in evidence-based trials. There is dispute as to whether adding these treatments to pharmacotherapy has a better outcome (Ollendick et al. 2008). For social skill interventions, none has been shown to reverse the deficits, which are more severe in the combined type of ADHD (McQuade and Hoza 2008). However, a recent non-randomized trial of a 2-week therapeutic summer camp program showed promise in improving ADHD symptoms, peer relationships and overall functioning (Hantson et al. 2012).

Other approaches

Neurofeedback has acquired some methodologically contested evidence base for ADHD (Butnik 2005, Arns et al. 2009, Gevensleben et al. 2009, Bakhshayesh et al. 2011, Lofthouse et al. 2012), but Vollebregt et al. (2014) found no evidence of benefit. Some research on sympathetic autonomic arousal and focused attention to task has suggested a potential role in Tourette syndrome (Nagai et al. 2009). Dietary methods (e.g. additive-free or oligoantigenic/elimination) have frequently been of interest to parents over the past 40 years but have minimal research-based support (Millichap and Yee 2012).

CONTROVERSIES AND SOURCES OF CONFUSION

A major source of confusion can arise when one uses descriptions from only one setting (home or school) rather than both, which is the clinical rule. Prior to the release of DSM-5, differing views of the diagnostic validity of ADHD appeared, including the question of categorical versus dimensional approaches, and fear that the new adult criteria may lead to overmedication. Preterm infants may have a higher risk of sensory hypersensitivity reactions and consequently tendencies to be overwhelmed by sensory stimuli, sometimes appearing as ADHD symptoms. Allergic rhinitis ('hay fever') can apparently produce symptoms mimicking ADHD (Brawley et al. 2004, Borres 2009), and can aggravate sleep problems (Léger et al. 2006).

Case example

When 'Bob' was 11 he reportedly slipped on ice when deliberately engaged in strangulation play (which was being practiced in his small rural community) and suffered a period of unconsciousness with anoxia. He was transferred by air ambulance to the regional children's hospital where he was ventilated for over 15 hours and then spent a week in a rehabilitation unit. Neuropsychological testing showed scatter: low-average Full-Scale IQ, strong nonverbal reasoning, weak verbal reasoning, slow written output, and complex learning difficulties. He showed facial tics, head-turning, and shoulder-shrugging, as well as making 'funny faces'. In school he was disruptive because of swearing; his head-turning was interpreted as an effort to cheat, and his tics had never been identified as such. His history showed both obsessive–compulsive behavior patterns and ADHD, along with an urge to engage in risky, impulsive behavior such as touching an electrified fence. He had been teased and bullied and was

---

socially unsuccessful.

> **Comment:** *Bob was embarrassed by his tics and his poor organizational ability. The nature of his problems was not known or investigated until the near-death incident.*

Obsessive–compulsive disorder (OCD)

> OCD is common in tic disorders and always requires exploration both in assessment and with heightened awareness as a child develops, because onset frequently follows onset of tics by several years. Even subthreshold symptoms of obsessive–compulsive behavior (OCB) can be significant. Symptoms can affect any area of functioning, at home, in the community, and in school, and may be more impairing than tics. Unlike tics they may not remit in late adolescence or early adult life. The distinction between complex tics and OCD is not always clear. Significant symptoms always affect others in the family in ways that mandate their involvement in treatment. Medication and cognitive–behavioral therapy (CBT) are often only partially effective in treatment; active research to provide better results is ongoing.

This is the second most common comorbidity in Tourette syndrome and is generally agreed to be genetically related to tics.

DEFINITION

Although there is some terminological confusion, OCD refers to a condition fulfilling DSM-5 criteria, while OCB refers to symptoms that do not meet those criteria, but are still of clinical significance. Sometimes 'OCS' (obsessive–compulsive symptoms) is used to refer to both. Recent research suggests that there are several overlapping clusters of symptoms or subtypes, rather than OCD being a single entity, though findings in different studies are inconsistent (Storch et al. 2008). This includes hoarding, a new separate disorder in DSM-5, discussed in the next section of this chapter. Since obsessive–compulsive patterns are a normal part of development, 'entity' is a misnomer — it is a matter of degree and any definition will be arbitrary. Illustrative of this point, in the *TIC* database, OCB associations are almost as robust in their reported effects as those of OCD.

The DSM-5 criteria include the presence of obsessions (recurrent unwanted thoughts, urges or images) and compulsions (repetitive behaviors or mental acts that the individual feels must be performed according to rigid rules, but are excessive and illogical). They are time-consuming and impairing, and specification must be made as to the extent of insight.

DIAGNOSIS (INCLUDING INSTRUMENTS AND FORMS)

Assessment and treatment effects have been tapped in quite a large number of assessment instruments. Each has its strengths and weaknesses for research and clinical purposes, and for diagnosis and treatment. These have been well reviewed by Merlo et al. (2005). In general, the criterion standard for assessment and research is the Children's Yale–Brown Obsessive–Compulsive Scale or C-YBOCS (Goodman et al. 1990, Scahill et al. 1997) and the adult YBOCS, both now available in revised versions by Goodman et al. (2006a). A general principle to keep in mind is that the history will most likely be incomplete: people will not tell you most (certainly not all) of their symptoms, even if they are self-aware and articulate, as some (despite explanatory attempts) may be too illogical and embarrassing. Substitutes, or lesser forms of the really big symptoms will probably be offered. This may or may not matter. For practical purposes, if time is available, it is often helpful to go through the C-YBOCS/YBOCS to identify additional symptoms.

Practice point

It is generally safe to assume that people will not tell you all of their symptoms, so it is good practice to go systematically through a list such as the C-YBOCS or YBOCS. Children should be interviewed individually (with the consent of their parents), not only in the presence of the parents.

PREVALENCE/EPIDEMIOLOGY

The prevalence is from 0.6% (full OCD) to 1.2% (including subthreshold OCB) but has frequently been cited as about 3% by late adolescence (Stein et al. 1997). There are two peaks of onset: one in puberty and one in early adulthood. A substantial number of cases become subclinical over time. OCD is highly familial, with risk in first-degree relatives of early-onset probands as high as 25% in some studies (do Rosario-Campos et al. 2005). An important recent study (Fullana et al. 2009) had some surprising findings, though. Apart from formal diagnoses of OCD, disturbing obsessions and compulsions were found to have a prevalence of 13% to 17% among adults without mental health disorders and 31% to 49% among those with disorders other than OCD. Obsessions caused more interference than compulsions: "obsessions and compulsions extend beyond the traditional nosological boundaries of OCD" (Fullana et al. 2009, p. 332). There was continuity between children reporting OCB at age 11 and meeting criteria for OCD 20 years later.

Practice point

Sub-threshold OCD symptoms are common in the general population.

PRESENTATION AND PHENOMENOLOGY

One must beware the common but mistaken idea that OCD equals general perfectionism: "My boy couldn't have that — you should see his room — it's a mess!" There is a problem in that for many patients with Tourette syndrome the symptom form is different from the classic description: there is less dread of danger to self or others, and more symmetry and 'just right' urges, the correction of which is insistent and repetitive (Leckman et al. 2010). Examples include combinations of having to arrange socks or shoelaces to feel exactly equal, to count, to arrange things symmetrically, or being bothered by not being able to get it right or achieve completion. Interference with schoolwork (e.g. handwriting/printing), homework or getting to school on time are all possible because of rituals, some of which are unlikely to be fully described or confessed to anyone.

The question of whether obsessive intrusive thoughts in OCD are just more of what the nonclinical population experiences (the continuum hypothesis) has been reviewed by Berry and Laskey (2012). They concluded otherwise: clinical obsessions are more violent/aggressive and bizarre, may be experienced without triggers, are re-experienced more often, and individuals have more distress because of them, including increased sense of personal responsibility, negative self-appraisals and use of avoidance responses.

In a study of college students, Sica et al. (2012) showed that "not just right experiences" or the "sensation of lack of rightness" play a role in OCD (and, it may be added, probably in many cases of Tourette syndrome where the boundary of obsessions and complex tics is blurred). Another study (Cougle et al. 2011) showed that distress intolerance was associated with OCD and indicated that interventions to improve tolerance might be useful therapeutically.

Children with OCD report worse social functioning, more fear of negative evaluation, more peer victimization, fewer friends, and difficulty making friends (Kim et al. 2012, Borda et al. 2013).

They may also show coercive behaviors that can be quite disruptive to families, a very good description of which has been provided by Lebowitz et al. (2011a,b,c), including the following situations where the patient forbids, or insists upon, certain actions by others, sometimes reacting badly or with rage if these are not adhered to:
- forbidding coughing, sneezing or sounds of chewing at the table (the last-named termed 'misophonia' and presented in detail in Chapter 12)
- forbidding changes in the household
- forbidding the performance of normal actions (e.g. saying particular words or sounds)
- forbidding the performance of actions on his or her behalf
- imposing strict rules of cleanliness or order on others
- asking never-ending questions (especially for reassurance)
- repeating actions or words and demanding that others listen
- depriving others of sleep.

A very important recent study has shown that attacks of rage (recurrent episodes of explosive anger or aggression triggered by minor provocations) are relatively common and contribute to functional impairment and to greater family accommodation in OCD (Stewart 2012, Storch et al. 2012). The highly pertinent finding for our purposes is that "young people with comorbid CTD [chronic tic disorder] were no more likely to have rage episodes than those without" (p. 589). It was the primary OCD, then, that accounted for the rage, not the tic disorder. In the *TIC* database, the term 'anger control problems' was used, in which category 'rage' would be a subset. The presence of OCD (only) increased the rate from 10% in TS-only to 16%, while the addition of ADHD (only) raised it to 25%, and both disorders to 40%. The Storch study did not analyze for ADHD. Another recent study (Krebs et al. 2012) showed that over a third of young people with OCD displayed temper outbursts, which was three times as common as in the comparison group. Children with OCD have a high risk of rage attacks, but so do children with ADHD.

> **Practice point**
> Children with OCD (as well as ADHD) have a high risk of 'rage' attacks; these are not characteristic of TS-only.

FAMILY ACCOMMODATION

It seems almost impossible under the onslaught of the coercive behaviors for family members not to be drawn into the rituals [Stewart et al. (2008) found it in 96.9% of their patients]. One mother described herself having to anticipate situations she felt she had to avoid or respond to 'just right' as: "I'm living in his mind." However, once this occurs the accommodation can be reinforcing of the obsessive–compulsive symptoms (Storch et al. 2007), and will need to be reduced as part of treatment. This also applies to the repeated giving of reassurance (Kobori et al. 2012) which some parents think they must do, when in fact no new information is being imparted: they are being recruited into a ritual that is perpetuated by negative reinforcement.

REPETITION, CHECKING, REASONING

Also of great importance is that this repetition (or checking) to try to achieve completion actually causes more uncertainty, which seems paradoxical (Giele et al. 2014). Repeated checking induces uncertainty about memory, prolonged staring induces uncertainty about perception, and obsessive–compulsive-like "step-by-step reasoning increases the probability of the feared outcome" (p. 37) in persons without OCD, too! This has obvious treatment implications.

COMORBIDITY AND COMMON ASSOCIATIONS

In the *TIC* database, several repetitive motor behaviors are associated with OCD: trichotillomania, skin-picking, nose-picking, joint-cracking, awake bruxism, self-cutting and -hitting, smelling non-food objects, spitting, and contrary urges. Contrary urges (see also Chapter 12) are a powerful urge to do something one is warned not to do, just because one has been warned (not because one is generally oppositional). In children without OCD the rate was 6%, but in those with OCD it was 23% (p<0.001, OR 4.8). Those with TS+OCD showed a higher rate of comorbidity than those without (Wanderer et al. 2012). The need for completeness, symmetry or other 'just right' feelings can result in what appears to be oppositional–defiant behavior and/or ADHD. Abramovitch et al. (2013) warn that overload of executive functions in OCD makes children inattentive or forgetful, similar to patients with ADHD, who may receive that diagnosis in error.

Practice point

Stress impacting rigid behavior patterns in OCD can result in an ODD-like clinical picture.

NATURAL HISTORY AND PROGNOSIS

Unlike most disorders, the symptoms can start at any age, and show relatively little developmental change in form (in contrast to tics). When OCD symptoms are present, their severity tends to co-vary with tic exacerbations (Lin et al. 2002). This is helpful to know in order to counsel patience before changing medication. Periods between major exacerbations varied from 4 to 10 months, and the average length of the exacerbation was 3.5 months. Some patients had no significant exacerbations. For persons with Tourette syndrome, the worst-ever OCD symptoms followed the worst-ever tics by about 2 years, and tended to persist (Bloch et al. 2006). A study of 50 children aged 11–17 years by Eddy et al. (2012) looked into effects on quality of life of those with TS+ADHD, TS+OCD and TS+ADHD+OCD, and found that there were more widespread negative effects of the triad, with somewhat different impacts of OCD and ADHD. In the study by Debes et al. (2010), comorbid OCD was associated with increased likelihood of teasing, avoiding social activities, and need for educational support in children with Tourette syndrome (similar to ADHD comorbidity).

A fascinating study of 1001 consecutive patients with OCD explored sensory phenomena (Ferrão et al. 2012). At least one type of sensory phenomenon was reported by 65% of patients preceding repetitive behaviors: 57% musculoskeletal sensations, 80% 'just right' perceptions, 22% 'energy release', and 37% 'urge only' phenomena. Comorbid Tourette syndrome and a family history of tics were associated with higher frequency and greater severity of sensory phenomena.

On follow-up of childhood-onset OCD, Bloch et al. (2009a) found that 44% had only subclinical symptoms. Those with tics had done better, while those with hoarding were less likely to improve. In another follow-up study, those with OCD+obsessive–compulsive personality disorder were more likely to relapse. In a 10- to 20-year follow-up (Bloch et al. 2013) most adults had not achieved remission, but initial positive treatment response showed a better course in 31%.

In the *TIC* database there were also additive effects of both of these comorbidities assessed separately as compared with TS-only (Freeman et al. 2000). Specifically, a history of anger control problems was reported in 10% of those with TS-only, 25% of those with TS+ADHD-only, and 16% of TS+OCD-only, but 40% in the triad-only (without any other comorbidity included). For sleep problem history the reported rate was 14% in TS-only, 19% in TS+ADHD-only, and 14% in TS+OCD-only, but 27% in the triad-only; and for coprophenomena, 6% in TS-only, 7% in TS+ADHD-only, and 9% in TS+OCD-only, but

TABLE 10.3
Children with and without OCD (*TIC* data, n=5245): selected variables

	Without OCD (n=4295)		With OCD (n=950)		*p*	Odds ratio
	n	*%*	*n*	*%*		
Female	695	16	174	18	ns	—
ADHD	2465	57	628	66	<0.001	1.4
Anxiety disorder	560	13	269	28	<0.001	2.6
Mood disorder	386	9	202	21	<0.001	2.7
SLD	982	23	246	26	0.047	1.2
Sleep disorder (now)	752	18	211	23	<0.001	1.4
Anger problem (now)	1114	27	321	36	<0.001	1.5
Coprophenomena (ever)	441	10	158	17	<0.001	1.7
SIB (ever)	472	11	199	21	<0.001	2.1
Inappropriate sexual behavior (ever)	136	3	54	6	<0.001	2.0

Excluded: intellectual disability, autism spectrum disorder and psychosis.
OCD, obsessive–compulsive disorder; ADHD, attention-deficit/hyperactivity disorder; SLD, specific learning disorder; SIB, self-injurious behavior; ns, non-significant.

TABLE 10.4
Adults with and without OCD (*TIC* data, n=1628): selected variables

	Without OCD (n=1117)		With OCD (n=511)		*p*	Odds ratio
	n	*%*	*n*	*%*		
Female	401	36	230	45	ns	—
ADHD	401	36	230	45	0.001	1.5
Anxiety disorder	209	19	156	31	<0.001	2.0
Mood disorder	317	29	201	39	<0.001	1.6
SLD	121	11	62	12	ns	—
Sleep disorder (now)	163	15	88	18	ns	—
Anger problem (now)	192	18	123	25	0.001	1.6
Coprophenomena (ever)	181	16	117	23	0.001	1.5
SIB (ever)	222	20	149	29	<0.001	1.7

Excluded: intellectual disability, autism spectrum disorder and psychosis.
OCD, obsessive–compulsive disorder; ADHD, attention-deficit/hyperactivity disorder; SLD, specific learning disorder; SIB, self-injurious behavior; ns, non-significant.

14% in the triad. The only behavior that was much more common in the total comorbidity group than in the triad-only group was social skill deficits.

Selected associations of children and adults with ADHD, anxiety and mood disorders, SLD, and other problems including sleep, anger control, SIB and coprophenomena are presented in Tables 10.3 and 10.4.

TREATMENT
There are two evidence-based treatments: CBT and medication. These have been reviewed by Goodman et al. (2006b), Heyman et al. (2006), Decloedt and Stein (2010) and Franklin

et al. (2010). The American Academy of Child and Adolescent Psychiatry has recently (2012) published a revised, extensive and very helpful practice parameter for OCD. Refractory cases may be helped by the thorough exposition by McKay et al. (2009). An important paper and commentary (Ressler and Rothbaum 2013) contests the currently recommended treatment for refractory cases, namely addition of an atypical antipsychotic drug. Exposure and response prevention is proposed as more effective. Selective serotonin reuptake inhibitors (SSRIs) and serotonin–norepinephrine reuptake inhibitors (SNRIs) are effective for only a subset of OCD patients, and may have a symptom suppressing effect, but emotional relearning (behavior therapy perhaps enhanced by D-cycloserine) appears to actually offer retraining of the brain. In the Mancuso et al. (2010) summary, CBT is first line for mild to moderate symptoms, CBT plus medication for more severe cases. Augmentation (as with an antipsychotic drug) for refractory (partially responsive) cases is considered less safe and effective in children than in adults.

An excellent and inexpensive handbook for parents and families, *Talking Back to OCD* (March and Benton 2007) is very helpful in understanding the disorder and its treatment, and comes from the experience of one of the master clinicians and researchers in the field.

Practice point

Anyone treating OCD would do well to read the Practice Parameter of the American Academy of Child and Adolescent Psychiatry (2012).

Medications used include the SSRIs and clomipramine (a serotonin reuptake inhibitor) (Goodman et al. 2006b, Watson and Rees 2008). Unfortunately, medication and CBT, separately or in combination, are not successful in all cases. Stimulant medication for ADHD may worsen OCD symptoms.

Quick discontinuation of medication (or stopping without careful tapering) may result in a 'discontinuation syndrome' as described in Chapter 15 (Hosenbocus and Chahal 2011). This typically presents with unpleasant side-effects: dizziness, nausea, lethargy and headache, more common with some drugs than others.

Practice point

Instruct parents and patients not to drop dosage or discontinue the medication without clinician approval. Clinicians should be aware of the risk of activation of the discontinuation syndrome.

Titration of dosage should be slow, since improvement may take up to 12 weeks. Support during this rather prolonged trial may be necessary to maintain collaboration. Activation by SSRIs or clomipramine (even conversion to mania) is more likely with pre-pubertal children (Martin et al. 2004).

Interest in alternative ways of disseminating CBT treatment more equitably and cost-effectively led to a trial of bibliotherapy and internet-administered treatment that showed comparable results with a waiting-list comparison group (Wootton et al. 2013). (This paper also provides a reference list for other studies of remote treatment for psychiatric disorders.)

To reiterate, it is essential to be aware that (1) significant OCD is almost always associated with parental (and often familial) accommodation to the symptoms, and (2) that this is hard to avoid, but that it is also a factor in reinforcing the behavior (Flessner et al. 2011). Higher parental anxiety is associated with higher levels of accommodation.

CONTROVERSIES AND SOURCES OF CONFUSION

Complex obsessive–compulsive behaviors may be mistaken for complex tics or psychotic symptoms (Palumbo and Kurlan 2007).

Case examples

'Ryan', a 6-year-old boy with a strong history of OCD and ADHD, manifested by needing to have everything said and done 'just right' and lack of confidence that he had performed an action adequately, had had a few tics, not enough for a diagnosis of Tourette syndrome. He also had skin-picking and several sensory hypersensitivities which improved as he matured. Over the course of the next 3 years the following took place: he developed a wide variety of new tics, including palilalia (repetition of his own words or phrases) and mental coprolalia, coughing and whooping, repeating questions, and an odd speech repetition of the last sound in a sentence (partial palilalia). He began chewing on his clothes and fingers. As school work became more demanding, his pre-examination anxiety increased and began to interfere with his performance; school adaptations were necessary. At age 13 he had episodes of excessive emotionality and sensitivity to any disappointment, but at age 15 his tics were not much of a problem and no new ones had emerged. His OCD symptoms had also become manageable without specific treatment.

Comment: He had a not uncommon progression of symptoms prior to puberty. During puberty his tics stabilized and lessened, and his other symptoms improved. Thus the clinical course, though discouraging in his early school years, moderated substantially, even without all disorders having received treatment.

'Arthur', first seen at age 7, showed multiple tics with onset at age 5, but no OCD features. Seven years later the two types of symptoms were intermixed and social anxiety had developed. He had to write certain words he heard in the air, and had to tap all four corners of a computer screen. Worse was a compulsion about completion and confirmation of communications: he would reply "OK" to a request made of him, but then he had to return, repeat the request that had been made, and hear the other person say "OK" again. A physical fight had led to an injured (but not fractured) nose, and subsequently he developed repeated checking because he felt his nose had become asymmetric. Response to sertraline was favorable.

> **Comment:** *This portrays the unpredictable but not unusual evolution of a number of symptoms of OCD in a young boy diagnosed with 'TS-only'. Body dysmorphic and social anxiety symptoms also emerged.*

There are two additional points of possible confusion that may arise. (1) The experience of tics following premonitory sensations may have a 'just right' quality that is compelling, even including creating just the right kind and degree of pain. Is this a feature of the tic or a compulsion? (2) An infrequent but clinically important and therapeutically difficult phenomenon occurs in a child who must have his or her parent (usually the mother) say things in a very specific way, avoiding or emphasizing certain sounds, voice tones, coordination with facial expressions, or number of repeats. This may require extreme parental accommodation to what seems to be a ridiculous or impossible-to-achieve demand, and the fine-tuning of the requirements may increase over time. In accordance with a recent study showing that hearing the voice tone accompanying a message has physiological effects on stress that are not conveyed by the message in a written form (Seltzer et al. 2012), it may be speculated that the system involved may be overactive.

The following case illustrates some of the problems.

Case example

'Glenn' was 14 when first seen. He had Tourette syndrome, ADHD, OCD and anxiety. He was socially popular with his peer group and doing well in school, though he had to erase his school work many times to get it just right, and had a light-switch ritual. He had sensitivity to sounds since early childhood, and gradually this became more of a problem because it led to a need for excessive reassurance and to family accommodation, built partly around sound. Mom was pressured to avoid certain sounds, or say things in certain ways and then wipe her mouth, or suffer a blow or verbal abuse. When he said something to her she had to respond with 'OK', he would then say 'OK' and then she would have to say it one more time or else he would become agitated. Medication had little effect on these symptoms and he was referred for CBT.

FINAL COMMENTS

OCD and even lesser levels than meet the full criteria (OCB) are very important in understanding and helping many persons with tic disorders. Even so, additional disorders and symptoms may be involved. It is a common clinical experience to observe a young child with TS-only or with TS+ADHD develop OCD a few years later and require new therapeutic strategies. Collaboration with schools and between primary care physicians and specialists as well as non-physician clinicians is always advisable. Competent CBT therapy may be difficult to obtain but is highly desirable for many children and young people. It is a favorable sign that in the future we will not be limited to pharmacotherapy alone and that refinements are being developed to be more effective with behavioral therapy. New studies of OCD treatment are described in the excellent newsletter of the International OCD Federation.

Practice point

As a child develops with OCD, symptoms may evolve, causing increased family accommodation and mandating increased collaboration with school and between all the clinicians and therapists involved.

Hoarding disorder

Hoarding is occasionally seen in young children, but it tends to have its onset in adolescence and can have comorbidity with anxiety disorders and OCD. Prevalence is estimated to be 2% to 4%. Unless its manifestations are extreme, early symptoms may not be spontaneously reported to clinicians. There may be a familial association with tics, but this is not well established.

In the DSM-5 hoarding is separated from OCD, but remains in association with it within the group of 'obsessive–compulsive and related disorders' (Leckman and Bloch 2008, Tolin et al. 2010). Mild hoarding tendencies appear in many children by age 6 years (Evans et al. 1997). There seems to be no significant association between tic disorders and hoarding disorder, although Saxena and Maidment (2004) reported that hoarding and tics are more common in first-degree relatives of hoarders.

Although hoarding is often thought to be a disorder of adulthood, individuals generally report an onset by early adolescence. The prevalence was 2% in a population-based study of adolescents by Ivanov et al. (2013) and 4% in a study of adults by Samuels et al. (2008). It was uncommonly associated with other neurodevelopmental disorders, but has a high comorbidity with social anxiety, generalized anxiety disorder and depression; about 20% also meet criteria for OCD, and in that group there are thought to be some unique clinical features (Pertusa et al. 2008). Frank et al. (2014) reported that hoarding symptoms were associated with an earlier age of OCD onset and a higher than expected rate of ADHD and anxiety symptoms.

Hoarding may not be reported spontaneously unless extreme. It is more likely to be revealed by systematic questioning in a structured assessment interview.

Anxiety disorders not related to obsessive–compulsive disorder

Anxiety, even if not much more common in persons with tics than in the general population, can affect many areas of functioning that may have an effect on quality of life. The most frequent comorbidity of an anxiety disorder is with another kind of anxiety disorder. Anxious children may interpret ambiguous stimuli as threatening; the result is that attentional bias affects further information processing, limiting the generation of appropriate responses. The readiness with which a person with tics enters into life activities is therefore essential to evaluate. Effective treatments are available with CBT and/or medication.

DEFINITION

Anxiety consists of a state of excessive worrying, uneasiness, and fear of future uncertainty, either continuous or episodic. There are several sub-categories in DSM-5: separation, selective mutism, social anxiety disorder, panic, agoraphobia, specific phobia, GAD, substance/medication-induced anxiety, and anxiety due to another medical condition. Post-traumatic stress disorder (PTSD) is now in the general category of 'trauma- and stressor-related disorders', and the 'overanxious disorder of childhood' of DSM-IV-TR is subsumed into GAD.

A good general text on all aspects of anxiety disorders is the book edited by Silverman and Field (2011).

DIAGNOSIS (INCLUDING INSTRUMENTS AND FORMS)

There are many questionnaires and checklists to aid in diagnosis and treatment effects: the Children's Manifest Anxiety Scale II, the Taylor Manifest Anxiety Scale, the Zung Self-Rating Anxiety Scale, and indicators on the Child Behavior Checklist (CBCL).

PREVALENCE/EPIDEMIOLOGY

Anxiety disorders are common (11% annual, 29% lifetime) in US community samples. Studies indicate a genetic component.

COMORBIDITY AND COMMON ASSOCIATIONS

Whatever the anxiety disorder subgroup, the most common comorbidity is another kind of anxiety disorder (Essau 2003), depression in 17% to 69%, and externalizing disorders in 8% to 69%. When an anxiety disorder is present, co-occurring OCD is likely to be more severe (Langley et al. 2010).

About 17% to 25% of those with ADHD meet criteria for an anxiety disorder, which may not be suspected in an overactive child (Spencer 2006). Panic disorder occurs in 6% and agoraphobia in 1.5%. There is evidence that anxiety is conducive to mood swings that are subthreshold for a bipolar diagnosis. Anxiety when comorbid also increases the risk of sleep-related problems in children with tics (Storch et al. 2009), confirmed by reports in the *TIC* database, where 28.4% of those with anxiety disorder had a sleep problem whereas without anxiety the rate was 17.9% (p<0.001, OR 1.8). The prevalence in the Storch report was 80.4% for at least one sleep disorder, and almost 20% of children experienced four or more kinds of sleep problems. Tic severity surprisingly was not correlated with sleep-related problems.

TABLE 10.5
Children with and without anxiety disorders (*TIC* data, n=5247[a])

	Without anxiety (n=4417)		With anxiety (n=830)		p	Odds ratio
	n	%	n	%		
ADHD	2574	58	520	63	0.019	1.2
OCD	681	15	822	32	<0.001	2.6
Mood disorder	416	9	172	21	<0.001	2.5
Sleep disorder (now)	738	17	225	28	<0.001	1.9
Anger problem (now)	1153	27	283	35	<0.001	1.5
SIB (ever)	491	11	180	22	<0.001	2.2
Social skill deficits (now)	649	15	189	23	<0.001	1.7
Coprophenomena (ever)	476	11	123	15	<0.001	1.4

[a]4378 males (83.4%), 869 females (16.6%).
Excluded: intellectual disability, autism spectrum disorder and psychosis.
ADHD, attention-deficit/hyperactivity disorder; OCD, oppositional–conduct disorder; SIB, self-injurious behavior.

NATURAL HISTORY AND PROGNOSIS

Anxiety disorders tend to be recurrent if not treated.

Anxiety is so common and so likely to interfere with quality of life that it should always be assessed. In the *TIC* database, the rate of diagnosed anxiety also increases from childhood into adulthood.

Practice point

Anxiety should always be assessed because it is highly likely to interfere with quality of life.

In a recent study of patients with chronic tic disorder (CTD), Specht et al. (2011) found ADHD in 26%, social phobia in 21%, GAD in 20%, and OCD in 19%. Their conclusion was that young people with a CTD seeking treatment should be evaluated for a non-OCD anxiety disorder in addition to the more obvious ADHD and OCD. Among their patients with anxiety disorder, 56% were diagnosed with ADHD.

In the *TIC* database, anxiety was reported in 15% to 16% of persons with Tourette syndrome, regardless of sex in children, but there was a significant difference in adults: males 20%, females 27% (p=0.002). In anxious children, significant increases were reported in those with mood disorder, OCD, SIB, sleep problems and social skill deficits, with lesser but still significant increases in those with anger control problems and coprophenomena. Details are in Table 10.5.

ATTENTIONAL BIAS IN ANXIETY DISORDER

Some children with Tourette syndrome may be socially anxious about their tics (perhaps due to bad experiences or the unpredictable arrival of new tics), what might be called

'noticing/noticing', namely embarrassed by the feeling that anyone looking at them is noticing their tics. Perhaps partly because their control is limited, anxious children preferentially
attend to threat-relevant stimuli, which biases their subsequent information processing and
results in their missing a more balanced interpretation of the situation (Mico et al. 2013).
Teasing tends to be interpreted as malicious (Nowakowski and Antony 2013).

TRICHOTILLOMANIA IN ANXIETY DISORDER

In anxiety disorders a relatively high rate of trichotillomania (10.2%) was recorded in the
TIC database, and because it is not always spontaneously mentioned (especially when its
manifestations are intermittent) it should be routinely questioned. Conversely, 41% of those
with trichotillomania have an anxiety disorder (vs 20% without), so ask.

> **Practice point**
> In assessment of an anxiety disorder, routinely question symptoms of hair-pulling.

TREATMENT

Tics can generate embarrassment and social anxiety, due to individual sensitivity, the nature
of the particular tics, and teasing. When this starts, it is advisable to look into the situation
early, before the pattern becomes more persistent and impairs quality of life.

> **Practice point**
> The start of significant anxiety symptoms is an indication for urgent intervention.

Treatment options (including for PTSD), psychological and pharmacological, have been
reviewed by Rapp et al. (2013). Trials of computer-based and computer-assisted treatments
have been completed or are underway and may offer increased accessibility and lower cost.
Online interventions have proven helpful in recent studies (Christensen et al. 2014), and
Nowakowski and Antony (2013) have made recommendations for treatment of social anxiety that involve cognitive restructuring and psychoeducation about how to use humor when
teased.

Traditionally, anti-anxiety agents have been the mainstay of treatment, though now
forms of psychotherapy such as CBT have become first-line. Connolly and Bernstein (2007)
provided a practice parameter. Identification of contributing environmental factors and their
minimization is an important first step. First-line evidence-based treatment is CBT, an SSRI
such as sertraline, or the combination, the choice depending upon treatment availability,
cost, and family preference (Piacentini et al. 2014). For CBT, comorbidity does not appear
to have an effect on therapeutic outcome (Ollendick et al. 2008). A recent long-term follow-
up study by Saavedra et al. (2010) compared group and individual exposure-based CBT
for childhood anxiety disorders and followed up their status 8–13 years later. Long-term

remission was found for both therapeutic approaches and, surprisingly, also for secondary outcomes (other anxiety disorders, depressive disorders, substance use disorders). The individual approach showed small but significant gains.

It is possible that use of an SSRI in children can cause activation, so clinicians should be aware of the clinical signs, which include increased activity level, impulsivity, insomnia, or disinhibition without mania, and hypomanic features not typical of that patient (Safer and Zito 2006, Reinblatt et al. 2009).

A more common complication, often overlooked, is the 'discontinuation syndrome' (Hosenbocus and Chahal 2011), discussed elsewhere in this chapter. Rapid reduction of dosage or discontinuation of SSRIs can produce unpleasant side-effects, commonly dizziness, nausea, lethargy and headache, more common with some drugs than others (paroxetine and venlafaxine most, fluvoxamine, sertraline and citalopram intermediate, and fluoxetine the least), though research on children and adolescents is not extensive. The message is to instruct parents and patients not to drop dosage or discontinue the medication on their own without clinician approval.

Practice point

Clinicians should be aware that SSRIs occasionally cause activation in children and adolescents, manifested by increased activity level, insomnia and disinhibition. Too-quick reduction of SSRI or SNRI dosage can produce unpleasant side-effects; dosage should not be quickly reduced without clinician approval.

Case example

'Gary' is a 9-year-old boy with tics from age 7 and a recent history of severe separation anxiety, manifested by difficulty going to school (where he is doing very well academically), stomach aches, and fears that something bad will happen to his parents. His mother lies with him to get him to go to sleep. He needs to know where she is, even in the home, and is upset if parental plans to pick him up at school change in the slightest way. He can leave the house when he initiates it, but becomes very anxious if he is left at home while his parents go out. His father had some similar fears as a child. Surprisingly, 'Gary' has friends and is good at public speaking and acting, in which activities he seems to have no unusual anxiety.

Comment: Somatic symptoms can lead to reinforcement of anxiety by facilitating the child going home instead of staying at school, and sleeping with the child also can be strongly reinforcing. He was referred for a trial of CBT. (Note a seeming discrepancy when he initiates a separation versus when it is initiated by others.)

Mood disorders

> Whether rates of mood disorder are higher in tic disorders or not, or intrinsic to the condition or secondary to it, exploration of mood is important. Mood states can affect tic severity and the impairment conferred by co-occurring disorders. Tic increases can worsen mood.

DEFINITION

Disturbances in mood have a complex set of criteria for subtypes, discussed in the DSM-IV-TR (APA 2000) and more recently in DSM-5. Sleep disorder and other vegetative symptoms, cognitive changes, difficulty concentrating, irritability, and changes in energy, motivation, interest and self-esteem are typically seen.

DIAGNOSIS

Depressed children may experience irritability rather than the depressed mood familiar in adults. Persistent depressive disorder (DSM-5, formerly dysthymic disorder in DSM-IV-TR) may be easily missed because the individual with a chronic low mood may come to feel "I'm just this way" and not report it. The required duration for diagnosis is 1 year for children and 2 years for adults (Kovacs et al. 1994). The diagnosis of bipolar disorder in children is controversial (Taylor 2009a, Towbin et al. 2013). One should be cautious about diagnosing a formal mood disorder such as bipolar disorder from mood lability in children and adolecents. The introduction of a new DSM-5 category, 'disruptive mood dysregulation disorder', with diagnosis below age 18 and onset at or before age 6, is also controversial and although introduced to distinguish many children from being overdiagnosed with bipolar disorder has been criticized for possibly extending the number of children likely to receive medication.

DIFFERENTIATION FROM OPPOSITIONAL–DEFIANT DISORDER AND BIPOLAR DISORDER

Mania in children is often manifested by irritability or explosive mood, decreased sleep, racing thoughts, thrill-seeking and over-talkativeness, but can be hard to differentiate from ADHD and conduct disorder (Spencer 2006). In disruptive mood dysregulation disorder the mood disturbance is non-episodic, unlike that in bipolar disorder.

PREVALENCE/EPIDEMIOLOGY

About 10% of preadolescent children show depressed mood, but only about 0.5% would meet DSM-IV-TR depression criteria. In adolescence the prevalence rises to 1% to 3% for major depressive disorder (MDD), with girls at twice the rate of boys. Unipolar disorders have a reported prevalence of 1.5% to 8%, common but often unrecognized (Thapar et al. 2012). However, in the Gorman et al. (2010) study, the rates for MDD in adolescence were much higher (61.5% in Tourette syndrome, 26.2% in a matched community comparison group) with additional proportions with bipolar disorder (6.2% vs 0%) and persistent depressive disorder (10.8% vs 4.6%) for a total mood disorder rate of 78.5% vs 30.8%. These results with sophisticated methodology are surprising, providing a rate of 56.9% of psychiatric disorder other than OCD for the comparison group. Contrast this with our results from the *TIC* database: the mean for all patients was 20% for all mood disorders, with rates from 2% to 47% reported from different sites. If we examine only rates for adolescents (first seen at ages 18–20) the range is 5% to 23%. These ranges suggest complexity in criteria and assessment.

PRESENTATION AND PHENOMENOLOGY

Perhaps of more frequent importance is the child who shocks or worries parents by talking of suicide or of wishing never to have been born, usually in the context of increased tic frequency and severity. This usually is due not to the onset of a depressive process but rather to the feeling of loss of control and self-esteem, social frustration, teasing, or worries about becoming increasingly different. Sometimes this occurs when treatment seems ineffective and tics are still increasing. Parents may be shocked when their young child voices suicidal thoughts or wishes; they need to know that this is a common result of frustration and discouragement. In general, only about one in 100 suicide threats leads to suicide, but they require attention, nevertheless.

Case example

Ten-year-old 'Derek' had obvious multiple tics and a dysfunctional family situation. He was doing poorly in school and showed some defiance, irritability, and constant whining and complaining. After several years of rather irregular unsuccessful attempts to draw him out and limit silliness there was a surprise: he asked to be seen and confessed to feeling sad, discouraged, and without motivation of any kind. A history could finally be obtained and it showed that he had had an absence of pleasure and energy for several years, and that he had frequent thoughts of suicide. He responded well initially to low-dose SSRI and satisfied criteria for dysthymic disorder. At age 16 he had matured, developed a realistic appraisal of his life and other people through a job, expressed a wide range of normal emotions and had been off all medication.

*   **Comment:** The change in attitude may have been due to maturity, but he also was able to describe his emotional state, which helped understand his previous uncooperative, disengaged behavior and establish a therapeutic alliance for the first time. The role of medication in his further improvement was hard to assess. Clinicians are fortunate to have an experience of this kind and should never forget it as a potential in any patient.*

COMORBIDITY AND COMMON ASSOCIATIONS

There is substantial comorbidity within the affective disorder group. About 75% also have an anxiety disorder at some point, with ADHD in 0% to 57%, and ODD/conduct disorder

TABLE 10.6
Children in *TIC* database (n=5656) with and without mood disorders

	Without mood disorder (n=4615)		With mood disorder (n=581)		*p*	Odds ratio
	n	*%*	*n*	*%*		
Medication for tics (ever)	2084	45	387	67	<0.001	2.4
ADHD	2666	57	424	72	<0.001	1.9
OCD	748	16	202	34	<0.001	2.7
Anxiety	657	14	172	29	<0.001	2.5
ODD/conduct disorder	582	13	138	24	<0.001	2.1
SIB (ever)	548	12	123	21	0.001	2.0
Anger problem (now)	1189	26	246	45	<0.001	2.3
Social skill deficits (now)	694	15	144	25	<0.001	1.9
Sleep disorder (now)	826	18	137	24	<0.001	1.5
Coprophenomena (ever)	509	11	90	15	<0.001	1.5

Excluded: intellectual disability, autism spectrum disorder and psychosis.
ADHD, attention-deficit/hyperactivity disorder; OCD, oppositional–conduct disorder; ODD, oppositional–defiant disorder; SIB, self-injurious behavior.

in 0% to 79%. In one large study half of the children with a mood disorder had at least one concurrent non-mood disorder. Depression is the most common complication of OCD (Robertson and Orth 2006). Among children with ADHD, 10% to 30% meet criteria for MDD. MDD occurs in 1% to 2% of elementary schoolchildren and 5% of adolescents in the general population. Comorbidity with ADHD is 15% to 75% in different samples, including epidemiologic ones. On ADHD follow-up, 11% were diagnosed with mania (Robertson and Orth 2006, Spencer 2006).

In the *TIC* database, there are significant increases in odds ratios for comorbidity with OCD (2.7), anxiety (2.5) and ODD/conduct disorder (2.2), and increases in anger control problems (2.3), self-hitting (2.5) and SIB (2.0): see Table 10.6 for details. Note that children with mood disorder are more likely to receive medication for tics than those without.

NATURAL HISTORY AND PROGNOSIS
The majority of cases of depression remit within a year, but in follow-up studies 50% to 70% recur within 5 years. An episode may herald a chronic or relapsing disorder with a broad range of additional difficulties (Thapar et al. 2012).

TREATMENT
Evidence-based psychological interventions considered first-line are CBT and various interpersonal therapies such as dialectical behavior therapy (Bohus et al. 2004, Harvey and Rathbone 2013). Medication for depression in children (typically SSRIs) is of questionable efficacy and can have problematic interactions with some medications (first generation antipsychotics) used for tics. Medication for bipolar disorder is also difficult and should be managed by an expert. Comorbid anxiety disorder reduces the outcomes of treatment for

mood disorder (Ollendick et al. 2008). In adults, only about one-third respond fully to anti-depressants, but a recent study showed very substantial benefit for adjunctive CBT for those whose depression is refractory to medication (Wiles et al. 2013). Unfortunately such treatment is often hard to access.

<small>Controversies and sources of confusion</small>
The diagnosis and therefore cited rates of bipolar disorder remain controversial (Berthier et al. 1998).

Oppositional–defiant disorder and conduct disorder

> ODD and conduct disorder are prevalent and very costly to society. Although often discussed together, their outcomes are sufficiently divergent to merit separate study. Comorbidity is common, of both internalizing and externalizing kinds, and a variety of complex situations can foster behavior similar to ODD. Special caution applies for persons from an ethnic group different from that of the clinician, who may not be fully aware of varying standards of behavior. Treatment is generally based on social learning theory.

<small>Definition</small>
ODD is described as a pattern of persistent negativistic, hostile, vindictive, defiant behavior (Spencer 2006), often associated with verbal threats and physical acts. Conduct disorder is more severe, with aggression, destruction, lying, stealing or truancy. A thorough review of the field has been well presented in the practice parameter of the American Academy of Child and Adolescent Psychiatry (2007b), and a comprehensive summary of the subject, with clinical recommendations and a review of current evidence, is available from the UK's National Institute for Health and Care Excellence (NICE 2013). Most adolescents with conduct disorder would have qualified for a diagnosis of ODD as a child; those whose symptoms started in adolescence have more extreme problems as adults and a worse outcome.

> **Practice point**
> In DSM-5, irritability has been included as a characteristic of the ODD pattern. Both emotional and behavioral features have been found to be important. Children reported as meeting criteria by both parents and teachers were more impaired, and cross-situationality may become a useful index of severity.

<small>Diagnosis</small>
Caution in making the diagnosis of ODD should be exercised because some situations can mimic the pattern, and one must distinguish it from some common age-related developmental

patterns, such as can be seen in the so-called 'terrible twos' (and threes) and early adolescence. Children with internalizing disorders (anxiety or depression) may react defensively with oppositional behavior when feeling overwhelmed. Inability to get one's own or one's parent's actions 'just right' in OCD can also result in such a presentation, and ODD-like reactions are common in ASD. Children who sense their inability to cope due to deficient skills (academic or social) may react with anger, defiance and 'challenging behavior' (Greene 2008).

Practice point

Several situations or other disorders can mimic ODD. Caution is advised.

In DSM 5 the new diagnosis of 'disruptive mood dysregulation disorder' (included under mood disorders) has some similarities in that the criteria include severe 'out of proportion' temper outbursts with persistently irritable or angry mood between episodes. This diagnosis cannot coexist with ODD, intermittent explosive disorder or bipolar disorder, and the age of occurrence must be between 7 and 18 years. Only about 15% of children with ODD are expected to meet the chronic mood criterion of disruptive mood dysregulation disorder, and the usefulness of this category is still unclear.

An important study by Roy et al. (2013) showed that in children referred for impairing temper outbursts these symptoms did not indicate early bipolar disorder, rather comorbidity (often ADHD, ODD, anxiety and/or depression), and demonstrate deficits in expression of positive emotions and weak frustration regulation.

PREVALENCE/EPIDEMIOLOGY

ODD with conduct disorder is reported to occur at a rate of 2% to 16% in different studies. (In the ICD-10, ODD is subsumed under conduct disorder.)

ETIOLOGY

A single cause is very unlikely, and causal links have not been well established. Aggressive children have been shown to underutilize social cues, to misattribute hostile intent to peers, and to generate fewer problem-solving solutions. Genetic factors are believed to contribute.

COMORBIDITY AND COMMON ASSOCIATIONS

There is an overlap of ODD with ADHD in 30% to 50% (Rowe et al. 2005). Conduct disorder and ADHD are related but independent dimensions. Depression was diagnosed in 2% to 46% in different studies, and anxiety disorder in 5% to 55% (Ollendick et al. 2008). Of those with a lifetime diagnosis of ODD, 92% had at least one other lifetime disorder, so it is highly comorbid.

In the *TIC* database, with ASD, intellectual disability and psychosis cases excluded, the following are impressive reported differences. Of the children with ADHD, 21% were diagnosed with ODD, whereas only 4% of those without ADHD were so categorized (p<0.001, OR 6.1); for those with anger control problems at the time registered, the respective figures were 28% versus 7% (OR 5.2); for inappropriate sexual behavior, 39% versus 12% (OR 4.5); and for coprophenomena, 28% versus 12% (OR 2.9). The only other disorder with a major difference was mood (24% vs 13%, OR 2.2). Highly significant differences in adults were for ADHD, SLD, anger control, coprophenomena, social skills deficits and sexually inappropriate behavior.

NATURAL HISTORY AND PROGNOSIS

ODD features often begin in the late preschool or early school years, and earlier onset is associated with a poorer prognosis. ODD and conduct disorder follow a divergent course: 30% to 40% of children with conduct disorder progress to adult antisocial personality disorder. Of children with ADHD with ODD, the latter persists in 17%; most do not progress to conduct disorder; nevertheless, their adult course is compromised compared with those without ODD (Biederman et al. 2008). About two-thirds of children with ODD show a significant reduction of symptoms on follow-up. Much research still remains to be done.

TREATMENT

A wide variety of behavioral treatments have been applied with greater success in recent years, now that multi-faceted approaches have been implemented and studied (Greene 2005, 2008; Greene and Ablon 2006; Barkley and Robin 2008; Kazdin and Rotella 2008; Kazdin 2010; Lochman et al. 2010; Webster-Stratton and Reid 2010). An excellent manual for CBT for anger and aggression has been produced by Sukhodolsky and Scahill (2012). Comorbidity has not been shown to cause poorer outcome of treatment (Ollendick et al. 2008).

CONTROVERSIES AND SOURCES OF CONFUSION

Children with OCD may become oppositional because their parents cannot accommodate successfully to their needs (which, because of disorder-related features, may sometimes seem insatiable). Clinicians also need caution in making this diagnosis on children from cultures and ethnic groups that may have different standards of obedience and methods of parenting. Children with ODD, when interviewed, may deny symptoms and patterns of behavior described by adults. They tend to justify their behavior by the circumstances that surround it.

Practice point

Children and adolescents with ODD tend to deny symptoms and behavior patterns or justify them by circumstances.

Case example

'Matthew' was 10 when first seen 28 years ago. He had multiple tics since age 3 as well as ADHD. Many clinicians had been uncertain about the Tourette syndrome diagnosis,

though in retrospect he certainly qualified. The diagnosis initially was 'habit spasms', despite a history of echolalia and palilalia and the subsequent start of coprolalia. Psychological testing showed no learning disability but a need for a structured learning environment. An annoying spitting tic developed and he took his medication only irregularly. There were obvious family problems and his behavior worsened. His schoolwork deteriorated. Omnipotent, self-centered attitudes were evident, but it was unclear how much of his attitude was due to the family situation and how much to his worsening pathology. He was seen only occasionally but by age 16 he had been in trouble with the law and seemed uncaring about others. Drug abuse began and he did not always come home. His mother became desperate. The final episode was when he stole a car, tried to evade a police roadblock, flipped the car and was killed.

Comment: Matthew's Tourette syndrome was not the cause of his demise. In his final years he appeared to best satisfy criteria for conduct disorder, but it had not been evident at age 10. It was never clear how much of his difficulty was attributable to his own pathology or to that of his family. This has been the only case with this outcome in over 40 years and was not associated with much of the comorbidity commonly encountered. It may be of interest that in the past clinicians were looking for much more severe tic symptoms before making what today would be an obvious diagnosis of Tourette syndrome, perhaps because of the initial absence of coprolalia

Autism spectrum disorder

Tics often develop in patients with ASD and may be impairing. Their occurrence is much more frequent than in the general population. Specialist initiation of treatment is advisable. Sleep problems are common and may need careful attention to prevent additional impairment. Sensory and movement differences may be all too easily seen as simply autistic behaviors to be treated, rather than understood in ways we are not familiar with from our own experiences. Knowledge about people aging with ASD and tics is lacking.

'Autism spectrum disorder' (Caronna et al. 2008) is the new DSM-5 overall term for the previous 'pervasive developmental disorder' in DSM-IV-TR. It consists of deficits in social–emotional reciprocity, nonverbal communicative behaviors, developing and understanding relationships, and restricted, repetitive patterns of behavior, interests or activities (Volkmar et al. 2014). A good review of evidence-based practice is now available (Anagnostou et al. 2014). Tourette syndrome is about six times more common in ASD than in the general population (Baron-Cohen et al. 1999a,b; Burd et al. 2009). Because "restricted, repetitive pattern of behavior" has been conflated in the diagnostic criteria, and stereotyped motor patterns are common in other disorders or in some children with typical development, children with tics or with stereotypic movement disorder may be misdiagnosed as having one of these ASD disorders (Freeman et al. 2010). Hand-flapping and smelling of non-food objects are especially likely to be equated with an ASD. It is very important to be aware of this bias and to warn parents about it if their child manifests one of these patterns.

Practice point

Parents should be made aware that hand-flapping and smelling are likely to be assumed to represent ASD, when such patterns are commonly found in other children, too.

Another complex issue is whether stereotypies in ASD occur without premonitory sensations or are 'purposeless'. Does the 'purpose' have to be articulated by the patient or be acceptable to the clinician? Is self-regulation a 'purpose' even if not described or claimed? Is a premonitory sensation an urge, or a need? "When we label aspects of a person's behavior as meaningless, we may miss opportunities to extend learning and develop our relationships" (Donnellan et al. 2013, p. 7).

The likelihood of Tourette syndrome in patients with an ASD (specifically Asperger syndrome) was studied for a small group of consecutive patients by Ringman and Jankovic (2000). Of eight persons diagnosed with Asperger syndrome, all showed stereotyped behaviors, seven had tics, and six of those met criteria for Tourette syndrome.

Case example

'Norman' was 15, with diagnoses of ASD and intellectual disability. He had no useful speech. His main behavioral problem was unpredictable aggression, for which he had been treated with risperidone for over 5 years. He had had a few tics or stereotyped movements during childhood. He then developed movements of his head and face that were thought by his pediatrician to be due to tardive dyskinesia. Benztropine was tried and had no effect. He had recently had extensive dental work done and it was concluded that the markedly increased tics were triggered by the changed sensations in his mouth.

Comment: Tardive dyskinesia is rare in Tourette syndrome and would be unlikely after years of an unchanging fairly low dosage of risperidone. Environmental changes or changes in sensation can be powerful factors in new symptoms, and should be considered as triggers in individuals with limited means of expression.

Some children with ASD have rather few behavioral problems until they are approaching or in puberty. Then they may develop OCD and/or tics as a significant therapeutic issue, and if they also have ADHD and a learning disability with or without intellectual disability, the challenges and complexities can be overwhelming (Anderson et al. 2011). There is an increasing appreciation that individuals with ASD often have an underlying motor coordination dysfunction (74% in a recent study by de Jong et al. 2011), such as posture, muscle tone, associated movement and fine motor problems, which may contribute to difficulty assessing movements.

The developmental trajectory of ASD into adulthood and in old age is poorly understood and little studied (Fombonne 2012). A high proportion appear to have other psychiatric disorders which may present with an unusual clinical picture (Anderson et al. 2011). Response to medication may be unpredictable and even paradoxical (Howlin and Moss 2012). Available research does not permit the development of rational services, despite the awareness that the increased number of diagnosed children and adolescents will present a very significant problem for governments around the world (Shattuck et al. 2012).

Case study

'Owen' was 15 years old and actively participating in an Applied Behavior Analysis (ABA) treatment program when he developed noises and other movements that were recognized by his workers and parents as probably not part of his usual behavioral repertoire. Indeed, he had multiple tics and then received the diagnosis of Tourette syndrome. The tics were significant enough to warrant treatment, so he was started on a modest dose of pimozide, which was successful for over 2 years, whereupon it seemed to lose its effect, necessitating a shift to aripiprazole (unsuccessful) and finally risperidone. The latter required several weeks of slow titration to demonstrate benefit. He developed occasional retching and vomiting that seemed to enable him to escape from difficult tasks. Vocal tics then worsened until they were continuous and interfered with all treatment and learning. No specific cause for the severe increase was identified. Finally a gastroenterologist diagnosed gastroesophageal reflux disorder, and after a proton pump inhibitor was tried, a dramatic drop of vocal tics almost to zero, cessation of retching and vomiting, and a return to his normal appearance and cooperation in treatment resulted and has been maintained. A new non-interfering pattern developed somewhat later: staring briefly but obviously at corners of rooms from specific locations.

***Comment:** This story is instructive. Owen's inability to describe his symptoms delayed the diagnosis and specific treatment, his retching/vomiting symptoms and related behavior could support a behavioral explanation. His impairing tics responded immediately to relief of physical discomfort, were unresponsive to tic-suppressing medication, and none of this invalidated the occasional development of a new tic as is so often seen in young persons with Tourette syndrome. All aspects of life may be relevant to management of tics.*

Early onset of ASD is expected for the diagnosis, but the assessment of general intelligence may be difficult, and if and when tics begin later, they may be mistaken for the stereotyped behavior of a person with intellectual disability.

When various developmental trajectories of children with ASD were studied by Fountain et al. (2012), stereotyped behavior tended to remain relatively stable after age 7, except in 15% (half of whom became worse and half improved).

Case study

'Danny' was born in Asia. As an infant he was taken to relatives in another country and then brought back again. When he started preschool he didn't seem interested in relating to other children. An ASD was suspected. His family moved to another country and he was assessed for the first time and declared to have a mild intellectual disability. The linguistic and cultural changes from living in three different countries were not taken into account. For a time he was home-schooled. Tics began around age 4 but were not recognized as such at that time. He had restricted interests and when enrollment in a public secondary school was sought, the school authorities insisted that he was too intellectually limited to attend a regular class. His parents obtained another assessment by a competent psychologist who found that, rather than intellectual disability, he had a nonverbal learning disability and a disorder of written expression. The school refused to accept that opinion (even with the psychologist present at the meeting), and suggested strongly that the parents were being unrealistic, that he would never graduate having fulfilled all requirements, and also that his loud and disruptive vocal tics made his presence in a regular class unfeasible. However, when he was started on risperidone the tics diminished. The specialist in ASD wrote a letter to the school and talked with the principal, requesting a better plan for inclusion. This was undertaken as a trial admission. In a short time he demonstrated that his capacity was much higher than the school had believed. He graduated, having met all requirements, and is now in a university program. He did well academically in his first year there, with the support of three approved accommodations: taking examinations alone, keyboarding instead of written submissions, and extra time for completion of examinations. At age 19 his tics are minimal and he has some friends, although his social skills are not at par with his peers.

Comment: Danny's experiences illustrate a number of points. Early psychological assessment is not fully adequate to predict later functioning, and results should not preclude later reconsideration; different cultural and linguistic experiences need to be taken into account; the effects of anxiety, ADHD and ASD also need to be considered; and obvious tics may compound the difficulties in that reconsideration. It is also possible that the presence of disruptive tics augmented the unwillingness of the school to open-mindedly consider the views of the parents and the psychologist.

TREATMENT OF OTHER SYMPTOMS/DISORDERS

Anxiety and ADHD occur commonly in ASD and may need treatment (Huffman et al. 2011). Originally ADHD was excluded by the ASD diagnosis; in DSM-5 the dual diagnosis is now allowed. Sensory over-responsivity is very common in ASD and when severe can contribute to family-life impairment (Ben-Sasson et al. 2013). Occupational therapists can help families to cope better with these peculiarities.

> **Practice point**
> Sensory problems are common in ASD and often cause difficulty that can be helped by occupational therapists, who have the most experience in their assessment and management.

SLEEP IN AUTISM SPECTRUM DISORDER

Sleep problems are frequent (40% to 80%), the most common being sleep-onset insomnia. The causative factors may be parental management of sleep problems, neurobiologically dysregulated systems (including circadian rhythm disorders), anxiety or mood disorder (Johnson et al. 2009). Because of their frequency and likelihood of impairing daytime functioning and increasing caregiver burden, sleep problems need to be screened for, and sleep hygiene problems improved before other interventions are considered.

> **Practice point**
> Sleep problems are common in ASD and can impair daytime functioning and caregiver burden, but are often modifiable. They should be routinely asked about.

Pharmacologically, melatonin is sometimes helpful and is considered safe. For parasomnias (sleepwalking, night terrors), clonazepam is usually recommended. Risperidone is approved in the USA for irritability or SIB in ASD and may be useful to aid sleep in conjunction with its employment to manage tics, but metabolic monitoring is necessary. A recent paper (Wink et al. 2014) found that the increasing effects on body weight of risperidone and aripiprazole treatment were equivalent.

Specific learning disability

> SLD is a common complication of tic disorders, especially when they are comorbid with ADHD, and a frequent cause of school-based problems, including school avoidance, aggravation of social anxiety, low self-esteem and early drop-out. Comorbid OCD and anxiety and mood disorders can also affect school performance and complicate the picture further. Careful screening of comorbidity and any other influencing factors is very important, and more so as task complexity and academic expectations increase with age.

There is a high rate (23%) of reported comorbid SLD in Tourette syndrome (Burd et al. 2005). Because of the substantial overlap with ADHD, children with TS+ADHD are at high risk for SLD. Detailed advice on assessment and management of SLD has been provided (American Academy of Child and Adolescent Psychiatry 1998).

Reading disability or dyslexia is a dimensional developmental problem with a strong familial tendency. When it occurs, especially in combination with psychosocial adversity and lack of school-based support, it can be a serious risk factor for reading avoidance and lowered self-esteem (Muter and Snowling 2009). Intervention to maximize opportunity and to lower risk via school support is necessary.

Reading disorder overlaps significantly with ADHD (Taylor 2011), and therefore children presenting with either problem should be screened for the other, and treatment plans should focus on both. The extent of the overlap has not been settled, studies varying widely in methodology and results (Sexton et al. 2012). There is some evidence for both medication and behavioral/educational treatments, but effect sizes are at best small to moderate. Full psychological testing by a competent psychologist is highly desirable but may not be available or affordable.

Practice point

Because of overlaps between ADHD and SLD, children with either disorder should be screened for the other, as well as for other disorders and symptoms, if possible with full psychological assessment.

Although little is said here about the specific relationship of tics to SLD, much more may be involved in learning processes because of the effects of comorbid disorders, symptoms, sensory peculiarities and other factors.

Tics can cause direct interference with reading, such as when eye-rolling causes losing one's place on the page, or hand or arm tics affect holding a book or paper, or severe tics are destructive to computer keyboards or mice.

Comorbid OCD can result in compulsive checking, excessive going over letters to get them to look right, or erasing them, which can greatly reduce efficiency.

Case example

'Duncan' is a 12-year-old boy with significant tics, obsessive–compulsive features and a mood disorder. For many years he has had sensory over-responsivity to the feel of paper. When he developed an eye-rolling tic he would lose his place on the page, but the usual simple way to cope with this (holding a straight edge under the line so that he would not have to visually locate the line and then his former position on the line) was unsuccessful without special equipment to avoid touching the paper surface. While he had this combination of interferences he needed official approval for the school staff to find a way to accommodate to his special need and to permit him to function adequately. Fortunately he had not yet started to dislike school.

***Comment:** Such bureaucratic approval might not be necessary in all school systems, but was in this one. Deviation from the strategies ordinarily employed may be necessary for children with tics.*

Many other creative solutions to unusual or unique problems can be found in the books by Dornbush and Pruitt (2008) and Packer and Pruitt (2010).

Intellectual disability (UK usage: learning disability)

Children and adults with intellectual disability are at greater risk for the development of repetitive behaviors, which are easy to confuse with each other. Tics may or may not be important in themselves or as confusing elements in a complex clinical picture that can include ASD, movement disorders and other kinds of repetitive behaviors. Comorbidity additional to Tourette syndrome with intellectual disability is very common, significantly more so than in those with typical development. In particular, coprophenomena, anger control problems and SIBs frequently occur and may become targets for intervention. Stereotypies are also more common in intellectual disability than in typically developing individuals.

'Intellectual disability' is the DSM-5 term, at least in North America, replacing the old 'mental retardation'. Onset needs to be during the developmental period. (The earlier proposal to include 'developmental' in the term was wise, but not followed.) Intellectual disability has a prevalence of about 2% to 3% in the general population. It is probably not much more common in persons with tics, but conversely persons with intellectual disability are more likely to have tics. There have been a few publications, mostly pointing out the risk of failing to diagnose Tourette syndrome, especially in moderate to severe intellectual disability, probably due to 'diagnostic overshadowing', in which symptoms are wrongly assumed to derive from the major diagnosis (Crews et al. 1993). Repetitive and stereotyped motor behaviors (sometimes self-injurious) are common in intellectual disability and can be confused with tics (Golden and Greenhill 1981). Their presence can add to the social stigma of intellectual disability. Psychiatric disorders are more common among those with intellectual disability than in persons with typical development, and therefore impairment is common (Dekker and Koot 2003, Chadwick et al. 2005, Hemmings et al. 2006).

At a time when Tourette syndrome was assumed to be rare, the combination of intellectual disability with Tourette syndrome would naturally have been thought rarer still, such instances thus meriting the publication of case reports. Now that the prevalence of tics and Tourette syndrome is known to be much more common, the co-occurrence is not by itself surprising, so case reports have dwindled. So what are the relevant questions?

• *Are there any syndromes or types of intellectual disability comorbid with tics, or raising any useful theoretical or etiological questions?* Probably not. Schneider et al. (2008) described the onset of multiple tics meeting criteria for Tourette syndrome in four patients with fragile-X syndrome and one with adult-onset tics. However, tic onset in all these cases was later than usual, and comorbidities were those of both fragile-X and Tourette syndromes. Kerbeshian et al. (1984) and Goldson and Hagerman (1992) also reported persons with fragile-X syndrome, but in the latter description the foul language was thought to derive from imitation of others. Lesch–Nyhan syndrome is reported to have coprolalia and spitting as part of the behavioral phenotype (Visser et al. 2000, Cif et al. 2007), interesting because of the association of coprophenomena and spitting found by Freeman et al. (2009). There was special interest in Down syndrome and Tourette syndrome (Barabas et al. 1986, Karlinsky et al. 1986, Karlinsky and Berg 1987, Collacott and Ismail 1988, Myers and Pueschel 1995, Kerbeshian and Burd 2000). Sedel et al. (2006) presented an instance of beta-mannosidase deficiency with atypical Tourette syndrome, suggesting screening for inborn errors of metabolism in atypical cases of Tourette syndrome. Finally, Simonic et al. (1997) presented instances of co-occurring Rett syndrome and Tourette syndrome, suggesting the possibility of neighboring circuit involvement.

• *Are there subtypes of intellectual disability in which tic disorders are more likely to be under-diagnosed? And if so, why?* It would seem that diagnosis is more difficult the more severe the degree of intellectual disability. This may be due to the person's limited language (restricting possibilities for differential diagnosis), a much greater likelihood of stereotypies that can be confused with tics, and the assumptions of diagnostic overshadowing (Golden and Greenhill 1981, Reid 1984, Goldman 1988).

• *Are there any studies of treatment of tics in people with intellectual disability who demonstrate differences from those with average IQ?* There are actually few studies of any kind of treatment, two with successful medication. Rosenquist et al. (1997) used haloperidol and King (1999) pimozide. Zarkowska et al. (1989) used a behavioral intervention. At this point there are no high-quality studies showing that medications to reduce tics are less successful in people with intellectual disability than in those of average intelligence, but theoretically that might be a possibility. The extent to which behavioral interventions can be successful is unknown, but modifications are likely to be important, and treatments such as CBIT requiring high levels of motivation and cooperation may not be feasible.

In the *TIC* database, 24% of 151 child patients with intellectual disability, compared with 2.9% of 5537 without, also had a diagnosis of ASD (vs 4% in others with Tourette syndrome). Significantly more common were the average number of comorbid disorders (3.3 vs 1.9), pre- and perinatal problems (33% vs 20%), neurological disorders (21% vs 5%) and seizures (25% vs 5%), strong indicators of the complexity of this subgroup. Psychosis was infrequent, but almost five times as often reported as in those without intellectual disability. SIB occurred more than twice as often, and coprophenomena were almost twice as common (18% vs 12%). It is of importance that a family history of tics was less common in those with intellectual disability (33% vs 52%, p<0.001), suggesting that factors such as abnormal brain development or insults play a larger role than in those without intellectual disability.

Practice point

Coprolalia, ASD, neurological disorders and seizures are more common in patients with intellectual disability than in those of average intellectual capacity.

Rates of 'difficult' behavior are significantly higher in persons with intellectual disability than in those without, and significantly higher still in those with comorbidities, so that it is vital to assess comorbidity and not attribute the problems solely to the intellectual disability or Tourette syndrome.

Practice point

Comorbidity is common and important to assess, since the behavioral picture should not be attributed solely to Tourette syndrome or intellectual disability or their combination.

Bodfish et al. (1995) studied co-occurrence of stereotypy and self-injury in adults with moderate to profound intellectual disability. They identified secondary stereotypies in 61%, SIB in 47% and compulsions in 40%; these three were also associated with each other. This concept of overlap has been taken further by Muehlmann and Lewis (2012), who describe shared phenomenology and pathophysiology.

Finally, it is necessary to repeat that the presence of tics can be a marker for other disorders and symptoms that could be significant in management, such as OCD. The need for careful differential diagnosis and assessment should be obvious.

Practice point

The presence of tics can be an indicator of other important symptoms or disorders, such as stereotypy and compulsions.

Co-occurrence of other types of repetitive movements is common, confusing, and may require consultation with a movement disorder specialist. However, apart from potential misunderstanding of tics, their presence might be trivial or of little importance in comparison with other problems and therefore not warrant specific intervention.

Case examples

'Michael' is 11 and was referred because of multiple tics from an early age, ADHD, irritability, moodiness, anxiety, and difficulty with transitions and minor changes in routines. The pregnancy was marked by maternal substance abuse. He complained of dry eyes and was rubbing saliva into them, causing infections. The rubbing of his eyes was performed symmetrically with the fifth fingers of both hands. The history revealed an unusually high number of repetitive motor behaviors (10, nine of them still present at the time of assessment, most of early onset, three of which were self-injurious), some obsessive–compulsive patterns, and psychological testing showed that in most areas he was functioning below the 2nd centile. Full-Scale IQ was in the mildly impaired range.

Comment: Here we have the early onset of both non-tic repetitive motor behaviors and tics, symmetry urges with a complex symmetrical tic related to a sensory annoyance causing eye infections, and a variety of other psychiatric symptoms.

'Shane', aged 12, had several SIB patterns: nail-biting, biting the skin of his arms, and head-banging. He picked at clothing. Full-Scale IQ was 64. He showed significant ADHD features and had been on stimulant medication. His speech was unusually rapid and loud, marked by irregularly recurring points of emphasis. Tics observed included eye-blinking, snorting and forced expiration.

Comment: *This boy's tics had not been identified as such, obscured as they were by several non-tic repetitive motor patterns, SIB, and the characteristic features of ADHD.*

'Larry', age 10, had had a 'cough' since age 6, thought by the allergist to be due to perennial allergic rhinitis, but it was not helped by steroids or asthma-type medica-tions. A psychiatric consultant put him on a very low dose of risperidone without apparent benefit. Testing showed functioning in the mild range of intellectual disability. The teacher reported odd movements and sounds. During a prolonged 2-hour examina-tion he demonstrated obvious facial grimacing and eyebrow-raising. More important, his 'cough' was always stereotypically the same. His father had had tics and a relative had been diagnosed with Tourette syndrome. Placed on a higher dosage of risperidone, his tics decreased.

Comment: *The stereotypic 'cough' unresponsive to treatment should have raised suspicion of a respiratory tic, obviating years of fruitless treatment. Tics additional to the 'cough' had not been identified so that the diagnosis of Tourette syndrome was not made. The dosage range of medication often needs to be explored before treatment failure is assumed.*

'Sheldon', aged 16, was seen because an intense eye-blinking pattern had interfered with his work-experience program; it had been at a less severe level since age 6. Full-Scale IQ was 60. He had seen an optometrist and ophthalmologist who had both diag-nosed 'dry eyes', but treatment based on that assumption had not helped. No other tics were seen or were described. He had marked sleep initiation difficulty. The therapeutic range of risperidone had not been explored.

Comment: *This is an example of a severe single tic, with a wrong diagnosis, com-bined with untreated insomnia and inadequate tic-suppressing medication.*

'Cody', aged 14, had been followed for mild congenital visual impairment with apraxic eye movements and nystagmus, hypotonia, very weak fine and gross motor coord-ination, autistic features not meeting a formal diagnosis, and moderate intellectual disability. Tics consisted of throat-clearing, facial grimacing, shoulder-shrugging, mouth-opening and tongue-rolling, all of which had recently increased. He also showed rocking, eye-rubbing, jiggling of objects, tactile hypersensitivity, auditory startle and many fears.

Comment: *This boy had a complex picture of developmental central nervous system impairment, visual impairment and sensory over-responsivity in more than one modality, with a variety of repetitive movements including multiple tics that had changed little over time.*

These vignettes indicate the wide variety of situations in which tics may be part of a complex clinical picture. There are several examples of missed diagnoses and inadequate exploration of the dosage range of medications for tics or ADHD. The tic disorder could be a persistent single tic, multiple motor tics without a vocal tic, or Tourette syndrome, all likely to present clinically when tics that had been present for years worsened or began to interfere with new activities or programs.

Borderline intellectual functioning can pose a significant risk for several reasons: services may be inadequate or inappropriate due to categorization ('not retarded enough' would have been the phrase many years ago), association with delayed diagnosis of learning and other problems, and poor adjustment to a frustrating school experience. In the midst of these and other factors, the role of tics may be quite unclear.

Case study

'Richard', 10 years old, was living in his fifth foster home and presented with barking, eye-blinking with blepharospasm, mouth-opening, coprolalia and copropraxia, but more importantly, impulsive, disruptive behavior that included aggression, lying, stealing, lack of response to behavioral consequences, and a diagnosis of ADHD. He was seen in his foster home and his mother was visited in her home. Family background included poverty, violence, physical abuse, alcoholism, parental divorce, rejection by his mother, and inability to handle his attention-seeking behavior, begun by age 5. At age 6 his tics began, blamed by the family on a stimulant drug. He was treated with haloperidol, 2mg daily, and later with pimozide, 4mg daily. When seen, he had rubbed his face in the area around his mouth until it was raw; he kept his jacket collar up so the area could not be seen, and cried about his separation from his father and a set of foster parents with whom he had bonded. Additional symptoms at times included pica (e.g. soap, toilet paper, shaving cream), enuresis, joint-cracking, bruxism, and rage outbursts at the slightest frustration. He was expelled from the class for the most behaviorally difficult children, and was removed from his foster home because of escalating behavioral problems. Medication was erratic due to parental beliefs. He was placed in an inpatient unit, where his behavior continued to be erratic. Psychological testing revealed borderline intellectual capacity and a language disorder. Tics were not seen as a problem, but his medication might have been responsible for a gradual excessive weight gain and limited exercise tolerance. At age 15 a report indicated that his tics were better.

*   *Comment: His tics were embedded in a pattern of multiple, unstable and destructive relationships and symptoms. His limited language, frequently changing parenting, and poor social and self-regulatory skills made the success of any practical plan for his future doubtful.*

Developmental coordination disorder (DCD) and handwriting problems

DCD is an important condition that should always be considered in an assessment of tic disorders, especially when there are co-occurring features of ADHD and/or problems of participation in school and community activities. Only recently, many clinicians have started to become aware of its importance and of the impressive increase of related research. The effects of poor coordination or written expression on social relationships and self-esteem can be extensive and directly or indirectly affect social skill development. Re-evaluation of the broader role of the cerebellum beyond motor coordination has contributed to the neurodevelopmental basis for this understanding. Handwriting problems are now subsumed under DCD and the cognitive component under Specific Learning Disorder in DSM-5, so they are considered in this chapter. It is vital to realize, however, that they occur outside of that diagnostic category, particularly in ADHD, which is the most common comorbid disorder in tic disorders. Poor handwriting or related skills can quickly make the early school experience frustrating and even humiliating, leading to anxiety, related somatic symptoms and school avoidance, and so must be considered for urgent exploration and intervention.

DCD occurs in about 2% to 6% of children (Lingam et al. 2009; Zwicker et al. 2009, 2012). In 1994 at an international gathering in London, Ontario, the term DCD was accepted for purposes of international usage. (The older term 'dyspraxia' still has some usage in the UK.)

Gillberg (2003) coined the acronym 'DAMP' to include children with *d*isorders of *a*ttention, *m*otor control and *p*erception (approximately equivalent to our current DCD+ADHD combination); it is an official diagnosis in Sweden. Following an international consensus conference in 2006, the European Academy for Childhood Disability published an elaborate (115 pages, 291 references) set of recommendations, including diagnosis, intervention and research needs (European Academy of Childhood Disability 2011, Blank et al. 2012), with a brief summary of that document for parents and teachers (Blank 2012).

The criteria are (1) motor skills are significantly weaker than those of the peer group; (2) this influences performance of activities of daily living or academic skills (using scissors, writing, play, dressing and use of cutlery); and (3) the difficulties are not explicable by physical, neurological or behavioral disturbances.

It was formerly believed that 'clumsiness' was not very important because children would 'grow out of it'. We now know that this is largely incorrect. The follow-up study by Rasmussen and Gillberg (2000) shows that a substantial proportion of patients not only continue to have problems with coordination (Cousins and Smyth 2003), but also are at risk for emotional and behavioral problems, ADHD, low self-esteem and lower quality of life (Dewey et al. 2002, Cairney et al. 2010, Barnett et al. 2013, Zwicker et al. 2013, Tal-Saban et al. 2014). Lingam et al. (2012) found that children with probable DCD had a significantly increased risk of psychiatric problems at 10 years of age. Schoemaker et al. (2013) found that comorbidity was positively associated with poorer motor coordination. Studies by Rigoli et al. (2012) and Wagner et al. (2012) suggested that the link between coordination

and emotional functioning could be the result of negative self-perceptions and peer problems. Other studies have shown that DCD is associated with a higher risk of psychopathology (Green et al. 2006); sleep disorder (Barnett and Wiggs 2011); low levels of physical
activity (Barnett et al. 2013); general health problems, anxiety and depression (Kirby et al.
2014); and risk of obesity in boys but not girls (Cairney et al. 2005). There is a significant
association with reading disability, ADHD and speech/language impairment (Flapper and
Schoemaker 2013), and current thinking implicates the cerebellum and possibly the corpus
callosum, parietal lobe and basal ganglia (Zwicker et al. 2009, Bejerot 2011).

DCD can be screened for by using a simple parent questionnaire, the DCDQ'07, a modification of the original DCDQ (Wilson et al. 2007, 2009; Rivard et al. 2014). However, it
is important to remember that a screening instrument is not diagnostic, and further evidence
must be provided, preferably from a full occupational therapy assessment. Unfortunately,
awareness of DCD is still lacking in many physicians (less than half in the survey by Wilson
et al. 2013, and only 9% in survey undertaken in a Canadian city by Gaines et al. 2008).

In the *TIC* database, a number of disorders and symptoms were found to be significantly
more likely to be reported in a group of 134 children with DCD (94% of whom were male)
than in others without it. The most robust differences were the increase in ADHD, SLD,
ASD, social skill deficits and sleep problems. These original data, in conjunction with what
is already known, suggest that DCD should always be considered in Tourette syndrome,
especially when combined with ADHD.

Although the sample base is smaller than for tics at present and more diverse in different centers, DCD seems to be common in SMD, justifying DCD screening for gross and
fine motor and graphomotor components (Mahone et al. 2014).

Teasing and bullying are possible consequences of DCD, as well as avoidance of competitive sports and an increased risk of obesity (the latter especially in boys). Furthermore,
there are also sensory relationships, evident in the *TIC* database data. The DCDQ'07 score
correlates with six of seven domains on the Short Sensory Profile, and has a strong correlation with the Total Score on the latter (0.607 on Spearman's rho).

Practice point

DCD should always be considered in a comprehensive assessment of a child or adult
with Tourette syndrome or persistent tic disorder, especially when ADHD is comorbid.

STUDENTS IN FURTHER AND HIGHER EDUCATION WITH DEVELOPMENTAL COORDINATION
DISORDER

Kirby et al. (2008) surveyed 93 students who had reported motor difficulties present since
childhood, compared with a group with reading difficulties ('dyslexia'). Two thirds reported
continuing motor problems in adulthood. The combination with ADHD was associated with
more problems. Half of the students reported continuing difficulty with handwriting, and more
with DCD were still living with their parents. Support from staff familiar with DCD was rare.

TREATMENT

Treatment of DCD involves attention to task-specific components of the function(s) concerned (Wilson PH et al. 2013). The other, often underappreciated, features associated with DCD require a broad concept of helpful intervention, including an opportunity for the young persons to talk about their experiences and ways of coping (Kirby et al. 2011, Lingam et al. 2013, Smits-Engelsman et al. 2013).

A study of the effects of treatment with methylphenidate in 23 children with combined ADHD+DCD showed significant improvement in both the ADHD and DCD symptoms in 18 (Flapper and Schoemaker 2008).

HANDWRITING AND PRINTING PROBLEMS

Handwriting and printing problems, which include combinations of fine motor control, grip, visual perception, visual–motor integration, motor planning, proprioception, sustained attention, sensory awareness, efficiency, force, speed and posture (Feder and Majnemer 2007), are common and can — if not recognized — quickly lead to the child realizing that he or she cannot keep up with peers, maybe becoming subject to unwanted attention from teachers, and not wanting to go to school, with associated somatic complaints on school mornings (but not on weekend days). In DSM-5 the previous Disorder of Written Expression is now a specifier in *Specific Learning Disorder, with Impairment in Written Expression*. This covers the cognitive–linguistic aspect of expression, while the physical motoric component is covered in the DCD diagnosis. Thus the former implies the ability to put ideas into sentences and paragraphs (a person with this problem may be competent in oral conversation). However, it should be noted that handwriting problems in children with ADHD who do not qualify for DCD are also common and require equal attention (Racine et al. 2008, Langmaid et al. 2014). Unfortunately, too little attention has been paid to this clinically very important cluster of problems and their consequences. Research on graphomotor problems is ongoing. There is no criterion standard way of assessing the process, although one known as the ETCH-C has been assessed as having reliability and validity (Duff and Goyen 2010). Therapeutic practice may lead to improvement (Denton et al. 2006).

In spite of the statements by Feder and Majnemer (2007) that "legible handwriting remains an important life skill that deserves greater attention" (p. 312), and by Cermak and Bissell (2014) that "proficient handwriting is an essential component of literacy and an important foundation needed to support a child's academic success" (p. 296), at the time of writing some US states have abandoned teaching cursive writing and reading, asserting that electronic devices will render it redundant; similar actions are downgrading its importance in other jurisdictions. How this change will affect students generally and those with DCD specifically is unclear.

The complexity of involved factors is illustrated by the following example.

Case study

'Ian' was 6 when first seen. He had a 3-year history of complex tics and a positive family history. He had many exquisite sensory sensitivities, including to his clothing

and in many other domains, and a number of repetitive patterns that were sometimes self-injurious. His pencil drawing was known to be poor before he entered school. OCD symptoms began, along with a sleep disorder and great difficulty with transitions. At age 8 he was hospitalized for a manic episode and diagnosed with bipolar I disorder. Psychological assessment showed that he was above average in all areas, but functioning at a much lower level in school. His written output was slow and tortured, but complicated not only by a perfectionistic approach with frequent erasures but a strong aversion to his skin touching paper, resulting in a very awkward writing grip. His sleep disorder and bipolar symptoms were well controlled at age 10 with medication, CBT and adaptations in school.

Comment: This child demonstrates the evolving complexity of symptoms (including very early-onset bipolar disorder), some of which have improved, but the graphomotor disability is impacted by a combination of his sensory over-responsivity (SOR) and his perfectionism. The course of this SOR is unpredictable.

Trichotillomania (hair-pulling)

Trichotillomania is relatively common, potentially quite impairing, and because often hidden, should be a focus of routine inquiry. Pulling can be automatic or focused. Aspects may be kept secret. Prevalence is about 3% to 6% in Tourette syndrome, considerably more in TS+ than in TS-only. Treatment with medication is of dubious efficacy; behavioral treatment has better evidence in its favor. Co-occurring conditions must also be assessed.

There is now a very substantial literature on hair-pulling (Woods et al. 2006; Bloch et al. 2007; Chamberlain et al. 2007; Bloch 2009; Franklin et al. 2011; Woods 2011, 2013), as well as professional and lay books (Stein et al. 1999, Keuthen et al. 2001, Penzel 2003).

DEFINITION

Trichotillomania is characterized by repetitive hair-pulling causing noticeable hair loss and resulting in significant distress or impairment. (The former criterion in DSM-IV-TR that required an urge to pull and relief after pulling was deleted in DSM-5.) Hair may be pulled from any area of the body, but most commonly involves the scalp and eyebrows. It often leads to social avoidance and reluctance to bring the problem to the attention of physicians or family.

DIAGNOSIS (INCLUDING INSTRUMENTS AND FORMS)

A number of measures to assess trichotillomania have been developed, reviewed by Diefenbach et al. (2005) and Duke et al. (2010).

PREVALENCE/EPIDEMIOLOGY

The true prevalence is not known, but is estimated at 0.5% to 3.9% with strict DSM-IV criteria including relief after pulling, but with DSM-5 criteria prevalence rates are 3.4% in females and 1.5% in males, though different studies present figures that range widely (Duke et al. 2010).

PRESENTATION AND PHENOMENOLOGY

Much hair-pulling is hidden. Even if it is admitted, some aspects may be denied, such as pulling pubic hair, eating removed hair, or pulling the hair on their own children or from dolls or pets. The pulling may be 'automatic' (done while doing something else and out of full awareness), or 'focused', such as occurs when hair feels different (e.g. split ends, an isolated kinky hair) or looks asymmetric or unsightly (Bloch 2009).

COMORBIDITY AND COMMON ASSOCIATIONS

In population studies there are high rates of co-occurring anxiety, OCD and mood disorder. In the *TIC* database, trichotillomania in children with Tourette syndrome is reported in 3.3% of females and 2.3% of males (a statistically insignificant difference); and in adults, in 5.5% of females and 2.4% of males (p=0.002, OR 2.3). There is no difference in the rate of family history of tics or in tic severity. However, it is much more common in TS+ (2.8%) than in TS-only (0.9%, p<0.001, OR 3.1). There is a significant difference in co-occurring children's anxiety disorders (4.3% vs 2.1%, p<0.001, OR 2.1).

NATURAL HISTORY AND PROGNOSIS

Hair-pulling with early childhood onset may subside on its own; with later onset it tends to be chronic or intermittent.

TREATMENT

Both pharmacotherapy and behavioral therapy have been advocated. Some studies report improvements on clomipramine or SSRIs, others none. A meta-analysis found clomipramine to be superior to placebo (Bloch et al. 2007).

There is some evidence from single studies that olanzapine and N-acetyl cysteine are superior to placebo. Behavioral treatment seems to provide superior results and outcome (Bloch 2009), but is less readily available. Co-occurring disorders may interfere with treatment. Information for patients, families and clinicians on trichotillomania and other body-focused repetitive behaviors is available from the Trichotillomania Learning Center, a well-organized service and research organization (www.trich.org) with a prestigious professional advisory board. They publish an excellent expert consensus set of free treatment guidelines for downloading from their website.

Substance use disorders (SUDs)

> Tourette syndrome by itself is not associated with substance abuse, but because of comorbidity, especially with ADHD, the risk needs to be kept in mind. Diversion of short-acting stimulants is an increasing problem and is now becoming acceptable to help friends who desire school-related performance enhancement, regardless of whether or not they have ADHD. Some patients have experimented with cannabis and claim that it calms their tics, which has been demonstrated in some short-term reports, but still carries a risk for adolescent brain development.

Tourette syndrome without comorbidities does not lead to substance abuse any more than for those without tics. However, childhood ADHD is itself a risk factor for nicotine usage and SUDs in adolescence and young adulthood (Charach et al. 2011), and it is well known that many people with Tourette syndrome also have ADHD.

ADHD itself poses a risk for later substance abuse (Wilens 2011); however, in properly diagnosed ADHD, stimulant treatment does not increase substance use (Faraone and Wilens 2007), and may decrease it. The possibility of diversion (reported to be on the increase) and misuse must always be kept in mind (Wilens et al. 2008). Individuals with and without ADHD may misuse stimulant medication. The immediate-release form is subject to misuse much more often than the extended-range forms. Misuse is frequently combined with the use of other drugs including marijuana and alcohol, and those involved are more likely to have conduct disorder or polydrug use. The usage is attributed to the need for performance enhancement and for euphorogenic effects.

> **Practice point**
> Treatment with short-acting stimulant drugs for ADHD carries a significant risk of diversion for either performance enhancement or euphorogenic effects, and questions should always be raised about it.

Self-medication can sometimes be used to calm tics. Limited study of marijuana use (including a randomized trial of tetrahydrocannabinol) has confirmed claims — at least on a short-term basis — that cannabinoids can improve tics (Müller-Vahl 2003, Müller-Vahl et al. 2003), but since marijuana is not a single drug, its effects can be highly variable, and, for some individuals, conducive to the development of psychosis as well as other adverse health effects (Hall and Degenhardt 2009, Pierre 2011, Evins et al. 2012, Volkow et al. 2014). With increasing legality or decriminalization (in the USA, for example), usage is certain to increase without sufficient knowledge of therapeutic effects or harms (9% of users becoming dependent, according to one estimate), so that research is urgently needed (*Nature Neuroscience* 2014).

An abstract by Lichter (2009) indicated that unreported cocaine abuse "should always be suspected as a possible contributing cause of severe tics and SIB (in youth or adults) with TS."

> **Practice point**
> For older children and adolescents, as well as adults, it is a good idea to routinely ask "Have you found that tobacco or other drugs have helped with your tics? How?"

REFERENCES

Abramovitch A, Dar R, Mittelman A, Schweiger A (2013) Don't judge a book by its cover: ADHD-like symptoms in obsessive compulsive disorder. *J Obsess-Compuls Relat Disord* 2: 53–61. doi: 10.1016/j.jocrd.2012.09.001.

American Academy of Child and Adolescent Psychiatry (1998) Practice parameters for the assessment and treatment of children and adolescents with language and learning disorders. *J Am Acad Child Adolesc Psychiatry* 37 (10 Suppl): 46–62S.

American Academy of Child and Adolescent Psychiatry (2007a) Practice parameter for the assessment and treatment of children and adolescents with attention-deficit hyperactivity disorder. *J Am Acad Child Adolesc Psychiatry* 46: 894–921. doi: 10.1097/chi.0b013e318054e724.

American Academy of Child and Adolescent Psychiatry (2007b) Practice parameter for the assessment and treatment of children and adolescents with oppositional defiant disorder. *J Am Acad Child Adolesc Psychiatry* 46: 126–41. doi: 10.1097/01.chi.0000246060.62706.af.

American Academy of Child and Adolescent Psychiatry (2012) Practice parameter for the assessment and treatment of children and adolescents with obsessive–compulsive disorder. *J Am Acad Child Adolesc Psychiatry* 51: 98–113. doi: 10.1016/j.jaac.2011.09.019.

American Psychiatric Association (2000) *Diagnostic and Statistical Manual of Mental Disorders, 4th edn, Text Revision.* Arlington, VA: American Psychiatric Association.

Anagnostou E, Zwaigenbaum L, Szatmari P, et al. (2014) Autism spectrum disorder: advances in evidence-based practice. *CMAJ* 186: 509–18. doi: 10.1503/cmaj.121756.

Anderson DK, Maye MP, Lord C (2011) Changes in maladaptive behaviors from midchildhood to young adulthood in autism spectrum disorder. *Am J Intell Dev Disabil* 116: 381–97.

Arcieri R, Germinario EAP, Bonati M, et al. (2012) Cardiovascular measures in children and adolescents with attention-deficit/hyperactivity disorder who are new users of methylphenidate and atomoxetine. *J Child Adolesc Psychopharm* 22: 423–31. doi: 10.1089/cap.2012.0014.

Arns M, de Ridder S, Strehl U, et al. (2009) Efficacy of neurofeedback treatment in ADHD: the effects on inattention, impulsivity and hyperactivity: a meta-analysis. *Clin EEG Neurosci* 40: 180–9.

Bakhshayesh AR, Hänsch S, Wyschkom A, et al. (2011) Neurofeedback in ADHD: a single-blind randomized controlled trial. *Eur Child Adolesc Psychiatry* 20: 481–91. doi: 10.1007/s00787-011-0208-y.

Barabas G, Wardell B, Sapiro M, Matthews WS (1986) Coincident Down's and Tourette syndromes: three case reports. *J Child Neurol* 1: 358–360. doi: 10.1177/088307388600100407.

Barkley RA, Robin AL (2008) *Your Defiant Teen: 10 Steps to Resolve Conflict and Rebuild Your Relationship.* New York: Guilford Press.

Barnett AL, Wiggs L (2011) Sleep behaviour in children with developmental co-ordination disorder. *Child Care Health Dev* 38: 403–11. doi: 10.1111/j.1365-2214.2011.01260.x.

Barnett AL, Dawes H, Wilmut K (2013) Constraints and facilitators to participation in physical activity in teenagers with developmental coordination disorder: an exploratory interview study. *Child Care Health Dev* 39: 393–403. doi: 10.1111/j.1365-2214.2012.01376.x.

Baron-Cohen S, Mortimore C, Moriarty J, et al. (1999a) The prevalence of Gilles de la Tourette's syndrome in children and adolescents with autism. *J Child Psychol Psychiatry* 40: 213–8. doi: 10.1111/j.1469-7610.00434.

Baron-Cohen S, Scahill VL, Izaguirre J, et al. (1999b) The prevalence of Gilles de la Tourette syndrome in children and adolescents with autism: a large-scale study. *Psychol Med* 29: 1151–9.

Bejerot S (2011) The relationship between poor motor skills and neurodevelopmental disorders. *Dev Med Child Neurol* 53: 779. doi: 10.1111/j.1469-8749.2011.04041.x.

Ben-Sasson A, Soto TW, Martínez-Pedraza F, Carter AS (2013) Early sensory over-responsivity in toddlers with autism spectrum disorders as a predictor of family impairment and parenting stress. *J Child Psychol*

Psychiatry 54: 846–53. doi: 10.1111/jcpp.12035.

Berry L-M, Laskey B (2012) A review of obsessive intrusive thoughts in the general population. *J Obsess-Compuls Relat Disord* 1: 125–32. doi: 10.1016/j.jocrd.2012.02.002.

Berthier ML, Kulisevsky J, Campos VM (1998) Bipolar disorder in adult patients with Tourette's syndrome: a clinical study. *Biol Psychiatry* 43: 364–70.

Biederman J, Petty CR, Dolan C, et al. (2008) The long-term longitudinal course of oppositional defiant disorder and conduct disorder in ADHD boys: findings from a controlled 10-year prospective longitudinal follow-up study. *Psychol Med* 38: 1027–36. doi: 10.1017/S0033291707002668.

Blank R (2012) Information for parents and teachers on the European Academy for Childhood Disability (EACD) recommendations on developmental coordination disorder. *Dev Med Child Neurol* 54: e8–e9.

Blank R, Smits-Engelsman B, Polatajko H, Wilson P (2012) European Academy for Childhood Disability (EACD): Recommendations on the definition, diagnosis and intervention of developmental coordination disorder (long version). *Dev Med Child Neurol* 54: 54–93. doi: 10.1111/j.1469-8749.2011.04171.x.

Bloch MH (2009) Trichotillomania across the lifespan. *J Am Acad Child Adolesc Psychiatry* 48: 879–83. doi: 10.1097/CHI.0b013e3181ac09f3.

Bloch MH, Peterson BS, Scahill L, et al. (2006) Adulthood outcome of tic and obsessive–compulsive symptom severity in children with Tourette syndrome. *Arch Pediatr Adolesc Med* 160: 65–9.

Bloch MH, Landeros-Weisenberger A, Dombrowski P, et al. (2007) Systematic review: pharmacological and behavioral treatment for trichotillomania. *Biol Psychiatry* 62: 839–46. doi: 10.1016/j.biopsych.2007.05.019.

Bloch MH, Craiglow BG, Landeros-Weisenberger A, et al. (2009a) Predictors of early adult outcomes in pediatric-onset obsessive–compulsive disorder. *Pediatrics* 124: 1085–93. doi: 10.1542/peds.2009-0015.

Bloch M, Panza KE, Landeros-Weisenberger A, Leckman JF (2009b) Meta-analysis: treatment of attention-deficit hyperactivity disorder in children with comorbid tic disorders. *J Am Acad Child Adolesc Psychiatry* 48: 884–93. doi: 10.1097/CHI.0b013c3181b26e9f.

Bloch MH, Green C, Kichuk SA, et al. (2013) Long-term outcome in adults with obsessive–compulsive disorder. *Depress Anx* 30: 716–22. doi: 10.1002/da.22103.

Bodfish JW, Crawford TW, Powell SB, et al. (1995) Compulsions in adults with mental retardation: prevalence, phenomenology, and comorbidity with stereotypy and self-injury. *Am J Ment Retard* 100: 183–92.

Bohus M, Haaf B, Simms T, et al. (2004) Effectiveness of interpersonal dialectical behavioral therapy for borderline personality disorder: a controlled trial. *Behav Res Ther* 42: 487–99. doi: 10.106/S005-7967(03)00174-8.

Borda T, Feinstein BA, Neziroglu F, et al. (2013) Are children with obsessive–compulsive disorder at risk for problematic peer relationships? *J Obsess-Compuls Relat Disord* 2: 359–65. doi: 10.1016/j.jocrd.2013.06.006.

Borres MP (2009) Allergic rhinitis: more than just a stuffy nose. *Arch Paediatr* 98: 1088–92.

Brawley A, Silverman B, Kearney S, et al. (2004) Allergic rhinitis in children with attention-deficit/hyperactivity disorder. *Ann Allergy Asthma Immunol* 92: 663–7. doi: 10.1016/S1081-1206(10)61434-2.

Brown TE, ed (2009a) *ADHD with Comorbidities: Handbook for ADHD Complications in Children and Adults.* Washington, DC: American Psychiatric Publishing.

Brown TE (2009b) Developmental complexities of attentional disorders. In: Brown TE, ed. *ADHD Comorbidities: Handbook for ADHD Complications in Children and Adults.* Washington, DC: American Psychiatric Publishing, pp. 3–22.

Burd L, Freeman RD, Klug MG, Kerbeshian J (2005) Tourette syndrome and learning disabilities. *BMC Pediatrics* 5: 34. doi: 10.1186/1471-2431-5-34.

Burd L, Li Q, Kerbeshian J, et al. (2009) Tourette syndrome and comorbid pervasive developmental disorders. *J Child Neurol* 24: 170–5. doi: 10.1177/0883073808322666.

Butnik SM (2005) Neurofeedback in adolescents and adults with attention deficit hyperactivity disorder. *J Clin Psychol* 61: 621–5. doi: 10.1002/jclp.20124.

Cairney J, Hay JA, Faught BE, Hawes R (2005) Developmental coordination disorder and overweight and obesity in children aged 9–14y. *Int J Obes (Lond)* 29: 369–72. doi: 10.1038/sj.ijo.0802893.

Cairney J, Veldhuizen S, Szatmari P (2010) Motor coordination and emotional–behavioural problems in children. *Curr Opin Psychiatry* 23: 324–9. doi: 10.1097/YCO.0b0113e32833aa0aa.

CADDRA (2011) *Canadian ADHD Practice Guidelines, 3rd edn.* Markham, Ontario: Canadian ADHD Resource Alliance (available free in French and English at: http://www.caddra.ca/).

Carlson GA, Potegal M, Margulies D, et al. (2009) Rages – what are they and who has them? *J Child Adolesc Psychopharmacol* 19: 281–8. doi: 10.1089/cap.2008.0108.

Caronna EB, Milunsky JM, Tager-Flusberg H (2008) Autism spectrum disorders: clinical and research frontiers. *Arch Dis Child* 93: 518–23. doi: 10.1136/adc.2006.115337.

Cermak SA, Bissell J (2014) Content and construct validity of Here's How I Write (HHIW): a child's self-assessment and goal setting tool. *Am J Occup Ther* 68: 296–306. doi: 10.5014/ajot.2014.010637.

Chadwick O, Kusel Y, Cuddy M, Taylor E (2005) Psychiatric diagnoses and behaviour problems from childhood to early adolescence in young people with severe intellectual disabilities. *Psychol Med* 35: 751–60. doi: 10.1017/S0033291704003733.

Chamberlain SR, Menzies L, Sahakian BJ, Fineberg NA (2007) Lifting the veil on trichotillomania. *Am J Psychiatry* 164: 568–74. doi: 10.1176/appi.ajp.164.4.568.

Charach A, Yeung E, Climans T, Lillie E (2011) Childhood attention-deficit/hyperactivity disorder and future substance use disorders: comparative meta-analyses. *J Am Acad Child Adolesc Psychiatry* 50: 9–21. doi: 10.1016/j.jaac.2010.09.019.

Charach A, Carson P, Fox S, et al. (2013) Interventions for preschool children at high risk for ADHD: a comparative effectiveness review. *Pediatrics* 131: e1584–e1604. doi: 10.1542/peds.2012-0974.

Christensen H, Batterham P, Calear A (2014) Online interventions for anxiety disorders. *Curr Opin Psychiatry* 27: 7–13. doi: 10.1097/YCO.0000000000000019.

Cif L, Biolski B, Gavarini S, et al. (2007) Antero-ventral internal pallidum stimulation improves behavioral disorders in Lesch–Nyhan disease. *Mov Disord* 22: 2126–9. doi: 10.1002/mds.21723.

Coffey BJ, Biederman J, Smoller JW, et al. (2000) Anxiety disorders and tic severity in juveniles with Tourette's disorder. *J Am Acad Child Adolesc Psychiatry* 39: 562–8. doi: 10.1097/00004583-200005000-00009.

Cohen-Zion M, Ancoli-Israel S (2004) Sleep in children with attention-deficit hyperactivity disorder (ADHD): a review of naturalistic and stimulant intervention studies. *Sleep Med* 8: 379–402.

Collacott RA, Ismail IA (1988) Tourettism in a patient with Down's syndrome. *J Ment Defic Res* 32: 163–6.

Connolly SD, Bernstein GA (2007) Practice parameter for the assessment and treatment of children and adolescents with anxiety disorders. *J Am Acad Child Adolesc Psychiatry* 46: 267–83. doi: 10.1097/01.chi.0000246070.23695.06.

Cortese S, Faraone SV, Konofal E, Lecendreux M (2009) Sleep in children with attention-deficit/hyperactivity disorder: meta-analysis of subjective and objective studies. *J Am Acad Child Adolesc Psychiatry* 48: 894–908. doi: 10.1097/CHI.0b13c3181ac09c9.

Cortese S, Brown TE, Corkum P, et al. (2013) Assessment and management of sleep problems in youths with attention-deficit/hyperactivity disorder. *J Am Acad Child Adolesc Psychiatry* 52: 784–96. doi: 10.1016/j.jaac.2013.06.001.

Cougle JR, Timpano KR, Fitch KE, Hawkins KA (2011) Distress tolerance and obsessions: an integrative analysis. *Depress Anx* 28: 906–14. doi: 10.1002/da.20846.

Cousins M, Smyth MM (2003) Developmental coordination impairments in adulthood. *Hum Mov Sci* 22: 433–59. doi: 10.1016/j.humov.2003.09.003.

Crews WD Jr, Bonaventura S, Hay CL, et al. (1993) Gilles de la Tourette disorder among individuals with severe or profound mental retardation. *Ment Retard* 31: 25–8.

Daley D, Birchwood J (2010) ADHD and academic performance: why does ADHD impact on academic performance and what can be done to support ADHD children in the classroom? *Child Care Health Dev* 36: 455–64. doi: 10.1111/j.1365-2214.2009.01046.x.

Dalgaard S, Damm D, Thomsen PH (2001) Gilles de la Tourette syndrome in a child with congenital deafness. *Eur Child Adolesc Psychiatry* 10: 256–9. doi: 10.1007/s007870170015.

Daughton JM, Kratochvil CJ (2009) Review of ADHD pharmacotherapies: advantages, disadvantages, and clinical pearls. *J Am Acad Child Adolesc Psychiatry* 48: 240–8. doi: 10.1097/CHI.0b013e318197748f.

Debes N, Hjalgrim H, Skov L (2010) The presence of attention-deficit hyperactivity disorder (ADHD) and obsessive–compulsive disorder worsen psychosocial and educational problems in Tourette syndrome. *J Child Neurol* 25: 171–81. doi: 10.1177/0883073809336215.

Decloedt EH, Stein DJ (2010) Current trends in drug treatment of obsessive–compulsive disorder. *Neuropsychiatr Dis Treat* 6: 233–42.

de Jong M, Punt M, de Groot E, et al. (2011) Minor neurological dysfunction in children with autism spectrum disorder. *Dev Med Child Neurol* 53: 641–6. doi: 10.1111/j.1469-8749.2011.03971.x.

Dekker MC, Koot HM (2003) DSM-IV disorders in children with borderline to moderate intellectual disability. I. Prevalence and impact. *J Am Acad Child Adolesc Psychiatry* 42: 915–22. doi: 10.1097/01.CHI.0000046892.27264.1A.

Denton PL, Cope A, Moser C (2006) The effects of sensorimotor-based intervention versus therapeutic practice on improving handwriting performance in 6- to 11-year-old children. *Am J Occup Ther* 60: 16–27.

Dewey D, Kaplan BJ, Crawford SG, Wilson BN (2002) Developmental coordination disorder: associated problems in attention, learning, and psychosocial adjustment. *Hum Mov Sci* 21: 905–18. doi: 10.1016/S0167-9457(02)00163-X.

Diefenbach GJ, Tolin DF, Crocetto J, et al. (2005) Assessment of trichotillomania: a psychometric evaluation of hair-pulling scales. *J Psychopath Behav Assess* 27: 169–78. doi: 10.1007/s10862-005-0633-7.

do Rosario-Campos MC, Leckman JF, Curi M, et al. (2005) A family study of early-onset obsessive–compulsive disorder. *Am J Med Genet B Neuropsychiatr Genet* 136B: 92–7. doi: 10.1002/ajmg.b.30149.

Donnellan AM, Hill DA, Leary MR (2013) Rethinking autism: implications of sensory and movement differences for understanding and support. *Front Integr Neurosci* 6: 124. doi: 10.3389/fnint.2012.00124.

Dornbush MP, Pruitt SK (2008) *Tigers, Too: Executive Functions/Speed of Processing/Memory*. Atlanta, GA: Parkaire Press.

Duff S, Goyen T-A (2010) Reliability and validity of the Evaluation Tool of Children's Handwriting-Cursive (ETCH-C) using the general scoring criteria. *Am J Occup Ther* 64: 37–46.

Duke DC, Keeley ML, Geffken GR, Storch EA (2010) Trichotillomania: a current review. *Clin Psychol Rev* 30: 181–93. doi: 10.1016/j.cpr.2009.10.008.

Eddy CM, Cavanna AE, Gulisano M, et al. (2012) The effects of comorbid obsessive–compulsive disorder and attention-deficit hyperactivity disorder on quality of life in Tourette syndrome. *J Neuropsychiatry Clin Neurosci* 24: 458–62. doi: 10.1176/appi.neuropsych.11080181.

Essau CA (2003) Comorbidity of anxiety disorders in adolescents. *Depress Anx* 18: 1–6. doi: 10.1002/da. 10107.

European Academy of Childhood Disability (2011) *EACD Recommendations (Long Version): Definition, Diagnosis, Assessment and Intervention of Developmental Coordination Disorder (DCD)*. Available online at http://www.eacd.org/publications.php.

Evans DW, Leckman JF, Carter A, et al. (1997) Ritual, habit, and perfectionism: the prevalence and development of compulsive-like behavior in normal young children. *Child Dev* 68: 58–68.

Evins AE, Green AI, Kane JM, Murray RM (2012) The effect of marijuana use on the risk for schizophrenia. *J Clin Psychiatry* 73: 1463–8. doi: 10.4088/JCP.12012co1c.

Faraone SV, Wilens TE (2007) Effect of stimulant medications for attention-deficit/hyperactivity disorder on later substance use and the potential for stimulant misuse, abuse, and diversion. *J Clin Psychiatry* 68 (Suppl 11): 15–22. doi: 10.4088/JCP.

Faraone SV, Biederman J, Mick E (2005) The age-dependent decline of attention deficit hyperactivity disorder: a meta-analysis of follow-up studies. *Psychol Med* 35: 1–7.

Feder KP, Majnemer A (2007) Handwriting development, competency, and intervention. *Dev Med Child Neurol* 49: 312–7. doi: 10.1111/j.1469-8749.2007.00312.x.

Ferrão YA, Shavitt RG, Prado H, et al. (2012) Sensory phenomena associated with repetitive behaviors in obsessive–compulsive disorder: an exploratory study of 1001 patients. *Psychiatry Res* 197: 253–8. doi: 10.1016/j.psychres.2011.09.017.

Flapper BCT, Schoemaker MM (2008) Effects of methylphenidate on quality of life in children with both developmental coordination disorder and ADHD. *Dev Med Child Neurol* 50: 294–99. doi: 10.1111/j.1469-8749.2008.02039.x.

Flapper BCT, Schoemaker MM (2013) Developmental coordination disorder in children with specific language impairment: co-morbidity and impact on quality of life. *Res Dev Disabil* 34: 756–63. doi: 10.1016/j.ridd.2012.10.014.

Flessner CA, Freeman JB, Sapyta J, et al. (2011) Predictors of parental accommodation in pediatric obsessive–compulsive disorder: findings from the Pediatric Obsessive–Compulsive Disorder Treatment Study (POTS) Trial. *J Am Acad Child Adolesc Psychiatry* 50: 716–25. doi: 10.1016/j.jaac.2011.03.019.

Fliers EA, Franke B, Lambregts-Rommelse NNJ, et al. (2010) Undertreatment of motor problems in children with ADHD. *Child Adolesc Ment Health* 15: 85–90.

Fombonne E (2012) Autism in adult life. *Can J Psychiatry* 57: 273–4.

Fountain C, Winter AS, Bearman PS (2012) Six developmental trajectories characterize children with autism. *Pediatrics* 129: e1112–20. doi: 10.1542/peds.2011-1601.

Frank H, Stewart E, Walther M, et al. (2014) Hoarding behavior among young children with obsessive–compulsive disorder. *J Obsess-Compuls Disord* 3: 6–11. doi: 10.1016/j.jocrd.2013.11.001.

Franklin ME, Freeman J, March JS (2010) Treating pediatric obsessive–compulsive disorder using exposure-based cognitive-behavioral therapy. In: Weisz JR, Kazdin AE, eds. *Evidence-based Psychotherapies for Children and Adolescents, 2nd edn.* New York: Guilford Press, pp. 80–92.

Franklin ME, Edson A, Ledley DR, Cahill SP (2011) Behavior therapy for pediatric trichotillomania: a randomized controlled trial. *J Am Acad Child Adolesc Psychiatry* 50: 763–71. doi: 10.1016/j.jaac.2011.05.009.

Freeman RD (2007) Tic disorders and ADHD: answers from a world-wide clinical dataset on Tourette syndrome. Tourette Syndrome International Database Consortium. *Eur Child Adolesc Psychiatry* 16 (Suppl 1): 15–23. doi: 10.1007/s00787-007-1003-7.

Freeman RD, Fast DK, Burd L, et al. (2000) An international perspective on Tourette syndrome: selected findings from 3500 individuals in 22 countries. *Dev Med Child Neurol* 42: 436–7. doi: 10.1111/j.1469-8749.2000.tb00346.x.

Freeman RD, Zinner SH, Müller-Vahl KR, et al. (2009) Coprophenomena in Tourette syndrome. *Dev Med Child Neurol* 51: 218–27. doi: 10.1111/j.1469-8749.2008.03135.x.

Freeman RD, Soltanifar A, Baer S (2010) Stereotypic movement disorder: easily missed. *Dev Med Child Neurol* 52: 733–8. doi: 10.1111/j.1469-8749.2010.03627.x.

Fullana MA, Mataix-Cols D, Caspi A, et al. (2009) Obsessions and compulsions in the community: prevalence, interference, help-seeking, developmental stability, and co-occurring psychiatric conditions. *Am J Psychiatry* 166: 329–36. doi: 10.1176/appi.ajp.2008.08071006.

Gadow KD, Sverd J (2006) Attention deficit hyperactivity disorder, chronic tic disorder, and methylphenidate. *Adv Neurol* 99: 197–207.

Gadow KD, Sverd J, Sprafkin J, et al. (1999) Long-term methylphenidate therapy in children with comorbid attention-deficit hyperactivity disorder and chronic multiple tic disorder. *Arch Gen Psychiatry* 56: 330–6.

Gadow KD, Nolan EE, Sprafkin J, Schwartz J (2002) Tics and psychiatric comorbidity in children and adolescents. *Dev Med Child Neurol* 44: 330–8. doi: 10.1111/j.1469-8749.2002.tb00820.x.

Gadow KD, Sverd J, Nolan EE, et al. (2007) Immediate-release methylphenidate for ADHD in children with comorbid chronic multiple tic disorder. *J Am Acad Child Adolesc Psychiatry* 46: 840–8. doi: 10.1097/chi.0b013e31805c0860.

Gadow KD, Nolan EE, Sverd J, et al. (2008) Methylphenidate in children with oppositional defiant disorder and both co-morbid chronic multiple tic disorder and ADHD. *J Child Neurol* 23: 981–90. doi: 10.1177/0883073808315412.

Gaines R, Missiuna C, Egan M, McLean J (2008) Educational outreach and collaborative care enhances physician's perceived knowledge about developmental coordination disorder. *BMC Health Serv Res* 8: 21.

Geller DA (2006) Obsessive–compulsive and spectrum disorders in children and adolescents. *Psychiatr Clin North Am* 29: 353–70.

Gevensleben H, Holl B, Albrecht B, et al. (2009) Is neurofeedback an efficacious treatment for ADHD? A randomized controlled clinical trial. *J Child Psychol Psychiatry* 50: 780–9. doi: 10.1111/j.1469-7610.2008.02033.x.

Gibbins C, Weiss M (2007) Clinical recommendations in current practice guidelines for diagnosis and treatment of ADHD in adults. *Curr Psychiatr Rep* 9: 420–6. doi: 10.1007/s11920-007-0055-1.

Giele CL, van den Hout MA, Engelhard IM, Dek ECP (2014) Paradoxical effects of compulsive perseveration: sentence repetition causes semantic uncertainty. *J Obsess-Compuls Relat Disord* 3: 35–8. doi: 10.1016/j.jocrd.2013.11.007.

Gillberg C (2003) Deficits in attention, motor control, and perception: a brief review. *Arch Dis Child* 88: 904–10. doi: 10.1136/adc.88.10.904.

Golden GS, Greenhill L (1981) Tourette syndrome in mentally retarded children. *Ment Retard* 19: 17–9.

Goldman JJ (1988) Tourette syndrome in severely behavior disordered mentally retarded children. *Psychiatr Q* 59: 73–8.

Goldson E, Hagerman RJ (1992) The fragile X syndrome. *Dev Med Child Neurol* 34: 826–32.

Goodman WK, Rasmussen SA, Riddle MA, et al. (1990) *Children's Yale–Brown Obsessive–Compulsive Scale (C-YBOCS).* Available from wayne.goodman@mssm.edu.

Goodman WK, Rasmussen SA, Price LH, Storch EA (2006a) *YBOCS-II: Clinical Version.* Available from: wayne.goodman@mssm.edu.

Goodman WK, Storch EA, Geffken GR, Murphy TK (2006b) Obsessive–compulsive disorder in Tourette syndrome. *J Child Neurol* 21: 704–14. doi: 10.2310/7010.2006.00169.

Gorman DA, Thompson N, Plessen KJ, et al. (2010) Psychosocial outcome and psychiatric comorbidity in older adolescents with Tourette syndrome: controlled study. *Br J Psychiatry* 197: 36–44.

Graham J, Banaschewski T, Buitelaar J, et al. (2011) European guidelines on managing adverse effects of medication for ADHD. *Eur Child Adolesc Psychiatry* 20: 17–37. doi: 10.1007/s00787-010-0140-6.

Green D, Baird G, Sugden D (2006) A pilot study of psychopathology in developmental coordination disorder. *Child Care Health Dev* 32: 741–50. doi: 10.111/j.1365-2214.

Greene RW (2005) *The Explosive Child*. New York: HarperCollins.

Greene RW (2008) *Lost at School: Why Our Kids with Behavioral Challenges are Falling Through the Cracks and How We Can Help Them*. New York: Scribner.

Greene RW, Ablon JS (2006) *Treating Explosive Kids: The Collaborative Problem-Solving Approach*. New York/London: Guilford Press.

Haddad ADM, Umoh G, Bhatia V, Robertson MM (2009) Adults with Tourette's syndrome with and without attention deficit hyperactivity disorder. *Acta Psychiatr Scand* 120: 299–307. doi: 10.1111/j.1600-0447.2009.01398.x.

Hall W, Degenhardt L (2009) Adverse health effects of non-medical cannabis use. *Lancet* 374: 1383–91.

Hamilton R, Gray C, Bélanger SA, et al. (2009) Cardiac risk assessment before the use of stimulant medications in children and youth: a joint position statement by the Canadian Paediatric Society, the Canadian Cardiovascular Society and the Canadian Academy of Child and Adolescent Psychiatry. *J Can Acad Child Adolesc Psychiatry* 18: 349–55.

Hantson J, Wang PP, Grizenko-Vida M, et al. (2012) Effectiveness of a therapeutic summer camp for children with ADHD: Phase I clinical intervention trial. *J Atten Dis* 16: 610–7. doi: 10.1177/1087054711416800.

Harvey P, Rathbone BH (2013) *Dialectical Behavior Therapy for At-risk Adolescents: a Practitioner's Guide to Treating Challenging Behavior Problems*. Oakland, CA: New Harbinger Publications.

Hemmings CP, Gravestock S, Pickard M, Bouras N (2006) Psychiatric symptoms and problem behaviours in people with intellectual disabilities. *J Intell Disabil Res* 50: 269–76. doi: 10.1111/j.1365-2788.2006.00827.x.

Herrero ME, Hechtman L, Weiss G (1994) Antisocial disorders in hyperactive subjects from childhood to adulthood: predictive factors and characterization of subgroups. *Am J Orthopsychiatry* 64: 510–21.

Heyman I, Mataix-Cols D, Fineberg NA (2006) Obsessive–compulsive disorder. *BMJ* 333: 424–9.

Hosenbocus S, Chahal R (2011) SSRIs and SNRIs: a review of the discontinuation syndrome in children and adolescents. *J Can Acad Child Adolesc Psychiatry* 20: 60–7.

Howlin P, Moss P (2012) Adults with autism spectrum disorders. *Can J Psychiatry* 57: 275–83.

Huffman LC, Sutcliffe TL, Tanner IS, Feldman HM (2011) Management of symptoms in children with autism spectrum disorders: a comprehensive review of pharmacologic and complementary–alternative medicine treatments. *J Dev Behav Pediatr* 32: 56–68.

Ivanov VZ, Mataix-Cols D, Serlachius E, et al. (2013) Prevalence, comorbidity and heritability of hoarding symptoms in adolescence: a population based twin study in 15-year-olds. *PLoS ONE* 8: e69140. doi: 10.1371/journal.pone.0069140.

Johnson KP, Giannotti F, Cortesi F (2009) Sleep patterns in autism spectrum disorders. *Child Adolesc Psychiatric Clin N Am* 18: 917–28.

Kadesjö B, Gillberg C (2001) The comorbidity of ADHD in the general population of Swedish school-age children. *J Child Psychol Psychiatry* 42: 487–92. doi: 10.1111/j.1469-7610.00742.

Karlinsky H, Berg JM (1987) Gilles de la Tourette's syndrome in Down's syndrome. *Br J Psychiatry* 151: 707.

Karlinsky H, Sandor P, Berg JM, et al. (1986) Gilles de la Tourette's syndrome in Down's syndrome — a case report. *Br J Psychiatry* 148: 601–4.

Kazdin AE (2010) Problem-solving skills training and parent management training for oppositional defiant disorder and conduct disorder. In: Weisz JR, Kazdin AE, eds. *Evidence-Based Psychotherapies for Children and Adolescents, 2nd edn*. New York: Guilford Press, pp. 211–26.

Kazdin AE, Rotella C (2008) *The Kazdin Method for Parenting the Defiant Child: With No Pills, No Therapy, No Contest of Wills*. New York: Houghton Mifflin.

Kerbeshian J, Burd L (2000) Comorbid Down's syndrome, Tourette syndrome and intellectual disability: registry prevalence and developmental course. *J Intellect Disabil Res* 44: 60–7.

Kerbeshian J, Burd L, Martsolf J (1984) Fragile X syndrome associated with Tourette symptomatology in a male with moderate mental retardation and autism. *J Dev Behav Pediatr* 5: 201–3.

Keuthen NJ, Stein DJ, Christenson GA (2001) *Help for Hair-Pullers*. Oakland, CA: Harbinger.

Kim KL, Reynolds KCV, Alfano CA (2012) Social impairment in children with obsessive compulsive disorder: do comorbid problems of inattention and hyperactivity matter? *J Obsess-Compuls Relat Disord* 1: 228–33. doi: 10.1016/j.jocrd.2012.06.005.

King R (1999) Comorbidity in Tourette's syndrome: pharmacological treatment in adults with a severe to profound handicap. *NADD Bull* 2: 3–7.

Kirby A, Sugden D, Beveridge S, Edwards L (2008) Developmental co-ordination disorder (DCD) in adolescents and adults in further and higher education. *J Res Spec Educ Needs* 8: 120–31. doi: 10.1111/j.1471-3802.2008.00111.x.

Kirby A, Edwards KL, Sugden D (2011) Emerging adulthood in developmental co-ordination disorder: parent and young adult perspectives. *Res Dev Disabil* 32: 1351–60. doi: 10.1016/j.ridd.2011.01.041.

Kirby A, Williams N, Thomas M, Hill EL (2014) Self-reported mood, general health, wellbeing and employment status in adults with suspected DCD. *Res Dev Disabil* 34: 1357–64. doi: 10.1016/j.ridd.2013.01.003.

Kobori O, Salkovskis PM, Read J, et al. (2012) A qualitative study of the investigation of reassurance seeking in obsessive–compulsive disorder. *J Obsessive-Compuls Relat Disord* 1: 25–32. doi: 10.1016/j.jocrd.2011.09.001.

Kovacs M, Akiskal HS, Gatsonis C, Parrone PL (1994) Childhood-onset dysthymic disorder: clinical features and prospective naturalistic outcome. *Arch Gen Psychiatry* 51: 365–74.

Krebs G, Bolhuis K, Heyman I, et al. (2012) Temper outbursts in paediatric obsessive–compulsive disorder and their association with depressed mood and treatment outcome. *J Child Psychol Psychiatry* 54: 313–22. doi: 10.1111/j.1469-7610.2012.02605.x.

Kurlan R, Como PG, Miller B, et al. (2002) The behavioral spectrum of tic disorders. A community based study. *Neurology* 59: 414–20.

Langley AK, Lewin AB, Bergman RL, et al. (2010) Correlates of comorbid anxiety and externalizing disorders in childhood obsessive compulsive disorder. *Eur Child Adolesc Psychiatry* 19: 637–45. doi: 10.1007/s00787-010-0101-0.

Langmaid RA, Papadopoulos N, Johnson BP, et al. (2014) Handwriting in children with ADHD. *J Atten Disord* 18: 504–10. doi: 10.1177/1087054711434154.

Lebowitz ER, Omer H, Leckman JF (2011a) Coercive and disruptive behaviors in pediatric obsessive–compulsive disorder. *Depress Anx* 28: 899–905. doi: 10.1002/da.20858.

Lebowitz ER, Vitulano LA, Mataix-Cols D, Leckman JF (2011b) Editorial perspective: when OCD takes over… the family! Coercive and disruptive behaviours in paediatric obsessive–compulsive disorder. *J Child Psychol Psychiatry* 52: 1249–50. doi: 10.1111/j.1469-7610.2011.02480.x.

Lebowitz ER, Vitulano LA, Omer H (2011c) Coercive and disruptive behaviors in pediatric obsessive compulsive disorder. *Psychiatry* 74: 362–71.

Leckman JF, Bloch MH (2008) A developmental and evolutionary perspective on obsessive–compulsive disorder: whence and whither compulsive hoarding? *Am J Psychiatry* 165: 1229–33 (editorial). doi: 10.1176/appi.ajp.2008.08060891.

Leckman JF, Denys D, Simpson HB, et al. (2010) Obsessive–compulsive disorder: a review of the diagnostic criteria and possible subtypes and dimensional specifiers for DSM-V. *Depress Anx* 27: 507–27.

Léger D, Annesi-Maesono I, Carat F, et al. (2006) Allergic rhinitis and its consequences on quality of sleep. *Arch Intern Med* 166: 1744–8.

Lichter D (2009) Substance use in adult Tourette syndrome. *Mov Disord* 24 (Suppl 1): S499 (abstract).

Lin H, Yeh C-B, Peterson BS, et al. (2002) Assessment of symptom exacerbations in a longitudinal study of children with Tourette's syndrome or obsessive–compulsive disorder. *J Am Acad Child Adolesc Psychiatry* 41: 1070–7. doi: 10.1097/00004583-200209000-00007.

Lin Y-J, Lai M-C, Gau S S-F (2012) Youths with ADHD with and without tic disorders: comorbid psychopathology, executive function and social adjustment. *Res Dev Disabil* 33: 951–63.

Lingam R, Hunt L, Golding J, et al. (2009) Prevalence of developmental coordination disorder using the DSM-IV at 7 years of age: a UK population-based study. *Pediatrics* 123: e693–700.

Lingam R, Jongmans MJ, Elklis M, et al. (2012) Mental health difficulties in children with developmental coordination disorder. *Pediatrics* 129: e882–91.

Lingam RP, Novak C, Emond A, Coad JE (2013) The importance of identity and empowerment to teenagers with developmental coordination disorder. *Child Care Health Dev* 40: 309–18. doi: 10.1111/cch.12082.

Lochman JE, Boxmeyer CL, Powell NP, et al. (2010) Anger control training for aggressive youths. In: Weisz JR, Kazdin AE, eds. *Evidence-based Psychotherapies for Children and Adolescents, 2nd edn.* New York: Guilford Press, pp. 227–42.

Lofthouse N, Arnold LE, Hersch S, et al. (2012) A review of neurofeedback treatment for pediatric ADHD. *J Atten Disord* 16: 351–72. doi: 10.1177/1087054711427530.

Mahone EM, Ryan M, Ferenc L, et al. (2014) Neuropsychological function in children with primary complex motor stereotypies. *Dev Med Child Neurol* 56: 1001–8. doi: 10.1111/dmcn.12480.

Mancuso E, Faro A, Joshi G, Geller DA (2010) Treatment of pediatric obsessive–compulsive disorder: a review. *J Child Adolesc Psychopharm* 20: 299–308. doi: 10.1089/cap.2010.0040.

March J, Benton C (2007) *Talking Back to OCD.* New York: Guilford Press.

Martin A, Young C, Leckman JF, et al. (2004) Age effects of antidepressant-induced manic conversion. *Arch Pediatr Adolesc Med* 158: 773–80.

McCabe SE, West BT (2013) Medical and nonmedical use of prescription stimulants: results from a national multicohort study. *J Am Acad Child Adolesc Psychiatry* 52: 1272–80. doi: 10.1016/j.jaac.2013.09.005.

McKay D, Storch EA, Nelson B, et al. (2009) Obsessive–compulsive disorder in children and adolescents: treating difficult cases. In: McKay D, Storch EA, eds. *Cognitive Behavior Therapy for Children: Treating Complex and Refractory Cases.* New York: Springer, pp. 81–113.

McQuade JD, Hoza B (2008) Peer problems in attention deficit hyperactivity disorder: current status and future directions. *Dev Disabil Res Rev* 14: 320–4. doi: 10.1002/ddrr.35.

Merlo LJ, Storch EA, Murphy TK, et al. (2005) Assessment of pediatric obsessive compulsive disorder: a critical review of current methodology. *Child Psychiatry Hum Dev* 36: 195–214.

Mico JA, Hirshfeld-Becker DR, Henin A, Ehrenreich-May J (2013) Content specificity of threat interpretation in anxious and non-clinical children. *Cogn Ther Res* 37: 78–88. doi: 10.1007/s10608-012-9438-7.

Millichap JG, Yee MM (2012) The diet factor in attention-deficit/hyperactivity disorder. *Pediatrics* 129: 330–7. doi: 10.1542/peds.2011-2199.

Mindell JA, Owens JA (2010) *A Clinical Guide to Pediatric Sleep: Diagnosis and Management of Sleep Problems, 2nd edn.* Philadelphia: Wolters Kluwer/Lippincott Williams & Wilkins.

Molina BSG, Hinshaw SP, Swanson JM, et al. (2009) The MTA at 8 years: prospective follow-up of children treated for combined type ADHD in a multisite study. *J Am Acad Child Adolesc Psychiatry* 48: 484–500. doi: 10.1097/CHI.0b013c31819c23d0.

Moyá J, Stringaris AK, Asherson P, et al. (2014) The impact of persisting hyperactivity on social relationships: a community-based, controlled 20-year follow-up study. *J Atten Disord* 18: 52–60. doi: 10.1177/1087054712436876.

Muehlmann AM, Lewis MH (2012) Abnormal repetitive behaviors: shared phenomenology and pathophysiology. *J Intell Disabil Res* 56: 427–40. doi: 10.1111/j.1365-2788.2011.01519.x.

Müller-Vahl KR (2003) Cannabinoids reduce symptoms of Tourette's syndrome. *Expert Opin Pharmacother* 4: 1717–25.

Müller-Vahl KR, Schneider U, Prevedel H, et al. (2003) Δ9-tetrahydrocannabinol (THC) is effective in the treatment of tics in Tourette syndrome: a 6-week randomized trial. *J Clin Psychiatry* 64: 459–65.

Muter V, Snowling MJ (2009) Children at familial risk of dyslexia: practical implications from an at-risk study. *Child Adolesc Ment Health* 14: 37–41.

Myers B, Pueschel SM (1995) Tardive or atypical Tourette's disorder in a population with Down syndrome? *Res Devel Disabil* 16: 1–9.

Nagai Y, Cavanna A, Critchley HD (2009) Influence of sympathetic autonomic arousal on tics: implications for a therapeutic behavioral intervention for Tourette syndrome. *J Psychosom Res* 67: 599–605.

Nature Neuroscience (2014) High time for advancing marijuana research. *Nat Neurosci* 17: 481 (editorial). doi: 10.1038/nn.3692.

Newcorn JH, Kratochvil CJ, Allen AJ, et al. (2008) Atomoxetine and osmotically-released methylphenidate for the treatment of attention deficit hyperactivity disorder: acute comparison and differential response. *Am J Psychiatry* 165: 721–30.

NICE (2008) Attention deficit hyperactivity disorder: diagnosis and management of ADHD in children, young people and adults. NICE Clinical Guideline 72 (available online at http://www.nice.org.uk/guidance/CG072).

NICE (2013) Antisocial behaviour and conduct disorders in children and young people: recognition, intervention and management. NICE Clinical Guideline 158 (available online at http://nice.org.uk/guidance/CG158).

Nigg JT, Lewis K, Edinger T, Falk M (2012) Meta-analysis of attention-deficit/hyperactivity disorder or attention-deficit/hyperactivity disorder symptoms, restriction diet, and synthetic food color additives. *J Am Acad Child Adolesc Psychiatry* 51: 86–97e8. doi: 10.1016/j.jaac.2011.10.015.

Nowakowski ME, Antony MM (2013) Reactions to teasing in social anxiety. *Cogn Ther Res* 37: 1091–1100. doi: 10.1007/s10608-013-9551-2.

Ollendick TH, Jarrett MA, Grills-Taquechel AE, et al. (2008) Comorbidity as a predictor and moderator of treatment outcome in youth with anxiety, affective, attention deficit/hyperactivity disorder, and oppositional/conduct disorders. *Clin Psychol Rev* 28: 1447–71. doi: 10.1016/j.cpr.2008.09.003.

Owens JA, Brown TE, Modestino EJ (2009) ADHD with sleep/arousal disturbances. In: Brown TE, ed. *ADHD Comorbidities: Handbook for ADHD Complications in Children and Adults.* Arlington, VA: American Psychiatric Publishing, pp. 279–91.

Packer LE, Pruitt SK (2010) *Challenging Kids, Challenged Teachers: Teaching Students with Tourette's, Bipolar Disorder, Executive Dysfunction, OCD, ADHD, and More.* Bethesda, MD: Woodbine House.

Palumbo D, Kurlan R (2007) Complex obsessive compulsive and impulsive symptoms in Tourette's syndrome. *Neuropsychiatr Dis Treat* 3: 687–93.

Pappadopulos E, Jensen PS, Chait AR, et al. (2009) Medication adherence in the MTA: saliva methylphenidate samples versus parent report and mediating effect of concomitant behavioral treatment. *J Am Acad Child Adolesc Psychiatry* 48: 501–10. doi: 10.1097/CHI.0b013e31819c23ed.

Penzel F (2003) *The Hair-Pulling Problem: A Complete Guide to Trichotillomania.* New York: Oxford.

Pertusa A, Fullana MA, Singh S, et al. (2008) Compulsive hoarding: OCD symptom, distinct clinical syndrome, or both? *Am J Psychiatry* 165: 1289–98. doi: 10.1176/appi.ajp.2008.07111730.

Piacentini J, Bennett S, Compton SN, et al. (2014) 24- and 36-week outcomes for the Child/Adolescent Anxiety Multimodal Study (CAMS). *J Am Acad Child Adolesc Psychiatry* 53: 297–310. doi: 10.1016/j.jaac.2013.11.010.

Pierre JM (2011) Cannabis, synthetic cannabinoids, and psychosis risk: what the evidence says. *Curr Psychiatry* 10: 49–57.

Pliszka SR (2009) *Treating ADHD and Comorbid Disorders: Psychosocial and Psychopharmacological Interventions.* New York & London: Guilford Press.

Posner K, Pressman AW, Greenhil LL (2009) ADHD in preschool children. In: Brown TE, ed. *ADHD Comorbidities: Handbook for ADHD Complications in Children and Adults.* Arlington, VA: American Psychiatric Publishing, pp. 37–53.

Racine MB, Majnemer A, Shevell M, Snider L (2008) Handwriting performance in children with attention deficit hyperactivity disorder (ADHD). *J Child Neurol* 23: 399–406. doi: 10.1177/0883073807309244.

Rapp A, Dodds A, Walkup JT, Rynn M (2013) Treatment of pediatric anxiety disorders. *Ann NY Acad Sci* 1304: 52–61. doi: 10.1111/nyas.12318.

Rasmussen P, Gillberg C (2000) Natural outcome of ADHD with developmental coordination disorder at age 22 years: a controlled, longitudinal, community-based study. *J Am Acad Child Adolesc Psychiatry* 39: 1424–31. doi: 10.1097/00004583-200011000-00017.

Reid AH (1984) Gilles de la Tourette syndrome in mental handicap. *J Ment Defic Res* 28: 81–3.

Reinblatt SP, dosReis S, Walkup JT, Riddle MA (2009) Activation adverse events induced by the selective reuptake inhibitor fluvoxamine in children and adolescents. *J Child Adolesc Psychopharm* 19: 119–26.

Ressler KJ, Rothbaum BO (2013) Augmenting obsessive–compulsive disorder treatment: from brain to mind. *JAMA Psychiatry* 70: 1129–31. doi: 10.1001/jamapsychiatry.2013.216.

Rigoli D, Piek JP, Kane R (2012) Motor coordination and psychosocial correlates in a normative adolescent sample. *Pediatrics* 129: e892–900. doi: 10.1542/peds.2011-1237.

Ringman JM, Jankovic J (2000) Occurrence of tics in Asperger's syndrome and autistic disorder. *J Child Neurol* 15: 394–400. doi: 10.1177/088307380001500608.

Rivard L, Missiuna C, McCauley D, Cairney J (2014) Descriptive and factor analysis of the Developmental Coordination Disorder Questionnaire (DCDQ '07) in a population-based sample of children with and without developmental coordination disorder. *Child Care Health Dev* 40: 42–9. doi: 10.1111/j.1365-2214.2012.01425.x.

Robertson MM, Orth M (2006) Behavioral and affective disorders in Tourette syndrome. *Adv Neurol* 99: 39–60.

Rosenquist PB, Bodfish JW, Thompson R (1997) Tourette syndrome associated with mental retardation: a single-subject treatment study with haloperidol. *Am J Ment Retard* 101: 497–504.

Rowe R, Maughan B, Costello EJ, Angold A (2005) Defining oppositional defiant disorder. *J Child Psychol Psychiatry* 46: 1309–16. doi: 10.1111/j.1469-7610.2005.01420.x.

Ruggiero S, Rafaniello C, Bravaccio C, et al. (2012) Safety of attention-deficit/hyperactivity disorder medications in children: an intensive pharmacosurveillance monitoring study. *J Child Adolesc Psychopharm* 22: 415–22. doi: 10.1089/cap.2012.0093.

Saavedra LM, Silverman WK, Morgan-Lopez AA, Kurtines WM (2010) Cognitive behavioral treatment for childhood anxiety disorders: long-term effects on anxiety and secondary disorders in young adulthood. *J Child Psychol Psychiatry* 51: 924–34. doi: 10.1111/j.1469-7610.2010.02242.x.

Safer DJ, Zito JM (2006) Treatment-emergent adverse events from selective serotonin reuptake inhibitors by age group: children versus adolescents. *J Child Adolesc Psychopharm* 16: 159–69.

Samuels JF, Bienvenu OJ, Grados MA, et al. (2008) Prevalence and correlates of hoarding behavior in a community-based sample. *Behav Res Ther* 46: 836–44. doi: 10.1016/j.brat.2008.04.004.

Saxena S, Maidment KM (2004) Treatment of compulsive hoarding. *J Clin Psychol* 60: 1443–54. doi: 10.1002/jclp.20079.

Scahill L, Riddle MA, McSwiggin-Hardin M, et al. (1997) Children's Yale–Brown Obsessive Compulsive Scale: reliability and validity. *J Am Acad Child Adolesc Psychiatry* 36: 844–52. doi: 10.1097/00004583-199706000-00023.

Scahill L, Williams S, Schwab-Stone M, et al. (2006) Disruptive behavior problems in a community sample of children with tic disorders. *Adv Neurol* 99: 184–90.

Schneider SA, Robertson MM, Rizzo R, et al. (2008) Fragile X syndrome associated with tic disorders. *Mov Disord* 23: 1108–12. doi: 10.1002/mds.21995.

Schoemaker MM, Lingam R, Jongmans MJ, et al. (2013) Is severity of motor coordination difficulties related to co-morbidity in children at risk for developmental coordination disorder? *Res Dev Disabil* 34: 3084–91. doi: 10.1016/j.ridd.2013.06.028.

Sedel F, Friderici K, Nummy K, et al. (2006) Atypical Gilles de la Tourette syndrome with β-mannosidase deficiency. *Arch Neurol* 63: 129–31. doi: 10.1001/archneur.63.1.129.

Seltzer LJ, Prososki AR, Ziegler TE, Pollak SD (2012) Instant messages vs. speech: hormones and why we still need to hear each other. *Evol Hum Behav* 33: 42–5.

Sexton CC, Gelhorn HL, Bell JA, Classi PM (2012) The co-occurrence of reading disorder and ADHD: epidemiology, treatment, psychosocial impact, and economic burden. *J Learn Disabil* 45: 538–64. doi: 10.1177/0022219411407772.

Shattuck PT, Roux AM, Hudson LE, et al. (2012) Services for adults with an autism spectrum disorder. *Can J Psychiatry* 57: 284–91.

Sibley MH Pelham WE, Gnagy EM, et al. (2012) Diagnosing ADHD in adolescence. *J Consult Clin Psychol* 80: 139–50.

Sica C, Caudek C, Chiri LR, et al. (2012) 'Not just right experiences' predict obsessive–compulsive symptoms in non-clinical Italian individuals: a one-year longitudinal study. *J Obsess-Compuls Relat Disord* 1: 159–67. doi: 10.1016/j.jocrd.2012.02.006.

Silverman WK, Field AP, eds (2011) *Anxiety Disorders in Children and Adolescents, 2nd edn.* Cambridge, UK: Cambridge University Press.

Simonic I, Gericke GS, Lippert M, Schoeman JF (1997) Additional clinical and cytogenetic findings associated with Rett syndrome. *Am J Med Genet* 74: 331–7.

Smits-Engelsman BCM, Blank R, van der Kaay A-C, et al. (2013) Efficacy of interventions to improve motor performance in children with developmental coordination disorder: a combined systematic review and meta-analysis. *Dev Med Child Neurol* 55: 229–37. doi: 10.1111/dmcn.12008.

Snyder G, Friman PC (2012) Habitual stereotypic movements: a descriptive analysis of four common types. In: Grant JE, Stein DJ, Woods DW, Keuthen NJ, eds. *Trichotillomania, Skin Picking, and Other Body-focused Repetitive Behaviors.* Arlington, VA: American Psychiatric Publishing, pp. 43–64.

Specht MW, Woods DW, Piacentini J, et al. (2011) Clinical characteristics of children and adolescents with a primary tic disorder. *J Dev Phys Disabil* 23: 15–31. doi: 10.1007/s10882-010-9223-z.

Spencer TJ (2006) ADHD and comorbidity in childhood. *J Clin Psychiatry* 67 (Suppl 8): 27–31.

Spencer TJ, Biederman J, Faraone S, et al. (2001) Impact of tic disorders on ADHD outcome across the life cycle: findings from a large group of adults with and without ADHD. *Am J Psychiatry* 158: 611–7. doi: 10.1176/appi.ajp.158.4.611.

Spencer TJ, Sallee FR, Dunn DW, et al. (2008) Atomoxetine treatment of ADHD in children with comorbid Tourette syndrome. *J Atten Disord* 11: 470–81. doi: 10.1177/1087054707306109.

Stein DJ, Christenson GA, Hollander E (1999) *Trichotillomania.* Washington DC: American Psychiatric Press.

Stein MB, Forde DR, Anderson G, Walker JR (1997) Obsessive–compulsive disorder in the community: an epidemiologic survey with clinical reappraisal. *Am J Psychiatry* 154: 1120–6.

Stewart SE (2012) Rage takes center stage: focus on an underappreciated aspect of pediatric obsessive–compulsive disorder. *J Am Acad Child Adolesc Psychiatry* 51: 569–71 (editorial). doi: 10.1016/j.jaac.2012.04.002.

Stewart SE, Beresin C, Haddad S, et al. (2008) Predictors of family accommodation in obsessive–compulsive disorder. *Ann Clin Psychiatry* 20: 65–70. doi: v10.1080/10401230802017043.

Storch EA, Geffken GR, Merlo LJ, et al. (2007) Family accommodation in pediatric obsessive–compulsive disorder. *J Clin Child Adolesc Psychol* 36: 207–16. doi: 10.1080/15374410701277929.

Storch EA, Stigge-Kaufman D, Marien WE, et al. (2008) Obsessive–compulsive disorder in youth with and without a chronic tic disorder. *Depress Anx* 5: 761–7. doi: 10.1002/da.20304.

Storch EA, Milsom V, Lack CW, et al. (2009) Sleep-related problems in youth with Tourette's syndrome and chronic tic disorder. *Child Adolesc Ment Health* 14: 97–103.

Storch EA, Jones AM, Lack CW, et al. (2012) Rage attacks in pediatric obsessive–compulsive disorder: phenomenology and clinical correlates. *J Am Acad Child Adolesc Psychiatry* 51: 582–92. doi: 10.1016/j.jaac.2012.02.016.

Suhr J, Zimak E, Buelow M, Fox L (2009) Self-reported childhood attention-deficit/hyperactivity disorder symptoms are not specific to the disorder. *Compr Psychiatry* 50: 269–75. doi: 10.1016/j.comppsych.2008.08.008.

Sukhodolsky DG, Scahill L (2012) *Cognitive–Behavioral Therapy for Anger and Aggression in Children.* New York: Guilford Press.

Tal-Saban M, Ornoy A, Parush S (2014) Young adults with developmental coordination disorder: a longitudinal study. *Am J Occup Ther* 68: 307–16. doi: 10.5014/ajot.2014.009563.

Taylor E (2009a) Managing bipolar disorders in children and adolescents. *Nat Rev Neurol* 5: 484–91.

Taylor E (2009b) Sleep and tics: problems associated with ADHD. *J Am Acad Child Adolesc Psychiatry* 48: 877–8. doi: 10.1097/CHI.0b013e3181af825a.

Taylor E (2011) Commentary: reading and attention problems – how are they connected? Reflections on reading McGrath et al. (2011). *J Child Psychol Psychiatry* 52: 558–9. doi: 10.1111/j.14697610.2011.02403.x.

Thapar A, Collishaw S, Pine DS, Thapar AK (2012) Depression in adolescence. *Lancet* 379: 1056–67.

Thapar A, Cooper M, Eyre O, Langley K (2013) Practitioner review: What have we learnt about the causes of ADHD? *J Child Psychol Psychiatry* 54: 3–16. doi: 10.1111/j.1469-7610.

Tolin DF, Meunier SA, Frost RO, Steketee G (2010) Course of compulsive hoarding and its relationship to life events. *Depress Anx* 27: 829–38. doi: 10.1002/da.20684.

Towbin K, Axelson D, Leibenluft E, Birmaher B (2013) Differentiating bipolar disorder – not otherwise specified and severe mood dysregulation. *J Am Acad Child Adolesc Psychiatry* 52: 466–81. doi: 10.1016/j.jaac.2013.02.006.

Visser JE, Bär PR, Jinnah HA (2000) Lesch–Nyhan disease and the basal ganaglia. *Brain Res Rev* 32: 449–75. doi: 10.1016/S0165-0173(99)00094-6.

Volkmar F, Siegel M, Woodbury-Smith M, et al. (2014) Practice parameter for the assessment and treatment of children and adolescents with autism spectrum disorder. *J Am Acad Child Adolesc Psychiatry* 53: 237–57. doi: 10.1016/j.jaac.2013.10.013.

Volkow ND, Baler RD, Compton WM, Weiss SRB (2014) Adverse health effects of marijuana use. *N Engl J Med* 370: 2219–27. doi: 10.1056/NEJMra1402309.

Vollebregt MA, van Dongen-Boomsma M, Buitelaar JK, Slaats-Willemse D (2014) Does EEG-neurofeedback improve neurocognitive functioning in children with attention-deficit/hyperactivity disorder? A systematic review and a double-blind placebo-controlled study. *J Child Psychol Psychiatry* 55: 460–72. doi: 10.1111/jcpp.12143.

Wagner MO, Bös K, Jascenoka J, et al. (2012) Peer problems mediate the relationship between developmental coordination disorder and behavioral problems in school-aged children. *Res Dev Disabil* 33: 2072–9. doi: 10.1016/j.ridd.2012.05.012.

Wanderer S, Roessner V, Freeman R, et al. (2012) Relationship of obsessive–compulsive disorder to age-related comorbidity in children and adolescents with Tourette syndrome. *J Dev Behav Pediatr* 33: 124–33.

Watson HJ, Rees CS (2008) Meta-analysis of randomized, controlled treatment trials for pediatric obsessive–compulsive disorder. *J Child Psychol Psychiatry* 49: 489–98. doi: 10.1111/j.1469-7610.2007.01875.x.

Webster-Stratton C, Reid JM (2010) The Incredible Years, Parents, Teachers, and Children Training Series: A multifaceted treatment approach for young children with conduct disorders. In: Weisz JR, Kazdin AE, eds. *Evidence-based Psychotherapies for Children and Adolescents, 2nd edn.* New York: Guilford Press, pp. 194–210.

Weiss MD, Wasdell MB, Bomben M, et al. (2006) Sleep hygiene and melatonin treatment for children and adolescents with ADHD and initial insomnia. *J Am Acad Child Adolesc Psychiatry* 45: 512–9. doi: 10.1097/01.chi.0000205706.78818.ef.

WHO (2010) *International Statistical Classification of Diseases and Related Health Problems, 10th Revision.* Geneva: World Health Organization (available online at: http://apps.who.int/classifications/icd10/browse/2010/en).

Wilens TE (2011) A sobering fact: ADHD leads to substance abuse. *J Am Acad Child Adolesc Psychiatry* 50: 6–8 (editorial). doi: 10.1016/j.jaac.2010.10.002.

Wilens TE, Adler LA, Adams J, et al. (2008) Misuse and diversion of stimulants prescribed for ADHD: a systematic review of the literature. *J Am Acad Child Adolesc Psychiatry* 47: 21–31. doi: 10.1097/chi. 0b013e31815a56f1.

Wiles N, Thomas L, Abel A, et al. (2013) Cognitive behavioural therapy as an adjunct to pharmacotherapy for primary care based patients with treatment resistant depression: results of the CoBalT randomized controlled trial. *Lancet* 381: 375–84. doi: 10.1016/S0140-6736(12)61552-9.

Wilson BN, Kaplan BJ, Crawford SG, Roberts G (2007) The Developmental Coordination Disorder Questionnaire 2007 (DCDQ'07). Alberta Children's Hospital Decision Support Research Team. Available online at http://www.dcdq.ca.

Wilson BN, Crawford SG, Green D, et al. (2009) Psychometric properties of the Revised Developmental Coordination Disorder Questionnaire. *Phys Occup Ther Pediatr* 29: 182–202. doi: 10.1080/01942630902784761.

Wilson BN, Neil K, Kamps PH, Babcock S (2013) Awareness and knowledge of developmental coordination disorder among physicians, teachers and parents. *Child Care Health Dev* 39: 296–300. doi: 10.1111/j.1365-2214.2012.01403.x.

Wilson PH, Ruddock S, Smits-Engelsman B, et al. (2013) Understanding performance deficits in developmental coordination disorder: a meta-analysis of recent research. *Dev Med Child Neurol* 55: 217–28.

Wink LK, Early M, Schaefer T, et al. (2014) Body mass index change in autism spectrum disorders: comparison of treatment with risperidone and aripiprazole. *J Child Adolesc Psychopharm* 24: 78–82. doi: 10.1089/cap.2013.0099.

Woods DW (2011) Trichotillomania: awareness and advances. *J Am Acad Child Adolesc Psychiatry* 50: 747–8. doi: 10.1016/j.jaac.2011.05.008.

Woods DW (2013) Treating trichotillomania across the lifespan. *J Am Acad Child Adolesc Psychiatry* 52: 223-4 (editorial). doi: 10.1016/j.jaac.2012.12.021.

Woods DW, Flessner C, Franklin ME, et al. (2006) Understanding and treating trichotillomania: what we know and what we don't know. *Psychiatr Clin North Am* 29: 487–501.

Wootton BM, Dear BF, Johnston L, et al. (2013) Remote treatment of obsessive–compulsive disorder: a randomized controlled trail. *J Obsess-Compuls Relat Disord* 2: 375–84. doi: 10.1016/j.jocrd.2013.07.002.

Zarkowska E, Crawley B, Locke J (1989) A behavioral intervention for Gilles de la Tourette syndrome in a severely mentally handicapped girl. *J Ment Defic Res* 33: 245–53.

Zwicker JG, Missiuna C, Boyd LA (2009) Neural correlates of developmental coordination disorder: a review of hypotheses. *J Child Neurol* 10: 1273–81. doi: 10.1177/0883073809333537.

Zwicker JG, Missiuna C, Harris SR, Boyd LA (2012) Developmental coordination disorder: a review and update. *Eur J Paediatr Neurol* 16: 573–81. doi: 10.1016/j.ejpn.2012.05.005.

Zwicker JG, Harris SR, Klassen AF (2013) Quality of life domains affected in children with developmental coordination disorder: a systematic review. *Child Care Health Dev* 39: 562–80. doi: 10.111/j.1365-2214.2012.01379.x.

11
STEREOTYPIC MOVEMENT DISORDER

Stereotypy is a very general term that often is used rather loosely. Stereotypic movement disorder (SMD) refers to a repetitive pattern in non-autistic persons that involves some impairment or interference in ordinary activities. (In the pediatric neurological literature it may be unofficially referred to as 'primary complex motor stereotypies' or 'secondary' if occurring in those with a neurological condition that may be considered strongly associated or causative.) If it is a target for intervention, the SMD diagnosis may also be applied to persons with intellectual disability. In the past and still in many books stereotypy (the general term) is assumed to be strongly associated with ASD and intellectual disability, and sometimes with blindness, where it is often referred to as 'blind mannerisms'. Stereotypies may be considered as normal in infants, but are assumed to resolve by age 4 years. The term is sometimes also applied to a wide variety of 'nervous habits'. [Because of heterogeneity of the topography and lack of clarity of category boundaries, this section should be read in conjunction with those on ASD and intellectual disability (Chapter 10) and repetitive motor behaviors and SIB (Chapter 12).] The causative factors are probably various, and there is often a positive family history.

Even when SMD is recognized, parents are often told that it will 'go away', which is often misleading, and they are usually given no way to understand the typical slow resolution of the social problem they fear. A substantial group of these children have a good outlook, and the clinical challenge is to facilitate tolerance of the pattern and minimization of misunderstanding before it evolves into a desirably private pattern. Habit reversal training has been reported to be helpful when impairment is significant. (There is a subgroup of adults whose history is similar to SMD and who may engage in fantasy to the point of substitution of other desirable activities. At present we do not have enough follow-up studies to know how many and to what extent, how to predict who they will be, and how to modify the excess when they are adults. This will be an important task for the future.) Another often overlooked point is that the presence of a stereotypy in persons with persistent tic disorders may be missed because tics, once identified, trump other kinds of movements. The reverse may also be true: tics may be 'lost' in identified SMD patterns. This has important implications for understanding, attitudes toward movement patterns, and treatment. The diagnostic distinction between tics and stereotypy based upon presence or absence of premonitory sensations is likely to be wrong (and a clinical example is presented).

A very significant problem persists with misunderstandings and misdiagnoses of persons with SMD as having autism or tic disorders, and generally a lack of clinician awareness and training. The mixture of stereotypies, either tics or ASD-associated, can present complex diagnostic and management challenges. In this very important section an unusually lengthy description and clinical implications are provided in an attempt to remedy the lack of readily available information and to identify points for further research and discovery.

SMD is an under-recognized and very important differential diagnosis for tics. It is only very recently that helpful information has been appearing in textbooks and some journal articles. Unfortunately, misdiagnosis is still rampant and most books about Tourette syndrome omit it entirely, therefore serious and extended attention will be paid to it here. We have published our work on this subject recently (Freeman et al. 2010) but the journal's length restrictions did not allow for a full discussion of all the clinical implications, which will be elaborated upon here. The most recent and arguably the best treatment of the subject is the book edited by Grant et al. (2012), which has a fine chapter on 'habitual stereotypic movements' by Snyder and Friman that is highly recommended.

Thanks are also due to the many parents who wrote in as a consequence of the Freeman et al. (2010) paper looking for answers and who helped by providing histories, descriptions, insightful questions, comments from the children, family patterns, and in some cases video clips of the movements.

Importance

(1) SMD is frequently misunderstood. (2) This misunderstanding may cause prolonged parental anxiety, conflict between parents as well as between parents and the school or clinician. (3) Unnecessary costs for assessment and ineffective treatments may result. (4) Tics and stereotypies can be misidentified or missed altogether, each in the other.

Definition

In the new DSM-5, previous criteria have been maintained, but provision is made for SMD to be diagnosed in conjunction with some other disorders provided the stereotypy is a focus for intervention. Two types are recognized: non-self-injurious and self-injurious. The main focus in this chapter is the non-self-injurious type.

A diagnosis or a symptom?

The field is confusing because stereotypic behavior is 'normal' at some point in everyone's life, has no strict criteria, may differ depending upon culture, co-exists with many other conditions and disorders or may stand alone, and varies in severity from trivial to catastrophic. Many different behaviors are termed 'stereotypic', with no general agreement (Rapp and Vollmer 2005a). In some instances (as with Tourette syndrome) the identification of a stereotypy is taken to explain other problematic behaviors. Partly for these reasons there has been a recent critique of the entire concept (Edwards et al. 2012).

Stereotypy (as a symptom) may warrant a separate diagnosis when other disorders of which it may be a part are not present or when it is impairing or damaging. Those other disorders are ASD, intellectual disability, early significant visual impairment and some neurological disorders (Barry et al. 2011). In the absence of other neurological disorders, Barry and colleagues suggest the term primary, and for those associated with or part of a neurological disorder, secondary. SMD should not be diagnosed when the pattern is not impairing (just different from behavior that those around the child are familiar with), but in practice this caveat is not always adhered to. One of the reasons may be that parents and teachers may be concerned or very anxious, but in that instance one needs to consider why that is the case before using it as the basis for a child's diagnosis.

Rarely, SMD is the result of brain injury. A 21-year-old man with a history of sickle cell anemia was reported by McGrath et al. (2002). He experienced a major subdural hematoma, and as his post-stroke condition developed he showed frequent chanting of phrases, body-rocking and teeth-clicking. These patterns gradually decreased on sertraline as his clinical condition improved.

The DSM-5 definition emphasizes that the motor behavior is "apparently purposeless", but significantly allows for exceptions, such as to "reduce anxiety in response to external stressors". Some medical texts have used lack of premonitory sensations as a distinction between tics and SMD, but this is probably incorrect. Here is a good example.

Case example

'Jack' was 14 when seen because of a prolonged (hours-long) pattern of winding string around his fingers, which had become almost completely private (done only with family members present) since beginning at age 4. He missed school because of not being able to perform the pattern there. He described a feeling of tension he would get in his wrists and a tingling in his fingers when he had not done his string-playing for a long time. Doing it clearly relieved these sensations. While doing it, he was running favorite videos or movies through his mind, and any worries he may have had were absent.

> *Comment: The function of the pattern is to enhance pleasant fantasy, and the specific premonitory sensations are evident. There is an associated sacrifice of other activities. We do not (cannot) understand the earlier 'choice' of the specific pattern, perhaps from experimentation with many different movements.*

This case exemplifies the argument that it is not true generally that tics can be distinguished from other movement disorders because they involve premonitory sensations while others (SMD and stereotypies associated with ASD and intellectual disability) do not. The generality of this challenge requires further research. Singer (2013), for example, states flatly: "Stereotypies, in contrast to tics, are not associated with premonitory urges, preceding sensations, or an internal desire to perform" (p. 24).

A summary of the critique by Edwards et al. (2012)

There has been 'differential diagnosis creep' with loose definitions, such as purposefulness, occurring at the expense of other movements, and as a result the following have sometimes been listed as stereotypies: drug-induced dyskinesia, mannerisms, restless legs syndrome, complex tics, akathisia and tardive dyskinesias. Is this helpful clinically? Does it define a cohesive group of conditions that may be linked pathophysiologically? Their answer is 'no' to both questions. The authors recommend *distractibility* as a necessary characteristic (this refers to the ease with which the person can be 'called out' of the pattern, typical of SMD, but not tics). There is another area of confusion with tics: movements characterized as 'stereotypies' in Rett syndrome (Temudo et al. 2007) would otherwise be classified as tics. After further discussion of difficulties, they recommend a unified definition as "a non-goal-directed movement pattern that is repeated continuously for a period of time in the same form and on multiple occasions, and which is typically distractible" (p. 4). This would exclude brief intermittent movements typical of tics, but include flapping and more severe repetitive movements dominating motor output at the expense of other movements. This paper is of great importance and represents a high level of thoughtfulness; it well repays several readings. Nevertheless, it should not be surprising that there are still problems. For example, there seems to be no place in their table of 'causes of stereotypy' for some cases of SMD. The detailed arguments about the adequacy of the proposed causes, however, are beyond the scope of this presentation.

Diagnosis (including instruments and forms)

There is a Stereotypy Severity Scale designed by the Hopkins group (Mahone et al. 2004), based upon the Yale Global Tic Severity Scale (YGTSS, presented in Appendix 5), which has recently been validated (Mahone et al. 2014).

Prevalence/epidemiology

The lower the patient's IQ, the more common stereotypies are, and they are seen in most individuals with intellectual disability and ASD, as well as in most of those with early-onset significant visual impairment (see Chapter 13). The prevalence of SMD in children without ASD or intellectual disability is unknown, although the text in DSM-5 cites 3% to 4% (without quoting a source for this). We do not know whether the neuroimaging differences found in a subgroup of six boys with SMD (two of whom also had ADHD) by the Hopkins group (Kates et al. 2005) will be replicated, and if so, what practical significance will emerge. The extensive clinical and follow-up experience that has informed our own study sheds no light on that question.

Presentation and phenomenology

What we do know is that there is a group of children who have pattern characteristics described by the parents and later by some children that are strikingly similar. A very early pattern is usually reported, often appearing in the first year of life. *It does not subside.* Others notice that it looks odd: different, more intense, more complex or more prolonged than ordinary patterns of repetitive motor behavior. Parents often spontaneously mention that it occurs at times of excitement or active imagination. The older child may ask for more or specific times to perform it. Almost uniformly the parents will say that their child is not unhappy with it — but they or a teacher are in distress or confusion, and worried about future social ostracism.

Caution should be exercised to not assume that this group's features are typical of *all* children with stereotypy. These features are best illustrated by a selection of descriptions by parents, as given below. (Names have been changed to ensure privacy, and either permission to publish has been granted or, as in some cases, the descriptions are derived from those in the public domain.)

We should not minimize the anxiety caused to the parents by going out in public with a child who periodically attracts attention because of a stereotypy, even after they have had what education the clinician can provide. (There is also a subgroup of unknown proportion who engage in excessive fantasy that may interfere with other activities; identification and study of these persons is very recent, but what little is known is presented below.)

There is another condition that has some features in common with SMD: *jactatio capitis nocturna* ('throwing the head at night') or the vaguer term *rhythmic sleep disorder*. It is poorly understood, may be confused with tics, and is reported to sometimes co-occur with more usual types of daytime stereotypies (Bonnet et al. 2010). This pattern of shaking, banging or rolling the head and/or body before sleep or sometimes during light sleep, often combined with vocalizations, is common in infants before the age of 3 years, but not after age 4 (Mayer et al. 2007). In a small number of cases the pattern persists into middle childhood or even adult life (Stepanova et al. 2005). There is no substantial case series that is informative, only a few case reports and small series. Clinicians unfamiliar with the pattern may suspect tics, ASD or sometimes epilepsy. Reports of associated disorders or problems (e.g. restless legs syndrome/ Willis–Ekbom disease) vary, as do recommendations for medications: clonazepam, imipramine or citalopram. Theories of etiology include persistence of self-soothing from intrauterine experience, abnormal neurology, reinforced learning patterns, and neglect. One of the differences from other forms of SMD is that it is said not to involve a desire or conscious need to do it (but this seems unlikely) (Muthugovindan and Singer 2009). It is also classified as a parasomnia in the sleep literature (Hoban 2004). In most instances a sleep study is not considered necessary and the case history is decisive for the diagnosis.

Differentiating tics and Tourette syndrome from stereotypic movement disorder
SMD starts earlier, often in the first year of life, usually by age 3; it is much less changeable and may be stable for years; the pattern tends to be rhythmic and prolonged, whereas tics usually are not, and subjectively the children like their SMD, but usually dislike or ignore their tics, and in SMD the children can be easily 'called out' of their pattern ('distracted'). In both there can be facial grimacing and vocalization, though it is only in tics that these occur on their own and not necessarily at the point of high excitement. In the recent paper by Ghosh et al. (2013) there were no cases out of 28 with 'phobic' stereotypy alone (but one wonders whether such cases would be referred to a tertiary neurology center).

TABLE 11.1
Distinguishing SMD from tics and ASD stereotypies

	SMD stereotypy	*Tics/TS*	*ASD stereotypies*
Age at onset	Usually before age 3	5–7 years	Early
Ease of distraction	Easy	Hard	May be hard
Pattern variability	Stable, few changes	Usually wildly unstable	Unstable
Comorbidity	About 85%	About 85% to 90% for TS	Common
'Just right' feeling	Unclear	Often very strong	Unknown
Premonitory sensations	Probably less frequent than in tics, but not rare	Yes	Unknown
Vocalizations	Common, not independent	Required for diagnosis of TS	Frequent
Facial grimacing	Common	Very common	Occasional
Attitude toward pattern	Like it, may seek it; may sometimes be excessive	Ignore, usually dislike, hate	Often ignore
SIB	Listed as subtype	~15%	Common
Ease of triggering new pattern	Difficult	Easy	Unknown

SMD, stereotypic movement disorder; ASD, autism spectrum disorder; TS, Tourette syndrome; SIB, self-injurious behavior.

Table 11.1 summarizes the differences between SMD and tics/Tourette syndrome, and they are considerable (but of course one can have both), as well as stereotypies in ASD.

Notice that our knowledge of patients with ASD is still incomplete or absent.

Importance of descriptions

The words or phrases used to describe stereotypies may be much too generic to be useful, and may obscure some significant characteristics. Just as the brief blepharospasm that typically accompanies an eye-blinking tic is rarely mentioned spontaneously by patients or parents, components of stereotypies (or RMBs) are often omitted in favor of a common generic label. Here is a good example.

Case example

A 3-year-old otherwise well-developing girl began 'hair-twirling' which received no interest when labeled 'hair-twirling' by physicians who did not observe the full pattern; they reassured her that it is common in children (true). Her mother always felt, though, that there was something more to it — and she was right. The twirling was done with one finger, with the other hand patting the hair at the same time, very frequently and for long periods of time, in preference to other activities. Three years later the intensity was reduced but the pattern was the same. This describes SMD. (And then a tic disorder was added.)

An important misunderstanding

Because SMD can be a diagnosed condition on its own, or with ADHD, OCD, Tourette syndrome, DCD or some other diagnoses, including intellectual disability if a focus of treatment, the place of the stereotypic behavior can easily be confusing. For example, parents report that their child engages in frequent hand-flapping when excited, and a clinician diagnoses SMD, so then they wonder why that child also has some developmental difficulty.

Comorbidity and common associations

We have found high rates of ADHD (36%) and tics (43%); of those with tics, 26% satisfy criteria for Tourette syndrome. As compared with the *TIC* database (Freeman et al. 2000) there is a higher proportion of females (29% vs 19%), an earlier onset age (mean 1.5 years vs 6.4 years), no OCD (vs 21%), only 6% OCB (vs 33%), 34% SLD (vs 21%), 11% anxiety (vs 17%), and 40% DCD (vs 10%) on screening with the 2007 revision of the Developmental Coordination Disorder Questionnaire (DCDQ). In 13% there were no co-occurring disorders. Sleep problems were reported at comparable rates in the two groups. In no case did the pattern develop into self-injurious behavior. Occasional accidents (to self or others) may occur from flailing limbs. Developmental coordination problems were common, as also reported by Mahone et al. (2014) in a group with minimal comorbidity.

Natural history and prognosis

There is often some gradual change in the SMD pattern, but overall much continuity. This is unlike childhood Tourette syndrome, where 'it's always changing'. There may be some increase in frequency and intensity as the very young child enters school, but the unselfconscious performance typically gives way gradually to what we have termed 'privatization': limitation to private or family-only situations. In one case series (Ghosh et al. 2013) the outcome was not so favorable and privatization was not described. In the case of 'Barry', below, other factors may have influenced the course.

Case study

Nine-year-old 'Barry' started his repetitive movements in his first year with hand-flapping but most prominent was rhythmical head-turning. He also had significant clumsiness. These continued into his middle childhood and seemed to the teacher to interfere occasionally with his focus on class activities. Unlike most children with stereotypy, he performed his head-turning almost continuously and apparently unselfconsciously when seen in the office. The pattern had become more intense and frequent in the previous 2 years. He described active imagination during his pattern. He had been assessed for ASD and was found not to meet the criteria. Why wasn't he showing some privatization? A possible clue was found in the history. He had to be reminded to eat because he did not seem to respond to hunger. He often did not respond to the urge to have a bowel movement until the last moment; his family members could guess at the approaching need by a change in the intensity and frequency of his head-turning. Socially he was fairly

---

competent but physically clumsy. Was there an association between difficulty in reading and not responding to these two body signals and his not seeming anxious to behave more like his peers? This was unclear.

Privatization, though desirable for social reasons, may have other values, some problematic (see below). Oakley et al. (2015) make the important point that impairment is unlikely compared with that from comorbid disorders and symptoms (much as in Tourette syndrome).

Etiology

The underlying function of motor stereotypy is not agreed upon; it may have many functions, one of which is regulation of the level of arousal. The factors present at onset and in later maintenance may be distinct. In the behavioral literature, stereotypy is seen as maintained by sources of automatic positive reinforcement (for discussion, see Rapp and Vollmer 2005a). Similarities have been advanced from the nonhuman literature (Mason and Rushen 2006). There appears to be a robust genetic component from clinical studies. Whatever may be different in the brains of persons with stereotypy, the pathways or circuits appear to be in the same general area (cortical–striatal–thalamo-cortical) as those associated with tics. Recently the potential neuroanatomic and neurotransmitter abnormalities have been extensively discussed and the literature on habit formation reviewed by the Hopkins group (Singer 2009, Gao and Singer 2013, Singer 2013). Their most recent study (Houdayer et al. 2014) has important implications. An ordinary voluntary movement is preceded by a movement-related cortical potential (MRCP). They found that the 10 children with SMD were not different from comparison children when performing an ordinary voluntary movement, but that their MRCP was absent from the SMD pattern initiation. This suggested that the stereotypy originates from the basal ganglia and activates a different pattern of sensorimotor loops. (Research implications are discussed below.)

Treatment

No treatment is usually necessary nor is there a strong evidence base to support it. Two children we have seen or been informed about complained about the pattern and openly asked that it be stopped; they had been frequently scolded by parents whenever they did it. Miller et al. (2006) did describe a subgroup that had behavior modification applied, with modest success (they did not describe why those cases were selected for treatment). Their work on this is ongoing (see below). Stereotypy can be induced by dopaminergic drugs and sometimes reduced by environmental enrichment. If pharmacological intervention can reduce stereotypy, behavioral intervention may ensure maintenance of that change, but further research is necessary (Rapp and Vollmer 2005b). No medication has so far been reported to be generally useful.

In cases of adults with excessive fantasy activity, treatment recommendations and outcome are as yet unsettled. Ricketts et al. (2013) have described behavior therapy in three patients with SMD who had some impairment (little time for other activities); two of them had premonitory sensations. This is a more detailed treatment description than that described by Miller et al. (2006). The Hopkins group has made a reasonable recommendation that behavioral approaches and advice to parents (such as to reinforce curtailing the pattern) are best applied in concert with a behavioral therapist (as is true for tics as well). The reason for this is that the tactics used are not always intuitive; they can be counterintuitive as well.

Management

If not specific 'treatment', then management is important. We have emphasized that the natural history of SMD is favorable because of privatization. Others have almost entirely ignored this factor and have portrayed the course as uncommonly improved. This leaves the parents with little to be optimistic about, and can reinforce a need for 'treatment'. But if our understanding is correct, because the stereotypy will become private (though probably continuing), no specific treatment should generally be necessary. There may of course be exceptions, some of which are discussed below under 'Excessive fantasy and imagery, some with stereotypy', and the proportion of those will eventually be determined. But what will help parents to tolerate the waiting? If their consultation with the clinician occurs between about ages 2–6 years, privatization may take some further 3–6 years! There is a possibility, other than mere follow-up, to sustain optimism. This is based upon a parallel aspect of childhood social development that most parents do not link to changes in stereotypy: common childhood patterns performed in public that need to be suppressed for social acceptance. These include the following examples that are well-known: crotch-grabbing, bottom-scratching, nose-picking and smelling/eating nasal mucus, wiping your nose on your sleeve, breaking wind, burping, sneezing or coughing with mouth uncovered, loud toilet-talk, swearing, commenting on stranger characteristics out loud, eating with open mouth, spitting, and so on. Some of these behaviors may be tolerated at home, to varying degrees, and they will vary by culture. But normally they are gradually successfully suppressed so as to become automatic (acculturated) and not require constant commands or reprimands, except under special circumstances. Stereotypies follow a similar but usually unacknowledged trajectory. Tracking these privatizations will provide an indication of a child's increasing social awareness so as to automatically distinguish among social situations in which certain behaviors are to be suppressed or allowed. A list can be provided and an inquiry made at follow-up. But mainly the parent can be helped to become aware of the similarity of developmental trajectories, a similarity that they will not usually make for themselves. Evidence that their child is making progress in this endeavor will provide confidence that the stereotypy can also become private. (It is important to see the parallel with what is allowed at home, for both the socially unacceptable patterns and stereotypy.) A first attempt at such a list is shown in Figure 11.1. However, an objection to drawing the parallel just mentioned may occur to the reader. The SMD pattern seems to be highly satisfying, whereas the to-be-suppressed behaviors described are not as distinctly and consciously pleasurable. Further work will be necessary to see if the parallel is in fact useful.

One additional feature relevant to privatization comes from follow-up on a 9-year-old boy whose parent noted that at times the child started his stereotypic pattern in public and was seen to quickly abort it by grabbing one hand with the other. This kind of progress in social suppression can be asked about on follow-up, is encouraging, and may not be otherwise valued by a parent.

Behavioral item	Date	Change (better, worse, example)	Never observed
Crotch-grabbing			
Breaking wind*			
Burping*			
Sneezing with mouth uncovered			
Coughing with mouth uncovered			
Buttock-scratching			
Comments about strangers out loud, in their presence			
Nose-picking (include actions with what is extracted)			
Coughing or sneezing with mouth uncovered			
Spontaneous action by child to abort or shorten pattern			
Other			

*Breaking wind and burping may not be completely suppressed; rather note apologies, change from total lack of awareness of effect on others, or from making a joke of it.

Note: Children with SMD often start out unselfconsciously performing their pattern anywhere, which can be embarrassing to family members, who realize that it looks strange. But stereotypy isn't the only kind of behavior you want to help become private (if not stop totally). Because privatization needs to become automatic and that requires time and awareness, we think that it should roughly follow what happens with other socially unacceptable patterns that parents and others gradually succeed in teaching children. This form is one way of documenting the course of this process and can be helpful to you, to teachers, and to involved clinicians.

Fig. 11.1. Sample form for parents of children with stereotypic movement disorder to record specific behaviors and track social shaping.

A school management issue

Can stereotypic patterns be ignored, and if so, should they be? This situation typically arises in preschool, kindergarten or the early school years. If a child is performing a pattern so as to bother another child (e.g. insert their pattern into another child's personal space, or prevent their normal activities) it is probably only a matter of time before children will complain to their parents who will complain to the school. At that point ignoring is no longer an option.

Here is some speculation on this question: (1) the child must learn to respect others' personal space and feelings (in general and with stereotypy), and increasing success should be reinforced; (2) gradually the notion of acceptable and unacceptable behaviors can be inculcated; and (3) lastly, there can be explanation about the need of all to follow school sequences and transitions (and reinforced by parents outside of school). Success with this approach will be gradual and irregular. An initial attempt at providing guidance to teachers may be found in Appendix 6.

Controversies and sources of confusion

There has been an unfortunate tendency to equate hand-flapping, the most common stereotypy, with ASD. One paper (Brasić 1999) has stated unequivocally that "hand-flapping … is uniquely seen in people with autistic disorder" (p. 49). This is clearly incorrect. Almost every parent of a child with stereotypy has had ASD mentioned to them as a diagnosis they should check out (by teachers and relatives), regardless of how socially competent the child may be. Less commonly, smelling objects other than food has also been equated with ASD.

Even the Medline Plus online medical encyclopedia service of the US National Library of Medicine (accessed July 26, 2012) lists as 'symptoms' of SMD nail-biting and mouthing of objects, which may well *not* be SMD, and confusingly states that "Tourette's syndrome and autism may also cause this disorder" (but ASD *excludes* the diagnosis of SMD!).

The diagnostic criterion for ASD, "restrictive and stereotyped patterns of behavior", causes confusion, because although this is true (by definition) one cannot logically reason backward to conclude that if a child meets one criterion, then that child has ASD, but that is what frequently happens. Here is a particularly obvious example.

Case example

'Florence' was 5 when first seen, had a typical stereotypy pattern with no comorbidity, good social development, and showed no unusual sensory patterns. In grade 1 at age 6, after being assessed by the head of pediatric neurology and by neuropsychiatry, and with good functioning in class reported by her teacher, and against the mother's wishes, the 'support teacher' nevertheless concluded that Florence might have an ASD, some neurological problem or ADHD, and should be seen by the school district's occupational therapist and psychologist (whose time was precious and in short supply).

An interesting example of a stereotypy was recently presented by Kim et al. (2013) in a rare genetic condition known as STXBP1 encephalopathy. Their three children developed one or more stereotypies after early childhood, often characterized by a 'figure of 8' head pattern that could result in muscle hypertrophy. The children did this when they were excited, happy, and sometimes bored or tired: "He often seemed happy when manifesting the stereotypy and vocalized with frequent hand sterotypies" (p. 770); "She appeared happy, smiling, and vocalizing…" (p. 771).

Case examples

'Alyssa' started prolonged body-rolling with humming vocalization in the supine position before sleep early in the first year. It could last half an hour. When seen at age 2 she could be easily called out of it. Her development was normal. Follow-up 2 years later at age 4 revealed that the pattern had completely subsided.

Comment: This is the most typical course of early body- or head-rolling or rocking. If not for the clinician's special interest becoming known, it is unlikely the pattern would have come to specialist attention.

'Emma' was 6 when first seen and had typical hand-flapping with occasional jumping when excited. Seen again at age 7 she was doing very well in school academically and was functioning well socially. She had an accepting and supportive teacher. The issue was that the stereotypy had increased and that fact was causing concern. It was not clear why there had been a change other than the increasing challenge at school. Emma wanted to talk about flapping. When asked what happened with the feeling the flapping produced if it was suppressed, she said that her mother had tried to get her to do so, and "it hurt". Her mother took this to mean a pain, but it seemed more like an unpleasant, unsatisfied urge. (The mother did not generally discourage the pattern, but recalled only that she had once tried to discourage the flapping when they had gone on a trip with some relatives.)

Comment: This case also illustrates the limited language of a young child in trying to describe feelings that are not usually the topic of discussion, and the caution that should be exercised in interpreting their explanations.

'Greg' started body-rocking well before his first birthday. At age 13 he would sometimes awaken during the night and engage in his pattern to help him fall asleep again, but have no memory of it in the morning. He would often sing phrases or parts of songs he liked while so engaged. When frustrated or excited during the day he might show some head-banging or head-shaking. Motor development had been normal and no ASD features were found on a specialized assessment. Seizures were ruled out. Although he had some oppositional behavior especially towards his mother, he showed no signs of psycho-pathology. He had recently been on sleepovers and at camp where no episodes were reported by others.

Comment: Although he did not report that he liked his pattern, the gradual pri-vatization in this case is also typical of many children with SMD, as is the absence of psychopathology.

'Glenda' developed body-rolling before sleep by age 1 year, and hand-flapping with wrist pronation/supination, finger mannerisms and facial grimacing a bit later. Possibly because of a slow-to-warm-up temperament, she was immediately suspected of ASD when she entered kindergarten. From the family aspect what was most interesting was a pattern of body-rolling or head-banging prior to sleep in the two older children and

a history of the same childhood pattern in the father, which in his case subsided in adult life.

'Joel', age 7, had a specific learning disability. At 18 months his parents had noticed repetitive movements: rubbing his hands and rotating and clenching his fists, at the same time making a hissing sound. These persisted. There were early questions about his range of emotional expression, coordination and thought processes. There was some hypotonia in toddlerhood. On psychological testing, he showed good verbal functioning but weak performance scores (35 point split). Electroencephalography showed right-sided spikes, but not an epileptic pattern. Spatial orientation was poor. The neurologist suggested 'mannerisms', not epilepsy. Confusing behavior, odd movements and learning patterns had been present for a long time. When excited during the assessment interview he showed tense movements of his hands behind his head or rotating his clenched fists in front of him. He commented that his parents didn't like them. (He showed the same patterns when watching TV.) Neither the parents nor clinicians knew how to understand these movements. They were concerned about possible teasing. (This was 25 years ago.)

  Comment: This is the story of a fairly typical SMD at a time when this was rarely recognized. The associated DCD is also common, but was not identified at that time.

'Noah', aged 11, had had cardiac surgery at age 1. At age 8 he was seen in another clinic and said to have had the onset of 'tics' at age 3, described as hand-flapping, spinning his body around, and finger-biting. He also showed some social anxiety, difficulty with focusing and clumsiness. Seen later on, and by video, he had obvious SMD that included bilateral pressing of his fists to his cheeks while waving his fingers, and he tended to bite a finger. These occurred mostly when he was excited, and did draw some attention to him. He was diagnosed with SMD, ADHD, DCD (including disorder of written expression) and social anxiety disorder. There was no evidence that he had ever had tics.

  Comment: This boy had a complex history both medically and in terms of confusing and overlapping diagnoses. The psychiatrist who first saw him missed the SMD and the DCD, but was correct about ADHD and anxiety. 'Noah' was relatively late in privatizing his stereotypies, but that may have been at least partly because his parents felt him to be more vulnerable medically and had been told that tics were involuntary.

The distinction between tics and SMD is so fundamental that there follow here a number of excellent first-person or parental descriptions that are in the public domain (lightly edited for clarity) from a non-password-protected website: www.sensory-processing-disorder.com/sons-hand-flapping-jumping-head-shaking.html#comments (accessed May 12, 2012). If you take a few minutes to read all these and to think about them, perhaps it would be useful to ask yourself: is it possible that these parents and adults have a higher level of observational capacity and conceptualization than in most available textbooks about child development, child psychiatry or neurology? Are they worth listening to? It seems that they contain many of the points made in the available literature, in a concise and believable manner. Such richness is out there, if we only look for it, on the internet and in our patients' lives.

Descriptions of SMDs in children

1. My son does do the hand flapping and jumping as well. He is 6 and is in Kindergarten. Due to the suggestion of a doctor, I have spoken to my son and advised it is ok for him to do this at home but at school he needs to work on controlling it. Kind of like burping and passing gas. This is behavior we try to control in front of people but is ok behind closed doors. I explained to him his hand flapping and jumping is not typical behavior at school. He understood and I do see he is working on controlling this. His teacher has noticed it as well. When he is at home I do let him do it but sometimes he gets too excited and I have to tell him to slow down with the jumping and hand flapping. I'm noticing it more again due to Christmas coming and all the fun and excitement happening.

2. My oldest daughter (7 years) who twirls her hair and sucks her tongue while playing or thinking or working hard at schoolwork also does the following behaviors simultaneously while playing with dolls, etc: grabs her hair near her face with her right hand, wiggles her fingers while shaking her hair, and stiffens up a bit. It is the same each time — very predictable, and she often makes a little stuttered utterance/noise while doing it. She also seems to lack a bit of control — or is it awareness? — of her noise level. The more she exhibits the behavior during a time of play, the louder she gets. It always occurs during imaginative play.

3. My 5 year old daughter has this thing that she flaps her arms and hands when excited (or sometimes I think it's random) and opens her mouth up really wide as she is flapping. I tell her "close your mouth" and she does. When she claps her hands, her mouth flies open again. It lasts usually a few seconds. Now she is old enough to get when I look at her, she closes her mouth. But she does it enough that it has concerned me. I have noticed this behavior since she was a year old. She is otherwise normal, very social, very artistic, funny, smart. It's just weird and I wanted to make sure it wasn't something I am missing or need to treat!

4. My son is 4 yrs old. I think it started around 11–12mo, or that's just when I first saw this repeating behavior. He sometimes gets hyper-excited, usually over a toy like his favorite Hot Wheels car. When he gets excited, he tucks his elbows in to his sides and quickly shakes his hands up and down, his eyes get wide, and his mouth opens wide as if he is screaming at the object. This usually only lasts for a few seconds, but can happen repeatedly every few seconds. He can stop if I call his name. Is this a condition with a name, or just something weird my son will grow out of?

5. My son turned 5 in September and had been "twisting his hands when raised" since he was 3½. He does it when excited or during imaginary play with toys such as GI Joe. If he is sitting he also shakes his legs. If I call his name he stops immediately. He tells me he is excited. He started kindergarten and some boy today told him he was a weirdo. It breaks my heart. I had him evaluated when he was 3 by the school district and brought him to a pediatric neurologist and they said it was "motor overflow" and he would grow out of it. He is an extremely bright, happy and social child. I am worried about his self-esteem when others tease him. I am a teacher and I know how cruel kids can be.

6. My son is 5 years old and is a twin. Last night he was getting ready to shower and I was watching him look at a reflection of himself in the glass. He kept flapping his arms and making this facial reaction that did not look normal. He has done this for almost 2 years now. When I ask him about it he tells me he likes to do it. His doctor says he has a tic. I believe it is not a tic. I have a video of him doing his homework and jumping up and down. He is a happy normal boy and very smart. So this is not affecting him with his schooling. He does this when he gets excited. I'm getting tired of the comments from people that say he is about to take off (like an airplane). I am sensitive to this because I'm not sure what it is and I don't know what to do.

7. We noticed my daughter hand flapping when excited around age 18 months. It didn't bother us until she was about 3 and had not stopped. I talked to the pediatrician, who suggested it was "just a habit she

would grow out of." Unfortunately this was not true. Although she is a very happy, sociable girl, she is still hand flapping when happy or excited at age 6. She has also begun contorting her face while flapping when she is VERY engrossed in her flapping pursuits! She can stop at any time you make her aware of what she's doing, but she says she likes doing it and doesn't want to stop. At age 5, she had physical/occupational therapy evaluations, and it was concluded that although she had some minor gross/fine motor delays, there was no neurological disorder present. She goes to physical/occupational therapy twice a week, and the therapists don't address the flapping at all. Her doctor still suggests she will grow out of it.

Descriptions of SMDs in adults

1. I'm a 19-year-old college student, and I've just realized that all of this applies to me, so I figured you worried parents would like some reassurance. When I was young, I would run across the room, mouth open and tongue flailing, shaking my wrists in front of my face. I would do it when I was very excited or wrapped up in my imagination. My grandmother convinced my parents to research autism, but I don't fit any other characteristics. I graduated summa cum laude in high school and I've always been plenty social. Now this is the tricky part: by "young" I mean at least through fourth grade. I went to a small private school, so no one bothered me about it, but I did it constantly and it was how I occupied myself during recess. My mind would go to some fantastic made-up world and my body had to express the energy somehow. So I flapped. My parents were understanding and didn't try to force any treatment on me, and eventually the symptoms went away. Or rather, they think they did. To be honest I realized that it was awkward and embarrassing and learned to control it. When I'm alone in my dorm, where I feel secure, I still pace and flap and go elsewhere mentally. I never told anyone that the flapping didn't stop, but the thing is, it didn't matter. I would advise you parents to let your kids go through it. I would not give up the flapping for anything; I'm an aspiring writer and it's how I create my worlds. To stop me would be like stopping the entire creative flow. I'm not saying that's a universal thing, but again, I would advise you not to worry, and most of all, not to let your child think there's something wrong with them because of it. My grandma thinking I was mental was the worst thing I'd ever felt.

2. I was a hand shaker when I got excited (and still do at certain times, I'm now 30). I would advise you just to let it be and just see it as a different side to his character. I've done it throughout my life and have had no problems interacting, making friends, I passed all my exams, have a good job etc etc and am now a father myself. I think parents are too ready to find "a cure" for something that really isn't important, to try and ensure the child is what other people perceive to be "normal".

3. My 20-year-old son has had these habits his whole life. He does a lot of pacing while he thinks, often flapping his hands and rubbing his head. When he goes to a movie he has repetitive behaviors (rubbing leg, head, eyes) during the action scenes. He is a junior in college and doing well. We did get him a single dorm room because his pacing can be extreme. This behavior doesn't bother him, just others, but he has friends and seems happy. He has learned to modify the behavior in public. I keep thinking it will lessen, but I don't see that. He has just learned to keep it more subdued in public. His older brother and younger sister had a little bit of the behavior as kids, but much less. They are all bright.

4. I thought I was the only one who did the "hand shaking" thing. For me, it was especially pronounced during my childhood. I still do it to this day (albeit privately) only when I get excited thinking about something really cool (usually car related)! I agree that it does help with deep thoughts, for sure. Usually when I'm thinking or day dreaming that I am actually there in my thoughts.

5. I'm reading this page with interest as someone who appears to have had Stereotypic Movement Disorder in my childhood or as I called it then "thinking". We had a large kitchen in which I used to run from one end to the other, shaking my hands and jumping on the spot for hours on end. Looking back I would describe the actions as a dynamo for my imagination. Whilst undertaking my "thinking" actions it seemed to enable me to think clearer, I would build houses [or] play football in my mind whilst running up and down the kitchen. No-one in the family could understand my "thinking" but accepted it and allowed me to get on with it. To put people's minds at rest I am now 30, married with a child on the way, have a bachelors degree and am a chartered Quantity Surveyor. I grew out of it but I still occasionally

shake my hands when I get excited but it is something I can control now and tend to do it when no-one is around.

6. The shaking definitely sounds a lot like what I experience. I am 23 years old now and consider myself to be normal besides the shaking. I can control it and I don't do it in public. It happens when I daydream and when I'm by myself… I actually like it because daydreaming is so much more intense.

7. To concerned parents, please don't worry. I am an attorney in my mid 20s and I, too, used to shake my fingers or other objects, like ribbons, in front of my face when I was a child. While doing this, I would often create stories in my mind and later write them down. It always felt like a creative outlet for me. My parents allowed me to do it within our home, but gently reminded me that other people may not understand it, and to refrain from "shaking" (my term for it) while in public. To this day, I still catch myself doing it sometimes, but not nearly as much as when I was young. For all the concerned parents out there, please do not think that these behaviors are automatically indicative of autism. My mother brought me to a psychologist when I was young and he determined that I was not autistic. Indeed, my "shaking" never hampered my social or intellectual growth. I am now happily married with a rewarding career. Good luck to all!

8. I do this thing with my fingers to where it looks like I'm putting a spell on you or something, LOL. Basically I put both hands and hold them a couple of inches in front of my mouth, point my fingers to where I'm looking and wiggle all my fingers really fast. Sometimes I'll even hold a pencil with my right hand's fingers and wiggle/shake it to what I'm looking at and while I'm doing this I'm imagining stuff, for example, I'll imagine me doing something cool, or beating someone up or winning the lottery or just fictitious scenarios. But I'm such a normal person, I'm 28 years old, Marine combat veteran, I'm married with 2 kids, almost done with my bachelors degree, and am on the road to becoming an officer in the military here soon. I only do it when I'm alone, my wife doesn't even know about it. I know for a fact that both of my older sisters used to do it as kids also, but I don't know if they still do or not. One of my sisters used to bounce her head face first into the pillow when she would go to bed, she would do it 20 or 30 times in a row. [Comment: a perfect description of jactatio capitis nocturna.]

9. I am a 21-year-old student at UC Berkeley. Since before I can remember, I have had a similar hand flapping experience where I close my eyes, put my hands behind my head, flap, and make weird noises. It only occurs now when I want it to in private. Usually I do it when I want to imagine something for fun (alien or ancient worlds, beautiful girls, tropical islands, etc) or when I am trying to solve something very puzzling (space, God, time, etc). When I was little I would do it while swinging in my back yard. It … brings me great comfort and therefore I see no need to change my behavior … for the most part I could be considered normal. I don't take any medication or anything and I am happier than most people I know. While your child might not be a genius, it is possible that he or she thinks better by visualizing things rather than using English words to solve problems or reflect. Of course this could be completely irrelevant to your child's situation, but none the less I would suggest that you treat your child as normal. My parents ignored my behavior, and I am very grateful. By making very little out of it, I believed that I was just like everyone else with the same opportunities.

10. I'm 22 and still do it. This blows my mind. Since I can remember, I've clenched my fists and shook them against my face whenever I got excited about something. I stopped doing it in public after being made fun of. But I grew up, learned piano and jazz by ear, went to college, made friends, learned to ski, learned to party, and moved on. That aside, I'm 22 and like everyone else here I still do it, but I can control it. I hide in my room, or lock myself in the bathroom to do it. Usually, when I get excited by something in a show, movie, book, or idea from class, I would feel so excited that I'd have to go do this and imagine it in another story I created. Example: while learning about the archaeological process in an anthropology class I took in college, I'd later imagine a very detailed story, almost a drama, about kids finding artifacts in the woods that would be complete with plot, setting, character personalities, emotion, etc.. Another example: when I first saw [futuristic movie] The Matrix, I went off and imagined a story about alternative realities, again, illustrated in my mind with full detail. Sometimes it's not about stories though. When I took some engineering classes I'd fantasize about building projects from start to finish. I'd even throw in complications that would arise that I couldn't solve until later in the fantasy.

All in all, it's a pleasurable experience. My doctor is convinced it's OCD. But I don't think it is because awhile back I saw my little cousin pace around in the backyard, clench his fist to his face, and mutter to himself. I KNEW what he was doing. He was imagining some sort of story. But since he wasn't even born when I stopped doing this in public, there's no way he could have copied my "ritual". I apologize for being long-winded, but the amount of people coming out and describing what I've been burdened with for all these years is a breath of fresh air. I'd love for this to not be labeled as ADHD or OCD. This HAS to be something different.

Practice point

One of the functions of stereotypy in persons with creative imagination seems to be to enhance their fantasy through altering their mental state. Most of them learn to keep it private and value its effects. To what extent this is similar in persons with intellectual limitations or ASD is at present unknown.

There may be no stereotypy that is pathognomonic of ASD, except perhaps using objects instead of one's own body (although adult vignette #7 above includes that feature), or atypical gazing at fingers or objects. The number of different stereotypic patterns may be higher, however, in ASD (Goldman et al. 2009).

There have been three excellent recent reviews by Singer (2009), Bonnet et al. (2010) and Singer et al. (2010). Earlier work was reviewed by us (Freeman et al. 2010), and original follow-up data on 42 children showed: (1) onset by age 3; (2) frequent confusion with ASD (especially because of hand-flapping) and Tourette syndrome (because of frequently co-occurring facial grimacing and vocalizations), occasionally with epilepsy; (3) in most cases the pattern remained largely the same over time, was associated with pleasurable excitement, and gradually became more private with maturation and therefore lost its possibly socially stigmatizing effects; (4) comorbidity was frequent, with ADHD and DCD being the most common (16/42), followed by tics (18/42). Eleven children met criteria for Tourette syndrome at some point. In almost one-third there was a positive family history of stereotypy. The Johns Hopkins Pediatric Neurology group has been especially active in this area. Mahone et al. (2004) focused on upper-limb stereotypies and later this team did a more extensive chart review (Harris et al. 2008). Imaging abnormalities were found in a subgroup of their cases and some were treated with behavioral methods (Miller et al. 2006). In 2010 they set up a website on the topic (www.hopkinsmedicine.org/neurology_neurosurgery/specialty_areas/pedsneuro/conditions/motor-stereotypies), which is probably the most elaborate and informative of any. It includes information for parents and clinicians about SMD [termed 'primary (non-autistic) motor stereotypies'] and their ongoing research projects.

Because of the importance of their work, it is appropriate here to mention some differences in their tentative conclusions and ours, to be resolved by means of ongoing research and follow-up. (Other than these, the majority of the descriptions and conclusions, arrived at independently, are identical.) Points of difference include

• Advisability of behavioural therapy: why, if the pattern is 'harmless'? Just because parents are anxious?

• Referral of children to a pediatric neurologist (expensive, limited access)

- No mention whatever of privatization, perhaps the most significant difference; and how that occurs (same as Ghosh et al. 2013)
- Inclusion of hearing impairment with visual impairment is wrong and based upon flawed reading of the very limited research reports
- They mention confusion with tics and OCD, but not with the very important ASD.

Aspects of SMD that were not considered in our SMD paper include: (1) variations in the intensity and frequency of the SMD pattern over time; (2) what else might be included under the broad category of SMD, other than flapping, pacing, running, bouncing, pressing and hand mannerisms; (3) relationship to sensory factors and DCD; (4) what to explain to schools (see Appendix 3); (5) the significance of comorbidity patterns (ADHD, SLD, etc.); and (6) a possible connection with adults who engage in excessive fantasizing (see below).

Excessive fantasy and imagery, some with stereotypy
After the first draft of this chapter was written, a paper was submitted by Robinson et al. (2014) about a subgroup of SMD children with "intense imagery" where the outcome may not be as positive as the examples presented in the chapter indicate. Based upon the possibility that some of these children may as adults become "compulsive fantasizers" as described by Bigelsen and Schupak (2011), they recommend preventive anticipatory interference with triggers or performance situations. This is an important consideration, but there is as yet no direct evidence to support this; only 79% of the Bigelsen and Schupak group of 90 self-selected adults had accompanying 'kinesthetic' movement patterns that seem like those described in this chapter, and 12% reported no distress or impairment. The patients in the submitted paper had normal MRI scans, which was not the case with those who were reported by the Johns Hopkins group (Miller et al. 2006). We do not yet know the relative proportion of either subgroup. Both Bigelsen and Schupak and Robinson and co-workers offer very significant insights and possibilities for the future. They both in complementary ways extend the work reported by us in Freeman et al. (2010). Commentary on these points has been presented (Freeman 2014). A last comment regards a different problem: who decides for others (still children) how much is too much and how their different activities should be apportioned? Some of the adults presented seem troubled not so much by impairment as by their own or anticipated attitudes of others, which could be culture- and time-bound. For example, one had a highly ambivalent attitude that the mental/emotional state he reached in fantasy was the best feeling and also the worst. It is possible that if we reach the point when we think we have enough knowledge to identify the subgroup of SMD children who are at risk of becoming 'compulsive' fantasizers we would face other difficult questions about whom to treat, when, for what reasons, and in what way. We should remember that there are other activities that can be excessive as judged by society, parents or clinicians (such as video gaming currently).

Aspects that may merit further research
There are many largely (or completely) neglected features of SMD that are appropriate targets for attention. Included here are possibilities arising from the Houdayer et al. (2014) research report.

- How and at what point in development can one's SMD be substituted in public by a common repetitive motor behavior?
- How successfully can children perform a truncated form of their pattern that is less visible to others in a social situation, or even done only in imagination?
- Further elaboration of 'need', 'urge' and other feelings associated, and changes over the course of development.
- How to best explain to your child the desirability of eventually privatizing the behavior, and the practical and unavoidable costs of not doing so, in such a way as to minimize feelings of rejection.
- Relationship with DCD.
- Comorbidity, its frequency and significance.
- At least seven subgroups could be compared: (1) older children who continue their pattern without impairment (not interfering with other desirable activities), and (2) the few who do have impairment; (3) cognitively normal blind children and adults who have privatized their stereotypy; and (4) those who have not and continue in public; (5) parents of children with SMD with a clear history of their own SMD and who continue it; and (6) those parents who no longer perform it; and (7) adults who are successfully creative now (musicians, writers, composers), whether they enhance their creativity with repetitive movements, and whether their movements are like anything they did in childhood. As Houdayer and co-workers indicate, similar study of 'secondary' stereotypies, as in ASD, is warranted. In addition to neurophysiologic procedures, standardized questions should be employed in taking histories and descriptions from (and about) these individuals.

Behavior therapy

An important paper (Ricketts et al. 2013) illustrates how behavior therapy can be applied in selected cases where interference with activities is significant and automatic reinforcement is postulated as maintaining the pattern. The treatment, beyond that described by Miller et al. (2006), included competing response training, as is also a component of CBIT for tics, and function-based assessment. The three case descriptions are very helpful in showing how the treatment can be applied, and also detailed the types of behaviors we have found (Freeman et al. 2010). During the treatment period, efforts by the patients to stop the pattern were observed, as well as substitution by a less obvious pattern. There were indications of a premonitory sensation or of a felt need to do it, but also a greater awareness after stopping the movements than before starting. A relevant question is whether those children who are aware of a premonitory sensation are easier to treat (perhaps because of a difference in motivation) than those who do not.

The combination of stereotypic movement disorder and tics

One final very important point needs to be made: *persons with persistent tic disorders may have other movement patterns, including SMD, which are obscured by the presence (and identification) of their tics.* This may occur because (as with RMBs) such a pattern (often single) is lumped in with tics. Once tics are identified and diagnosed, the tics tend to trump other patterns. The reverse is also sometimes true: *tics may be obscured and not recognized in persons with stereotypy.* The clinician may be unaware of this point, may not listen closely enough to the history, or may not ask the right questions. This might account for the persons with tics who report (when asked) that they *like* some of their 'tics'. More important, the stereotypy may not respond to either medication or CBIT therapy. This is an opportunity for further research.

Important concept and practice point

One or more stereotypy patterns of the SMD type may be mixed with tics and then missed as different from them. This may account for some treatment refractoriness and should always be considered as a possibility. The reverse may also occur.

REFERENCES

Barry S, Baird G, Lascelles K, et al. (2011) Neurodevelopmental movement disorders – an update on childhood motor stereotypies. *Dev Med Child Neurol* 53: 979–85. doi: 10.1111/j.1469-8749.2011.04058.x.

Bigelsen J, Schupak C (2011) Compulsive fantasy: proposed evidence of an under-reported syndrome through a systematic study of 90 self-identified non-normative fantasizers. *Consciousness Cogn* 20: 1634–48. doi: 10.1016/j.concog.2011.08.013.

Bonnet C, Roubertie A, Doummar D, et al. (2010) Developmental and benign movement disorders in childhood. *Mov Disord* 25: 1317–34. doi: 10.1002/mds.22944.

Brasić JR (1999) Movements in autistic disorder. *Med Hypotheses* 53: 48–9.

Edwards MJ, Lang AE, Bhatia KP (2012) Stereotypies: a critical appraisal and suggestion of a clinically useful definition. *Mov Disord* 27: 179–85. doi: 10.1002/mds.23994.

Freeman RD (2014) Treatment for stereotypic movement disorder: a case for Procrustes? *Dev Med Child Neurol* 56: 1139–40. doi: 10.111/dmcn.12538.

Freeman RD, Fast DK, Burd L, et al. (2000) An international perspective on Tourette syndrome: selected findings from 3500 individuals in 22 countries. *Dev Med Child Neurol* 42: 436–7. doi: 10.1111/j.1469-8749. 2000.tb00346.x.

Freeman RD, Soltanifar A, Baer S (2010) Stereotypic movement disorder: easily missed. *Dev Med Child Neurol* 52: 733–8. doi: 10.1111/j.1469-8749.2010.03627.x.

Gao S, Singer HS (2013) Complex motor stereotypies: an evolving neurobiological concept. *Future Neurol* 8: 273–85. doi: 10.2217/fnl.13.4.

Ghosh D, Rajan PV, Erenberg G (2013) A comparative study of primary and secondary stereotypies. *J Child Neurol* 28: 1562–8. doi: 10.1177/0883073812464271.

Goldman S, Wang C, Salgado MW, et al. (2009) Motor stereotypies in children with autism and other developmental disorders. *Dev Med Child Neurol* 51: 30–8. doi: 10.1111/j.1469-8749.2008.03178.x.

Grant J, Stein D, Woods D, Keuthen NJ, eds (2012) *Trichotillomania, Skin-Picking, and Other Body-Focused Repetitive Behaviors.* Arlington, VA: American Psychiatric Publishing.

Harris KM, Mahone EM, Singer HS (2008) Nonautistic motor stereotypies: clinical features and longitudinal follow-up. *Pediatr Neurol* 38: 267–72. doi: 10.1016/j.pediatrneurol.2007.12.008.

Hoban TF (2004) Sleep and its disorders in children. *Semin Neurol* 24: 327–40. doi: 10.1055/s-2004-835062.

Houdayer E, Walthall J, Belluscio BA, et al. (2014) Absent movement-related cortical potentials in children with primary motor stereotypies. *Mov Disord* 29: 1134–40. doi: 10.1002/mds.25753.

Kates WR, Lanham DC, Singer HS (2005) Frontal white matter reductions in healthy males with complex stereotypies. *Pediatr Neurol* 32: 109–12. doi: 10.1016/j.pediatrneurol.2004.09.005.

Kim YO, Korff CM, Villaluz MMG, et al. (2013) Head stereotypies in STXBP1 encephalopathy. *Dev Med Child Neurol* 55: 769–72. doi: 10.1111/dmcn.12197.

Mahone EM, Bridges D, Prahme C, Singer HS (2004) Repetitive arm and hand movements (complex motor stereotypies) in children. *J Pediatr* 145: 391–5. doi: 10.1016/j.peds.2004.06.014.

Mahone EM, Ryan M, Ferenc L, et al. (2014) Neuropsychological function in children with primary complex motor stereotypies. *Dev Med Child Neurol* 56: 1001–8. doi: 10.1111/dmcn.12480.

Mason G, Rushen J, eds (2006) *Stereotypic Animal Behavior: Fundamentals and Applications to Welfare, 2nd edn.* Wallingford (UK)/Cambridge, MA (USA): Commonwealth Agricultural Bureaux International.

Mayer G, Wilde-Frenz J, Kurella B (2007) Sleep related rhythmic movement disorder revisited. *J Sleep Res* 16: 110–6. doi: 10.1111/j.1365-2869.2007.00577.x.

McGrath CM, Kennedy RE, Hoye W, Yablon SA (2002) Stereotypic movement disorder after acquired brain injury. *Brain Injury* 16: 447–51. doi: 10.1080/02699050110113660.

Miller JM, Singer HS, Bridges DD, Waranch HR (2006) Behavioral therapy for treatment of stereotypic movements in nonautistic children. *J Child Neurol* 21: 119–25. doi: 10.1177/08830738060210020701.

Muthugovindan D, Singer H (2009) Motor stereotypy disorders. *Curr Opin Neurol* 22: 131–6. doi: 10.1097/WCO.0b013e328326f6c8.

Oakley C, Mahone EM, Morris-Berry C, et al. (2014) Primary complex motor stereotypies in older children and adolescents: clinical features and longitudinal follow-up. *Pediatr Neurol*, published online December 18. doi: 10.1016/j.pediatrneurol.2014.11.002.

Rapp JT, Vollmer TR (2005a) Stereotypy. I: A review of behavioral assessment and treatment. *Res Dev Disabil* 26: 527–47. doi: 10.1016/j.ridd.2004.11.005.

Rapp JT, Vollmer TR (2005b) Stereotypy. II: A review of neurobiological interpretations and suggestions for an integration with behavioral methods. *Res Dev Disabil* 26: 548–64. doi: 10.1016/j.ridd.2004.11.006.

Ricketts EJ, Bauer CC, Van der Fluit F, et al. (2013) Behavior therapy for stereotypic movement disorder in typically developing children: a clinical case series. *Cog Behav Pract* 20: 544–55. doi: 10.1016/j.cbprac.2013.03.002.

Robinson S, Woods M, Cardona F, et al. (2014) Intense imagery movements (IIM): a common and distinct paediatric subgroup of motor stereotypies. *Dev Med Child Neurol* 56: 1212–8. doi: 10.1111/dmcn.12518.

Singer HS (2009) Motor stereotypies. *Semin Pediatr Neurol* 16: 77–81. doi: 10.1016/j.spen.2009.03.008.

Singer HS (2013) Motor control, habits, complex motor stereotypies, and Tourette syndrome. *Ann NY Acad Sci* 1304: 22–31. doi: 10.1111/nyas.12281.

Singer HS, Mink JW, Gilbert DL, Jankovic J (2010) *Movement Disorders in Childhood.* Philadelphia: Saunders/Elsevier.

Stepanova I, Nevsimalova S, Hanusova J (2005) Rhythmic movement disorder in sleep persisting into childhood and adulthood. *Sleep* 28: 851–7.

Temudo T, Levy A, Barbot C, et al. (2007) Stereotypies in Rett syndrome: analysis of 83 patients with and without detected *MECP2* mutations. *Neurology* 68: 1183–7.

12
SYMPTOMS AND PATTERNS

A variety of behavioral patterns has been described and, probably because of comorbidity, some have become attached to the image of Tourette syndrome with or without good evidence. In those patients in the *TIC* database who have no comorbidity ('TS-only'), rates of problem behaviours are relatively low. With comorbidity ('TS+'), the picture changes: most patterns increase in direct relationship to extent of comorbidity (Freeman et al. 2000).

In Table 12.1, one can clearly see that there are marked increases in the proportion of TS+ versus TS-only children for anger control problems and sleep problems. TS+ children are about twice as likely to have received medication for tics and to have had pre- or peri-natal problems. Although not included in the table because patient numbers are insufficient, similar trends show increases in the TS+ group for SIB, social skill deficits and coprophenomena. In adults, the main differences are for SIB, anger control problems, social skill deficits, sleep problems and coprophenomena (numbers again being too low for statistical comparison).

Anger/'rage'/aggression

> Anger, 'rage' and aggression are not symptoms of TS-only, rather of TS+. This behavior is the one most strongly related to the extent of comorbidity. More common in those with anger control problems are: ADHD, conduct disorder/ODD, mood disorder, tricho-tillomania, coprophenomena, spitting, rocking, and sexually inappropriate behavior, indicating that those with anger control problems and aggression are likely to be further compromised by their other disorders.

Much has been made about 'rage' in Tourette syndrome. Some have claimed that 'tourettic rage' is special, but no one has been able to confirm this. The conventional description is of minimal provocation, sudden escalation of severe behavior, and long duration (up to 2 hours). Budman (2006), Budman et al. (2003, 2008) and Chen et al. (2013) have shown that this pattern is strongly related to comorbidity. Our own *TIC* study (Freeman et al. 2000) has demonstrated this as well (see Tables 12.1, 12.2).

In the *TIC* database, anger control problems in children at the time of registration were almost four times as likely to occur in TS+ as in TS-only (22% vs 5%). This was a highly significant finding (p<0.001, OR 3.7). Other strong associations are with conduct disor-der/ODD (OR 5.2), ADHD (OR 3.2), sexually inappropriate behavior (OR 4.1), social skill

TABLE 12.1

Differences between TS-only and TS+ children (*TIC* data, n=5197)

	TS-only (n=872)		TS+ (n=4325)		p	Odds ratio
	n	%	n	%		
Female sex	200	22.6	669	15.3	<0.001	1.5
Medication for tics (ever)	296	33.9	2175	50.3	<0.001	1.8
Pre-/perinatal problems	108	13.1	805	20.7	<0.001	1.6
Sleep problems (now)	81	9.3	883	20.8	<0.001	2.3
Anger (now)	76	8.7	1360	32.3	<0.001	4.1

Excluded: intellectual disability, autism spectrum disorder and psychosis.

TABLE 12.2

Anger control problems in children (*TIC* data, n=5083)

	Without problems (n=3647)		With problems (n=1436)		p	Odds ratio
	n	%	n	%		
Female sex	642	18	203	14	0.003	1.3
Medication for tics (ever)	1578	44	783	55	<0.001	1.6
Pre-/perinatal problems	593	18	278	22	0.008	1.2
TS-only	799	22	76	5	<0.001	3.7
ADHD	1856	51	1102	77	<0.001	3.2
OCD	577	16	321	22	<0.001	1.5
SLD	770	21	422	29	<0.001	1.6
Mood disorder	304	8	246	17	<0.001	2.3
Anxiety disorder	522	14	283	20	<0.001	1.5
CD/ODD	259	7	407	28	<0.001	5.2
Sleep problems (now)	537	15	426	30	<0.001	2.4
Sexually inappropriate behavior (ever)	72	2	118	9	<0.001	4.1
SIB (ever)	336	9	302	21	<0.001	2.6
Social skill deficits (now)	362	10	437	30	<0.001	4.0
Coprophenomena	312	9	251	18	<0.001	2.3

Excluded: intellectual disability, autism spectrum disorder and psychosis.
ADHD, attention-deficit/hyperactivity disorder; OCD, obsessive–compulsive disorder; SLD, specific learning disability; CD/ODD, conduct disorder/oppositional-defiant disorder; SIB, self-injurious behavior.
There were no significant associations with nail-biting, nose-picking, bruxism, joint-cracking, smelling or lip-licking.

deficits (OR 4.0), mood disorder (OR 2.3) and SIB (OR 2.6). Of all the symptoms investigated in Tourette syndrome, anger control problems have the steepest slope in association with degree of comorbidity. It is clear from these data that children with anger control problems are likely to have a variety of associated problems that will require attention. This is another example of a transdiagnostic symptom that does not 'belong' to any diagnostic category.

In adults, *TIC* database findings are similar to those in children, with a three times greater likelihood of comorbidity and strong associations with conduct disorder/ODD,

ADHD, sleep disorder, skin-picking, SIB, weak social skills and sexually inappropriate behavior.

Practice point

Children and adults with anger control problems have a high risk of other troublesome symptoms, mostly related to weak impulse control and self-regulation.

An interesting study by Carlson et al. (2009) showed that 'rages' were closely associated with ADHD comorbidity. When admitted to an inpatient psychiatric unit for this specific symptom, only half showed 'rages', suggesting that these behaviors might be context-specific. Bipolar disorder was not common among these. Their conclusion was that "the combination of impulsivity and low frustration tolerance from severe ADHD and the inability to process and express frustration because of learning and language problems initiate and perpetuate rages" (p. 286).

Similarly, the important study by Roy et al. (2013) showed that children referred for impairing temper outbursts did not have early bipolar disorder, rather comorbidity (often ADHD, ODD, anxiety and/or depression) with weak frustration regulation. Anger control problems overlap the new DSM-5 category of disruptive mood dysregulation disorder, which has stimulated some controversy because of its overlap with several other disorders (McGough 2014). Another way to think of it is as chronic non-episodic irritability in childhood (see the section on mood disorders in Chapter 10, and Roy et al. 2014).

TREATMENT

The clinician dealing with highly comorbid Tourette syndrome should expect a large proportion of such children to manifest anger control problems or aggression, including those that can be termed 'rage'. Pharmacologic treatment can be challenging, and a wide variety of medications have been used. The 'impulsive–affective type' is more likely to respond favorably to medication than those termed 'controlled–predatory' (Budman 2006).

An excellent manualized CBT program for excessive anger and aggression in children (including a detailed portion for parents) has been provided by Sukhodolsky and Scahill (2012). They had previously published a report on their treatment program for children with such problems (Sukhodolsky et al. 2009).

Another program with evidence of efficacy was developed by Hanisch et al. (2014) in Germany and is known as the PEP (Prevention Program for Externalizing Problem Behavior). In a randomized controlled trial, most effective in improving child behavior were reductions in dysfunctional parental reactions in difficult situations and improvement in their parenting skills.

Sleep problems

Sleep problems are a common complaint in Tourette syndrome, especially in children, but their relationship with tics is complex. Disturbed sleep can mimic or worsen ADHD and mood symptoms, and stimulant treatment of ADHD and use of TV or electronic devices can interfere with sleep initiation. These problems are especially important during the adolescent school years, when inadequate sleep is almost universal.

Although there is still a general idea that Tourette syndrome 'causes' sleep problems, it has been established long ago that this is largely attributable to comorbid ADHD (Allen et al. 1992). However, there are still some puzzles about the entire question of whether sleep problems are more common than in the general population. Surveys via parent questionnaires show that they are, but objective studies do not reliably confirm this, even for ADHD without tics. Methodological problems abound. In addition, do tics occur in sleep? Generally parents do not mention this, and if asked they say no. Objective sleep studies contradict this generalization. In this section we will overlook these unsettled issues and accept that sleep problems of some sort are very common generally, and ignore presently unreliable prevalence figures.

Up-to-date reviews of this entire problem have recently been published (Stein et al. 2012, Yoon et al. 2012), and include consideration of study methodology and sleep problems associated with pharmacotherapy. Factors in individual variation remain poorly understood. The relationship of sleep problems to ADHD (and therefore also to tic disorders) remains problematic. An excellent review of sleep disorders in general has been provided by Mindell and Owens (2010).

Recently a position statement of multiple organizations has comprehensively reviewed the field of pediatric sleep and provided access to questionnaires and handouts for clinicians, parents and adolescents (Gruber et al. 2014).

In ASD, sleep problems are highly prevalent (rates of 40% to 80%) (Johnson et al. 2009).

An important general population study of young children by Petit et al. (2007) has provided prevalence figures for parasomnias and dyssomnias. Difficulty falling asleep at night decreased significantly with age from 16% at age 3.5–4 years to 10% at age 5 and 7.4% at age 6. Somnambulism occurred in 14.5%, sleep terrors in 40%, bruxism in 45.6% and rhythmic movements (head-banging and body-rolling) in 9.2%. There is no reason to believe that the corresponding figures in Tourette syndrome would be any lower.

Practice point
Sleep problems are common and should be assessed in every evaluation and follow-up.

Storch et al. (2009) found that sleep-related problems were widely experienced (80% with at least one problem and 20% with four or more). Anxiety disorder was positively related

TABLE 12.3
Sleep problems related to diagnoses and behavior in children (*TIC* data, n=5112)

	Without problems (n=4148)		With problems (n=964)		p	Odds ratio
	n	%	n	%		
ADHD	2331	56	656	68	<0.001	1.6
OCD	703	17	211	22	<0.001	1.4
Anxiety disorder	583	14	225	23	<0.001	1.3
Mood disorder	424	10	137	14	<0.001	1.5
ODD/CD	524	18	168	17	<0.001	1.9
SLD	932	23	264	27	<0.001	1.5
Pre-/perinatal problems	668	19	207	23	<0.001	1.4
Medication for tics (ever)	1957	48	444	46	ns	—
Anger (now)	1008	25	426	44	<0.001	2.4
SIB (ever)	457	11	190	20	<0.001	2.0
Coprophenomena (ever)	461	11	117	12	ns	—
Social skill deficits (now)	586	14	224	23	<0.001	1.8
Sexually inappropriate behavior	131	4	59	6	<0.001	1.8

Excluded: intellectual disability, autism spectrum disorder and psychosis.
ADHD, attention-deficit/hyperactivity disorder; OCD, obsessive–compulsive disorder; ODD/CD, opposi-
tional-defiant disorder/conduct disorder; SLD, specific learning disability; SIB, self-injurious behavior; ns,
non-significant.

to sleep disorder, as were internalizing and externalizing behaviors.

During upsurges of tics sleep onset may be more difficult, especially if the tics are complex or involve large-amplitude movements. Children may be more likely to be upset about
their previous day's experience (including teasing), and some may have increased anxiety
or obsessive–compulsive symptoms co-occurring. Parents who are still unsure about or
inexperienced with their child's tics may not know how to comfort their children at night.

In the *TIC* database, sleep problems at the time of registration were reported to be 2.5
times as common in TS+ as in TS-only children (21.3% vs 9.4%, p<0.001, OR 2.3). At a
comorbidity score level of 5 the mean prevalence of sleep problems was 34%. In children
with sleep problems the strongest associations were with ADHD, non-OCD anxiety disorder,
neurologic disorder, anger control problems, SIB and social skill deficits. These findings
are summarized in Table 12.3. In adults, the strongest associations were with anger control
problems, SIB, trichotillomania, ADHD, non-OCD anxiety disorder, coprophenomena,
mood disorders, stuttering and specific learning disorder.

SLEEP PROBLEMS IN ATTENTION-DEFICIT/HYPERACTIVITY DISORDER

A quarter to a half of children and more than half of adults with ADHD are reported to
suffer from sleep problems. It is unclear whether sleep problems are intrinsic to ADHD,
comorbid with ADHD, or misdiagnosed (cause ADHD-like symptoms). Objective methods
have yielded inconsistent results in both children and adults. This enduring problem is due
to varied methodologies, study conditions, and the very nature of ADHD itself (Yoon et al.
2012). Of patients with ADHD, 20% to 37% suffer from depression and 32% from anxiety,

both of which can present ADHD-like symptoms. Memory consolidation can be impaired by sleep disorder. Inconsistency in studies complicates determination of the effects of ADHD medication on sleep. The relationship is highly complex.

In preadolescent children bedtime resistance is reported to occur in 27% and sleep-onset delays in 11%. In adolescence, the average length of sleep declines from 9 hours to 7.9 hours, and daytime sleepiness increases. Delayed bedtime on non-school nights and later waking time become much more common, and conflict with parents over timely awakening on school mornings increases. The common adolescent sleep restriction on school nights has been shown to worsen mood and decrease the ability to regulate negative emotions after only a few nights (Baum et al. 2014).

Before medication is considered, sleep 'hygiene' needs to be investigated, including bedtime routine, i.e. activities allowed close to bedtime, unrestricted use of computer or video games (especially in the bedroom), sleep schedule, sleep environment, and behavioral limit-setting (Hoban 2004).

Many children and families fail to report sleep problems because they are so used to the problems that they simply expect to put up with them. This can include mild cases of restless legs syndrome (see case example below).

RESTLESS LEGS SYNDROME (WILLIS–EKBOM DISEASE)

Restless legs syndrome — renamed Willis–Ekbom disease in 2011 — occurs in children and adolescents (about 3%) as well as adults (about 10%). In the following discussion, I use the old name as many clinicians may not be familiar with the new one. The symptoms may be difficult for children to describe. International criteria for children were established in 2003 and revised by integrating them with the adult criteria (Picchietti et al. 2013). Studies in ADHD have been reported (Picchietti et al. 1998, Chervin et al. 2002). Further epidemiologic information has been synthesized by Ohayon et al. (2012). Low serum ferritin levels may be a factor (Picchietti and Picchietti 2010). Current criteria are given in the box below, and further information may be found in Picchietti et al. (2013). RLS is more common in children with ADHD, and therefore may also be in Tourette syndrome because of the high rate of co-occurrence (Picchietti et al. 1998, Kotagal and Silber 2004). These symptoms may prevent sleep onset and be perceived as insomnia or a bedtime behavior problem (Yilmaz et al. 2011). A large population-based study (Picchietti et al. 2007) showed a prevalence of 2% in children and adolescents, without sex differences. In over 70% at least one parent had the same symptoms, and in 16% both parents. A history of 'growing pains' was obtained in 81%. This is an important study, for this condition is considered to be under-diagnosed.

Diagnostic criteria for restless legs syndrome/Willis–Ekbom disease

Restless legs syndrome, a neurological sensorimotor disorder often profoundly disturbing sleep, is diagnosed by ascertaining a syndrome that consists of all of the following features.

1. An urge to move the legs usually but not always accompanied by or felt to be caused by uncomfortable and unpleasant sensations in the legs.

2. The urge to move the legs and any accompanying unpleasant sensations begin or worsen during periods of rest or inactivity such as lying down or sitting.

3. The urge to move the legs and any accompanying unpleasant sensations are partially or totally relieved by movement, such as walking or stretching, at least as long as the activity continues.

4. The urge to move the legs and any accompanying unpleasant sensations during rest or inactivity only occur in the evening or at night, or are worse at those times than during the day.

5. The above features are not solely accounted for as symptoms primary to another medical or behavioral condition (e.g. myalgia, venous stasis, leg edema, arthritis, leg cramps, positional discomfort, habitual foot tapping).

Specifier for clinical significance of restless legs syndrome
The symptoms of RLS cause significant distress or impairment in social, occupational, educational, or other important areas of functioning by the impact upon sleep, energy/ vitality, daily activities, behavior, cognition or mood.

Specifier for clinical course of restless legs syndrome
• *Chronic–persistent RLS:* symptoms when not treated would occur on average at least twice weekly for the past year.
• *Intermittent RLS:* symptoms when not treated would occur on average less than twice per week for the past year, with at least five lifetime events.

Special considerations for the diagnosis of pediatric restless legs syndrome
• The child must describe the RLS symptoms in his or her own words.
• The diagnostician should be aware of the typical words children and adolescents use to describe RLS.
• Language and cognitive development determine the applicability of the RLS diagnostic criteria, rather than age.
• It is not known if the adult specifiers for clinical course apply to pediatric RLS.
• As in adults, a significant impact on sleep, mood, cognition and function is found. However, impairment is manifest more often in behavioral and educational domains
• Simplified and updated research criteria for probable and possible pediatric RLS are available.
• Periodic limb movement disorder may precede the diagnosis of RLS in some cases.

Case example
'Ethan' was 10 when first seen. Aside from numerous behavioral problems, Tourette syndrome, ADHD features, sleep problems and many sensory sensitivities, there was a family history of several neurodevelopmental difficulties. Later he was diagnosed with high-functioning ASD and DCD and there was a long history of losing energy after

brief activities. His mother has a history of RLS and iron deficiency. Referred for a biochemical disease consultation, 'Ethan' was found to have 'growing pains' and dyskinetic toes at rest, along with relatively low ferritin and normal iron. A trial of iron supplementation was instituted.

*   **Comment:** *The diagnosis of RLS is not always simple, and can even be missed by clinicians who are aware of it. In this case, the history of poor sleep, lack of energy and a family history suggestive of similar problems in his mother raises the possibility of this diagnosis.*

Looked at from the other side, how likely are children diagnosed with RLS to have psychiatric disorders? Pullen et al. (2011) reviewed 374 RLS cases and found 64% had at least one disorder: ADHD in 25%, mood disturbances in 29%, anxiety disorders in 11.5%, and behavioral disturbances in 10.9%.

Associations with Tourette syndrome are not yet well established. The most recent study (Lespérance et al. 2004) of a clinical group of 114 children showed a prevalence of RLS of 10% of probands with Tourette syndrome or persistent tic disorder, 21% of their mothers and 25% of their fathers. RLS was not correlated with the presence of ADHD or OCS, and the gender distribution was equal. It therefore seems that RLS should be considered a more than rare comorbidity of chronic tic disorders and inquiry should therefore be made.

PERIODIC LIMB MOVEMENTS IN SLEEP (PLMS)

These are frequent brief, repetitive jerks of the limbs during sleep, and may be associated with changes in cardiac function and blood pressure. Awareness of these may be absent until someone sleeps in the same bed with the patient. In a study by Gingras et al. (2011), 66 cases were identified out of 468 referred children (14%) in a single pediatric sleep practice. Correlations were found with disturbed sleep, leg discomfort, parasomnias, and family history of RLS. This condition is still relatively under-studied in children. Voderholzer et al. (1997) used polysomnography to study a group of seven children with Tourette syndrome, finding PLMS in five of them. What are often called 'growing pains' may be a form of PLMS (Wong et al. 2014).

Practice point
Children have a hard time describing their uncomfortable sensations, so they may term it 'pain', reported as such by their parent. But if given the choice between 'pain like other pains' and 'weird feelings' at bedtime, they typically choose the latter.

TREATMENT

Given the many forms that sleep disorders can take, a generalization is that assessment should be first, with medication a last resort (melatonin may be an exception, and may need to be tried in a desperate situation before a complex picture can be fully understood;

melatonin is not patentable as a drug, and in the USA is not regulated by the Food and Drug Administration. Disorders and medical problems that may co-occur with sleep disorders need to be taken into account. Environmental factors, significant previous ways of dealing with sleep problems, and habits that can be involved should be identified. Useful books for children's problems include that by Owens and Mindell (2005), and a companion pair of therapist guide and parent workbook by Durand (2008a,b). The latter workbook for parents includes a sleep diary, sleep scale, behavior log forms and bed-wetting recording sheet forms.

Social skill deficits

Social skill deficits are a very common complaint, but it is not easy to determine and analyze the causative factors, which must be many. Weak social skills with peers may not be evident when a child relates to an adult. The disorders most associated with weak social skills are ADHD, ODD, mood and anxiety disorders, SLD and DCD, as well as the obvious ASD and moderate intellectual disability. Thus, social skill deficits are 'transdiagnostic', not limited to any diagnostic category. Anger control problems and sexually inappropriate behavior were most strongly correlated. In the *TIC* database, only 4% of TS-only children were rated as having weak social skills, compared with 19% of those with TS+. There are many social development programs but none is acknowledged as pre-eminent.

This is one of the most difficult areas of work with young people. Complaints of poor social skills abound, examples being rejection by peers, not knowing how to enter a group, going too far, and poor reading of social cues. As adults, we may find a child or adolescent engaging and even delightful when his or her peers do not. The very qualities that provoke positive reactions in adults may be negative for peers, but can we actually understand the components involved, developmentally? Can we derive helpful information, as adults, from other adults (parents, teachers), that can shed light on the problem? Are therapeutic or social skills groups doing more than offering socialization opportunities (specifically, providing diagnostic information)? There are no good general answers to these questions.

Aside from ensuring socialization opportunities, reasonable nonspecific measures include preventing or expeditiously reducing adverse influences such as teasing, bullying and misunderstandings by working with parents and school staff.

In the *TIC* database (Freeman et al. 2000, Freeman 2007), social skill deficits were noted to be over five times as common in children with TS+ as in those with TS-only (19% vs 4%, p<0.001, OR 5.1). As was previously noted, these deficits are much more commonly found in association with the comorbid disorders of conduct disorder/ODD, ADHD, mood and anxiety disorders, SLD and DCD. The associated behaviors are inappropriate sexual behavior, anger control problems, rocking, skin-picking and spitting, followed closely by coprophenomena and SIB: details are given in Table 12.4.

Carter et al. (2000) found that TS+ADHD accounted for more of the internalizing and externalizing behavior problems as compared with TS-only. Kim et al. (2012) and Borda et

TABLE 12.4
Social skill problems in children (*TIC* data, n=5247)

	Without problems (n=4409)		With problems (n=838)		*p*	Odds ratio
	n	*%*	*n*	*%*		
Female sex	766	17	103	12	<0.001	1.5
Medication (ever)	2019	46	452	55	<0.001	1.4
Pre-/perinatal problems	739	19	174	24	<0.001	1.4
ADHD	2421	55	673	80	<0.001	3.3
OCD	740	17	210	25	<0.001	1.7
SLD	894	20	334	40	<0.001	2.6
Mood disorder	444	10	144	17	<0.001	1.9
Anxiety disorder	641	15	189	23	<0.001	1.7
CD/ODD	476	11	244	29	<0.001	3.4
Sleep (now)	740	17	224	28	<0.001	1.8
Anger (now)	999	23	437	55	<0.001	4.0
SIB	504	11	167	20	<0.001	1.9
Sexually inappropriate behavior	110	3	80	11	<0.001	4.1

Excluded: intellectual disability, autism spectrum disorder and psychosis.
ADHD, attention-deficit/hyperactivity disorder; OCD, obsessive–compulsive disorder; SLD, specific learning disability; CD/ODD, conduct disorder/oppositional-defiant disorder; SIB, self-injurious behavior.

al. (2013) found that children with OCD had poorer social skills and consequently poorer peer relationships. Lewin et al. (2012) found that adult women who still had symptoms of Tourette syndrome (as compared with men) suffered from reduced quality of life including impaired social functioning and relationships.

A question still remains as to whether social impairment in persons with persistent tic disorders is due to a neurologic abnormality or their experiences of social rejection and stigmatization.

Coprophenomena

> The anticipatory fear parents have of future coprophenomena is often worse than the reality. This is because moderating factors aren't sufficiently appreciated and are not mentioned in most internet entries. Coprolalia is three times more common than copropraxia. Each form occurs more frequently in association with higher rates of comorbidity. Coprophenomena are both more common and more diverse than currently stated, but there is a need for more longitudinal research. One common belief is that coprophenomena are 'not to be taken personally', i.e. are not directed, but this is not necessarily so, an example of the diversity of the phenomenon.

One of the enduring peculiarities of Tourette syndrome is that while people associate coprolalia (involuntary emission of unacceptable words or phrases) and copropraxia (similar for gestures) with Tourette syndrome (often their only known piece of information), the patterns are infrequent. But they are not rare! While Gilles de la Tourette assumed that all cases (and his were severe) would eventually develop coprophenomena, in recent times these patterns were downplayed along with the emphasis upon the predominance of mild cases, now in the majority. If not actually termed 'rare', figures of 1%, 2%, 5% or at most 10% have been commonly cited. Often the description includes shouting of obscenities, as if this is typical. In fact, as will be seen below, the situation is more complicated and one should use caution in making or accepting general statements about coprophenomena. One reason coprophenomena may be so well known is that the pattern represents a contrast with normal socially controlled behavior of ordinary people. If it emerged from the mouth of a drunk or a person with a mental illness it would not have the same impact.

Although coprophenomena occur most often in Tourette syndrome, they can occasionally be encountered in patients who have had a stroke, a neurological degenerative disease, or in autism where a strange, narrow fascination can be elaborated and talked about regardless of the listener (such as we have seen with feces and penises, for example).

Another important category was first described in detail by Kurlan et al. (1996) as 'NOSI' or the blurting out of *non-obscene socially inappropriate* patterns, such as "Shut up!" or "You're boring!"

Despite the importance of coprophenomena, not much is known about their course and associated features. The few studies on the clinical course of Tourette syndrome say little about it. Is it intermittent, more common in males, associated with tic upsurges, often a first tic at onset? Is it as responsive to medication or behavioral intervention as other tics? Is it more likely to occur in those with prominent vocal tics, or in those with an urge to do the wrong thing? Can patients substitute one pattern for another, and if so, to what extent?

Another aspect is sometimes mentioned: the presence of *mental coprolalia*. This obviously indicates an urge to utter something inappropriate, but the expression may be inhibited (partially or completely). A recent paper by Eddy and Cavanna (2013) reported that all their 39 adult patients with obscene (overt) coprolalia had mental coprolalia, but only the presence of more severe tics was related to outbursts of obscene vocal tics. Half of the patients reported mental coprolalia, two-thirds of those expressed overt obscene coprolalia, but only half of the total sample did so. Ten always were able to suppress the coprolalic urge. Quality of life was poorer for those with overt coprolalia, but not for those with mental coprolalia only. (There was no comparison group to report the prevalence of NOSI in those without Tourette syndrome.)

For all coprophenomena, there is the problem of what defines the boundary of social unacceptability, especially when no one sees or hears it. A teenager who has (and likes to have) a foul mouth may use swear words in the presence of persons who do not approve, or are shocked by it. That may be a problem sometimes, but isn't necessarily coprolalia. Is someone who is angry or frustrated, blurting out obscenities when by themselves, performing coprolalia? Then we come to the even more difficult problem of mental coprolalia: what is the rate in the general population? We still do not know, despite the additional information provided by Eddy and Cavanna (2013) mentioned above. Without that information, the concept is not very useful. Someone who never wants to swear but finds themself shocked by doing it in their mind without having any reason to do so seems to be suffering from something very like an obsessional 'horrific thought' or urge.

Another less often mentioned concept is coprographia, made notorious by claims that its most famous practitioner was Wolfgang Amadeus Mozart in letters to his mother. After the initial publicity about this claim, it was criticized because at that time scatological language in one's parting phrases in a letter was said to have been quite common. [If I may interject a personal opinion here, I agreed with this criticism after reading some of the letters shown in the first (English) paper on this subject. However, after reading the much more extreme German samples in Müller-Vahl's book (2010) I now have doubts about my earlier skeptical conclusion.]

In the *TIC* database, coprophenomena are 2.5 times more likely to occur in TS+ as in TS-only (18.1% vs 7.5%, p<0.001, OR 2.5). In terms of increasing comorbidity, the reported history of coprophenomena increases from 10% at a score of 1 to an impressive 33% at a score of 5 disorders. The implication is that for our most complex children, coprophenomena are common, not rare as is often stated. However, in many cases the coprophenomena are intermittent or subside.

One important association is with SIB: in the *TIC* database, 33% of children with SIB have had coprophenomena (compared with 10% in those without SIB), and 36% of adults (compared with 14% without SIB). These are highly statistically significant differences (p<0.001, OR for children 4.4; OR for adults 2.8).

Here are the main conclusions from our recent study (Freeman et al. 2009).
- Lifetime reports of coprolalia: males 19.3%, females 14.6%; mean age at onset 11 years, 5 years 4 months after tic onset (SD 5y 10mo).
- Lifetime reports of copropraxia: males 5.8%, females 4.9%; mean age at onset 11 years, 4 years 10 months after tic onset (SD 5y 5mo).
- In half of child cases, coprophenomena had ceased or were intermittent. When coprophenomena had been present, it was coprolalia without copropraxia in 71%, the reverse in 9%.
- Those with coprophenomena had a mean comorbidity score of 2.31; those without had a score of 1.62.
- In TS-only, 10% reported coprolalia and 2.4% copropraxia; in TS+ the figures were 21% and 6.7%, respectively. Coprolalia is approximately three times as frequent as copropraxia.
- The number of non-tic repetitive behaviors was strongly associated with coprophenomena (3.24 with, 1.87 without).
- Behavior patterns strongly associated in children were sexually inappropriate behavior (OR 3.0), spitting (OR 5.4), smelling non-food objects (OR 3.0), SIB (OR 4.4) and anger control problems (OR 2.3); in adults, spitting (OR 4.4), SIB (OR 2.7), sexually inappropriate behavior (OR 2.6), and smelling things (OR 2.1).
- In a bootstrapping statistical procedure, non-tic repetitive behaviors and spitting were the two most frequently selected variables, followed next by inappropriate sexual behavior.

Complex associations reported in children in the *TIC* database are shown in Table 12.5. The significance of most associations in children applies also in the adult sample (details

TABLE 12.5
Coprophenomena in children (*TIC* data, n=5246)

	Without coprolalia (n=4647)		With coprolalia (n=599)		*p*	Odds ratio
	n	*%*	*n*	*%*		
Female sex	779	16.8	90	15.0	ns	—
Medication for tics (ever)*	2053	44.6	417	70.2	<0.001	2.9
Pre-/perinatal problems	786	18.7	127	24.6	0.002	1.4
ADHD*	2684	57.8	409	68.3	<0.001	1.6
OCD*	791	17.0	158	26.4	<0.001	1.7
SLD	1062	22.9	165	27.6	0.012	1.3
Mood disorder*	497	10.7	90	15.0	0.002	1.5
Anxiety disorder	706	15.2	123	20.5	0.001	1.4
CD/ODD*	552	11.9	160	28.0	<0.001	2.9
Sleep problems (now)*	846	18.7	117	20.2	ns	—
Anger (now)*	1185	26.2	251	44.6	<0.001	2.3
Social skill deficits (now)*	687	14.8	150	25.0	<0.001	1.9
SIB (ever)*	471	10.1	199	33.2	<0.001	4.4
Sexually inappropriate behavior (ever)*	140	3.4	50	9.5	<0.001	3.0

Excluded: intellectual disability, autism spectrum disorder and psychosis.
ADHD, attention-deficit/hyperactivity disorder; OCD, obsessive–compulsive disorder; SLD, specific learning disability; CD/ODD, conduct disorder/oppositional defiant disorder; SIB, self-injurious behavior; ns, non-significant.
[a]Significant association also found in adults (n=1628).

for the latter not shown). In general children and adults with coprophenomena are a more complex group with more comorbidity and behavioral problems.

DIAGNOSIS

Coprolalia is not having a 'foul mouth', or for emphasis, or due to pain or frustration. It often has a different voice quality, volume, cadence and tempo, and may be inserted into a sentence at seemingly random points or truncated. It also occurs in private, not only in conversation. It may be combined with other words or word-fragments, as a young child might do.

NATURAL HISTORY

The onset of coprophenomena is highly variable. An unmodified assumption is often made: that once it occurs, you're stuck with it, one of the reasons parents are so afraid of it. This is often incorrect. In many persons it subsides, maybe to return; or it may go underground, reduced in volume or truncated so that it is hardly noticeable. One of Gilles de la Tourette's own cases ('SJ') had his coprolalia and some other features spontaneously subside (Kushner 1995). An important feature in some patients is that the coprophenomena cannot be substituted by something neutral: the urge can only be briefly relieved by something strong, and a neutral word or gesture does not suffice. At the same time, some patients (especially young ones) may be embarrassed and remorseful about their symptom. But if the felt need or impulse must be strong, how is it that sometimes the outburst can be low or truncated? At this point we do not know.

IMPACT

Although it is generally assumed that coprophenomena have a significant negative social impact, this is not necessarily so. Of those with the pattern, a significant proportion were reported not to have impairment in the family or in school. Sometimes a disgusting behavior such as spitting, licking or play with saliva may accompany and aggravate the social impact. Some adolescents report that their classmates aren't bothered by their coprolalia.

REACTIONS

Although coprophenomena aren't necessarily impairing, when it takes the form of obvious expletives, assumptions may be made that a bad mouth makes for bad behavior. A recent case in the UK involved a child custody dispute: it was claimed that a cursing father would be a noxious influence on his children's development (without any further factors being considered).

TREATMENT

What can be done? First, persons with a 'need to know' should have an explanation. Second, the young person's willingness to try to modify the behavior should be assessed. This includes blocking the offensive words by putting something in the mouth when in a risky situation. A classic example of this is told about a white man in a subway car in New York City who looked around and suddenly realized that everyone else present was black. He immediately developed an overwhelming urge to yell "nigger!" but prevented a possibly dangerous situation by stuffing something in his mouth. (The urge was not based upon racist feelings, rather the awareness and temptation of risk.) As a last resort, medication may be considered (but there are no studies on whether the efficacy of treatment is the same as with other types of tics). With CBIT therapy (see Chapter 15), we do not yet have comparative efficacy rates.

DIRECTED, OR NOT?

It is often said that coprophenomena are both involuntary and not to be taken personally. This may be an oversimplification. It seems more likely that sometimes the socially un-acceptable utterance is personal (i.e. targeted), but its usual extent of inhibition is reduced. An obvious example comes from a conference with some persons with Tourette syndrome present. Part way through a speaker's presentation a loud "Boring!" was heard from the audience (which may have been a legitimate comment).

A HISTORICAL DILEMMA

Howard Kushner (2012, personal communication) has warned that there is a danger in the current trend of portrayals of mild Tourette syndrome. With the broadening of the criteria (e.g. distress and impairment removed in DSM-IV-TR), most patients coming to attention have mild cases mostly without coprophenomena, while patients with really dramatic, persistently severe coprophenomena may be (and feel) marginalized.

It may be seen, then, that coprophenomena are variable along several dimensions and that much more study is needed to characterize them. Individual variations in subjective experience are still to be adequately described in Tourette syndrome, and compared with other conditions (relatively rare) in which coprophenomena also may occur. The remission and recurrence of coprophenomena in relation to other factors and symptoms need to be explored longitudinally. This is one glaring lack in our understanding of tics.

Spitting

> Spitting in Tourette syndrome is a copropraxia-equivalent. However, there are several other causes or factors: a compulsion, a phobia, delusion, or a consequence of sexual molestation. It is most closely associated with contrary urges, coprophenomena, anger control problems, SIB, sexually inappropriate behavior and nose-picking. No data are available on a specific treatment.

Spitting as a copropraxia-equivalent was touched on in the previous section. But there is more to be said about it. Spitting was once socially acceptable in North America (at least), good aim being prized as a skill for men (spittoons placed in the corner of a room) until the cause of tuberculosis was discovered. Spitting in public then became a punishable offence, and 'No Spitting' signs were commonly to be seen. We apparently have no information on how spitting fitted into the symptoms of persons with Tourette syndrome in those days. Now that spitting is socially disgusting, and spitting at a person is taken as a seriously hostile act, we must consider its place in a disorder.

Teenagers may spit casually as they may swear casually, not caring how others (usually adults) regard their behavior. This is not spitting as a symptom of a disorder, but can sometimes be confused with it.

Assessing spitting requires that the following be determined:
• Where it occurs, and where it does not.
• When it occurs, and when not (and what was happening when it started).
• What has been tried (and by whom) to control it, and what is said about it.
• Has it occurred before, and then subsided?
• Whether, around the time it started, other symptoms or symptom changes also occurred.

It is possible that the spitting, if done randomly throughout the day, and not just outside, is a tic, strongly tic-like, or a compulsion. Sometimes it occurs only in certain places, at certain times, or with certain persons. It can also be done because of a phobia or delusion, or as a consequence of a sexual molestation or provocation. It may be combined with other behavior patterns, such as smearing saliva. The patient may describe the feeling of having an excess of saliva, saliva that tastes bad, and/or a fear or aversion to swallowing or choking. The changed taste of saliva may have no objective basis, may be used as an excuse, or may be present due to conditions in the mouth, upper gastrointestinal tract or nasopharynx, or rarely due to a brain-based alteration. Hearing about, seeing, or experiencing oral sex may occasionally be a trigger that may not be readily identified. The factors involved may thus be many. During a local epidemic (e.g. influenza), spitting, like sneezing or coughing, may be strongly sanctioned as an indication of dangerous contagion.

Associations with other patterns are many and important; in the *TIC* database (Freeman et al. 2000) the following patterns co-occur: coprophenomena (OR 5.4), anger (now) (OR 2.8); SIB (OR 2.9), sexually inappropriate behavior (OR 4.3), nose-picking (OR 4.8), smelling things (OR 3.6), rocking (OR 4.8), trichotillomania (OR 4.4), and highest of all, contrary urges (OR 8.7). Spitting is significantly more common in children with TS+ than TS-only (OR 2.1), with OCD being the most strongly associated (OR 5.3).

We may not find out anything causative, but should try. Unfortunately, very little research has been done on this specific topic. If the symptom is significantly impairing, treatment may be considered, but is unlikely to be successful with tic medication if it is not a tic. An effort should be made to see whether some control can be exerted in situations that are likely to be especially unacceptable. CBIT (behavioral) treatment may be worth trying, but no reports of results have so far been published.

Case example

'Cindy' was 10 years old and had Tourette syndrome and ADHD. She started spitting, both in and out of her home, but mostly on mornings of days when her mother was going to work the afternoon shift, which meant that they would not see each other till the next day; it never happened on the days another relative got her ready for school.

Comment: *This is an illustration that situational factors may be operating.*

Repetitive motor behaviors

- RMBs or stereotyped behaviors of many kinds tend to be lumped together, sometimes with SMD, compulsions or ASD, as well as tic disorders. They often change during development, but why and when is variable and not well understood.
- The lack of a full and recognized nosology of different patterns of repetitive behaviors is hindering understanding and often confuses diagnosis.
- In all cases it is advisable to go beyond automatic labeling of a pattern as supportive of any one diagnosis.
- If RMBs are not observed, parental or individual labeling of the pattern and its description often omit component parts that may be important. Video recording can often solve this problem.

• Findings in the *TIC* data show that there is a correlation between number of RMBs and extent of comorbidity and problems of behavior.
• RMB exploration is a non-threatening entry into the more personal habits and functioning of individuals and their family context.

How many hugs with back-slaps is normal?

Observations while waiting in the arrivals area of our airport led to the conclusion that when people are greeted they often hug and then slap or pat each other's backs. Obvious, you may think. But the remarkable fact is that the average number of slaps is within a very narrow range, namely two or three. Thinking that this might be of some importance, school-age children were asked what they would expect if they were observing at the airport, and the typical answer was, two or three! They were not taught this in school or by their parents; they 'just know', and in knowing, they 'know' that slapping five or more times would look weird. (It might be of interest to ask blind children the same question, since they have not watched this activity.) This means that for this repetitive pattern a 'normal' range has been established without our knowing how or why. In a recent newspaper horoscope entry for Scorpio: "You'll gain energy from hugs. When you hug, hold for three breaths. Then the hug becomes more than a greeting or parting gesture; it becomes an act of healing." (The repetition number has meaning.)

RMBs are an ill-defined group of patterns that all infants and most adults engage in at different times, with differing degrees of self-awareness, intensity, stereotypy, triggers and persistence. Helpful information about the causes, prevalence, associations and ways of modifying them is sparse. Some are accorded their own diagnoses (e.g. trichotillomania, excoriation), most are not (joint-cracking, nail-biting, nose-picking) but may have Greek names (e.g. rhinotillexomania for pathological nose-picking) and rating scales (e.g. Skin-Picking Scale). This messiness can be quite confusing. Thus, 'stereotyped behavior' is very heterogeneous when part of the criteria for an ASD, and can complicate the definition of SMD and descriptions of intellectual disability and many genetic syndromes (e.g. Rett syndrome). A commonly used but misleading term is 'stimming', related to the idea that the RMB is a response to overstimulation. But overstimulation may be only one possibility or factor, since general self-regulation in either direction may be involved. Some of the patterns have a fuzzy boundary with SMD, OCD and SIB.

A major and under-recognized problem is that the terms used to label individual RMBs are too general. There are typically several patterns with different features lumped under one term. Complexity and specific and important associations may thereby be missed (Rapp and Vollmer 2005a,b).

> **Practice point**
>
> Labels used for problem behaviors are too general; more detailed descriptions are often more helpful; this includes both stereotypies and RMBs.

Body-focused repetitive behavior disorder (BFRBD) is another term often used, "an umbrella term for debilitating, repetitive behaviors that target one or more body regions" (McGuire et al. 2012, p. 855). These authors have provided an exhaustive analysis of the status of instruments to assess BFRBs, concluding that one reason for the lack of useful research in children is the absence of reliable and valid methods of assessment. They include under this rubric compulsive skin-picking (dermatillomania, excoriation disorder), trichotillomania and (perhaps surprisingly) chronic tic disorders. An excellent free set of treatment guidelines for BFRBs as well as trichotillomania and skin-picking is available from the Trichotillomania Learning Center as a free download (www.trich.org). For a good general overview, there is a recent book by Grant et al. (2012). Note, however, that not all RMBs fit into the category of BFRBDs (e.g. contrary urges, spitting) considered here. (SIB is considered in the following section.)

Lip-licking dermatitis may result from a tic or RMB due to excessively dry skin from low humidity (especially in homes with forced-air heating in winter). It is often unclear whether there is a tic component to this pattern.

> **Case example**
>
> *A boy with a long tongue had a pattern termed 'lip-licking' that included licking the tip of his nose and also head-turning; the parents initially described the licking, but not the head-turning.*

BRUXISM

Bruxism can occur when awake or in sleep, and consist of lateral or forward-and-back grinding, clenching of the teeth, clicking of the teeth, popping of the temporomandibular joint, and chewing on pencils, pens or other objects such as pieces of ice, or combinations of these. Pain may result. Multiple factors are probably involved, including dental malocclusion, altered sensations from dental or orthodontic work and broken teeth. Suggestions of causes include stress, occlusal irregularities, and abnormally low arousal thresholds during sleep. Reported prevalence rates have varied widely, from 8% to 21%.

The causes of bruxism are not well established; dentists deal with the results of the physical wear on the teeth, regardless of when the pattern occurs (Lobbezoo et al. 2013). There is a popular belief that bruxism is closely related to anxiety and tension, probably derived from awareness of clenching with stress. However, we have some reason to separate bruxism in sleep from that when awake in our large Tourette sample. It is awake bruxism that has an association with anxiety and OCD, not sleep bruxism. This becomes clear when the following *TIC* database percentages are viewed. Awake bruxism is reported in 11% of the total group of 607 patients. In TS-only, however, the rate is only 5%, versus 13% in ADHD, 17% in anxiety, 21% in mood disorder, and 17% in OCD. Thus the rate is increased in comorbid disorders. Sleep bruxism is reported in 20% of the total group, but in 17% to 24% of the clinical disorders just mentioned, thus not significantly increased over that in TS-only. Additional disorders are not associated with a significant increase. In sum, the data from the *TIC* database suggest that awake bruxism has significantly more associated symptoms and problems than does sleep bruxism.

A very extensive study in Sweden (Egermark et al. 2001) followed 402 children into adult life, obtaining data from 80% of them at the final point. Thirteen percent reported at least one symptom of temporomandibular disorder, including pain, but associations were weak and severe symptoms were rare. Research by Manfredini et al. (2005) suggested some subclinical associations between bruxism and some anxiety symptoms, but the evidence is not strong. De Laat and Macaluso (2002) concluded that sleep bruxism is "an exaggerated manifestation of an otherwise normal occurrence of rhythmic masticatory muscle activity" (p. S69) with multifactorial causation. The publications of many researchers in the dental field tend to agree that the factors involved are multiple and the outcome variable, as is the response to various interventions (Manfredini and Lobbezoo 2010).

> **Case example**
> *After a flight a patient had a persisting sensation of blocked eustachian tubes and frequently attempted to unblock them by contortions of her temporomandibular joint as well as repeated swallowing.*

Treatment of bruxism is still rather poorly defined and the efficacy questionable, possibly because the pattern is heterogeneous. Yüce et al. (2013) reviewed the effects of some drugs, and especially atomoxetine, in causing or worsening bruxism. Citalopram and other SSRIs as well as antidopaminergic drugs (Micheli et al. 1993) have also been reported to provoke bruxism in a small number of cases (Ellison and Stanziani 1993, Wise 2001).

It may be unclear whether an RMB is a tic. If an individual with one or more tics later develops significant nail-biting, lip-licking or joint-cracking, is that a tic, because they have tics? If considered thus, is this used to validate the necessary criterion A for Tourette syndrome ('multiple motor…')? Could a person with no tics or one tic be given the diagnosis of Tourette syndrome because of a few RMBs? Yes, it can happen!

> **Practice point**
> Confusion of RMBs with tics can sometimes lead to false-positive diagnoses of tic disorders.

There is also a lack of clarity as to whether a repetitive behavior is 'tic-like' or

'OCD-like'. In a complex study by a consortium of 23 French investigators on 166 consecutive patients aged 16–68 years, Worbe et al. (2010) classified patterns as one or the other, or neither. A majority of patients (64%) had what were termed repetitive behaviors, 24% tic-like (characterized as touching, counting, just-right and symmetry patterns), 21% OCD-like (washing and checking), 13% mixed, and 6% unclassifiable. However, their methods of distinguishing these categories and the involved assumptions seem unclear. Furthermore, they assert that repetitive smelling (classified as a ritual) is rare, contradicting our findings of 20%. Why 'counting' is classified as tic-like is also unclear, as also with the inclusion of intrusive thoughts or images as 'unclassifiable'. Finally, no account is taken of comparative base rates of repetitive behaviors in persons with typical development, i.e. not all repetitive behaviors need to be understood as tic- or OCD-like, since everyone has some repetitive behaviors.

Unfortunately, although the *TIC* database has data on RMBs in persons with Tourette syndrome, there are no truly comparable data to indicate whether RMBs are more or less prevalent in those without Tourette syndrome or tics, or those with ADHD or OCD; all we may have is some unrelated study of an RMB in more typical groups, with all the associated problems of definition, intensity and duration. Nevertheless, some associations occurring more commonly in TS-only patients are presented here from an as yet unpublished study by the *TIC* Consortium. (Note that these data were elicited by asking about whether a pattern had ever been noticeable, not necessarily considered a problem.)

Skin-picking is four times as common in those with OCD and social skill deficits as in TS-only; awake bruxism four times as common with OCD; smelling three times as common with coprophenomena and twice with social skill deficits; rocking three times as common with ADHD, four times with anger control problems and almost five times with social skill deficits; and finally spitting is three times as common in those with social skill deficits. With the exception of asleep bruxism, persons with TS-only have significantly fewer RMBs than those with TS+.

Smelling

Smelling non-food objects is interesting, as it is reported in about 20% of our *TIC* children, and wrongly seen by some as pathognomonic of either ASD or Tourette syndrome. It should not be considered pathognomonic of ASD! Some children very briefly smell almost any object that passes their face (or they at least pass the object under their nose); others smell their fingers repeatedly (or after some specific activity), and still others smell their mothers (arms, hair, armpits or clothing). They may 'graze' along their mother's body in front of the clinician. Children who do this don't seem to be thinking about how this looks to their peers. They almost never smell their fathers or siblings. From available data, this type of smelling is strongly associated with OCD. Older children may be able to describe the sensations or urges that precede or accompany the pattern so as to classify it and determine its associations. (One may wonder whether this difference is related to the difference in accommodation to the OCD between mothers and fathers.) In children with Tourette syndrome and comorbid ASD a smelling pattern is more common (about 50%) and may have a more bizarre quality.

In the *TIC* database, smelling is significantly associated with coprophenomena (36%), OCD (33%) and social skill problems (23%).

Case example

'Dawson', an 11-year-old boy, frequently put his hands inside his pants and smelled his fingers when he removed them. He said that he was feeling his anus and that he liked the smell.

*   **Comment:** *Not surprisingly, this was highly aversive to his classmates. What was decisively important to him was his own perception, not that of others.*

Other patterns in the *TIC* database significantly associated with OCD in children are trichotillomania, skin-picking, nose-picking, awake bruxism, self-cutting and -hitting, joint-cracking, spitting and contrary urges.

NAIL-BITING

Nail-biting is a general descriptive term. It can consist of specific patterns of biting finger-nails, toenails, cuticle, or skin of finger-tips, or actually picking these rather than biting, or any combination. Typically the activity stops when observed by others. In an interesting paper, Ghanizadeh (2008) reported that it occurred in 14% of 450 children referred to a psychiatric clinic. The strongest associations were with ADHD (75%), ODD (36%), separation anxiety disorder (21%), enuresis (16%), tics (13%), and OCD (11%). Other prevalence estimates range widely from 12% to 60%. Nail-biting is uncommon before age 3, increases thereafter to age 7, remains level through age 10, rises and peaks at onset of adolescence, then declines to below 10% at age 35 (Snyder and Friman 2012). Complications include secondary infections and social stigmatization. In the *TIC* database, 32% of children were reported to be (or to have been) nail-biters. Nail-picking seems to be associated with other BFRBs. Snorrason and Woods (2014) presented a case with moderate benefit from acceptance-enhanced behavioral treatment (willingly experiencing urges to pick without reacting to them). Successful behavioral treatment has been described by Bate et al. (2011).

There may be other consequences, rarely considered.

Case example

'Emily' was a 14-year-old girl with mild Tourette syndrome and OCD. Only after several years was it discovered that her puzzlingly recurrent bouts of pinworms were due to her re-infecting herself by frequent nail-biting.

THUMB-SUCKING

Thumb-sucking was not a commonly reported pattern in the *TIC* database, but should be mentioned here. The prevalence is not well established but has been cited as about 25% in

5-year-olds, but almost nonexistent in 14-year-olds. As children mature its practice may become private. Effects on dentition are well-known, but there is also the possibility of skin infections. It is not clear that there is any association with psychopathology; thumb-suckers may be negatively regarded, however.

ROCKING

Rocking is often observed in blind children and also is the one identified pattern (nocturnally) in deaf children (Bachara and Phelan 1980). Pre-sleep rocking in dormitories was observed in 17% of deaf children between the ages of 5 and 9 years, 12% in the age range 10–13 years, and 10% in age range 13–16 years. The duration of the pattern ranged from 15 minutes to 2 hours and 25 minutes. The authors stated that such patterns started in the first year of life and usually stopped by age 3, occurring in 19% to 21% of infants with typical development. It was not clear (in the absence of matched comparison children) that pre-sleep rocking was more common in deaf children than in those with normal hearing. Some of these cases with pre-sleep patterns may have fit the description of jactatio capitis nocturna (body-rolling type), discussed in Chapter 11.

JOINT-CRACKING

Some joint-cracking is done only occasionally, like stretching, and not in a complex, stereotyped way. Others engage in frequent complex patterns, often in a rigid way, running through a sequence that must be performed by a rule, or if missed, started again and repeated until 'just right'. This can involve one or several joints (often of the hands) or a sequence of joints. This rigid pattern can seem compulsive or tic-like to some observers. Different cultures have different beliefs about the consequences of joint-cracking. In North America and some other countries it is believed to lead to arthritis and practitioners are warned (without any good evidence) about future ugly, distorted, enlarged joints. An excellent example in literature from an Indo-Canadian author, quoted here, is as good as the subjective aspect gets.

> Confused by what had happened, he sat on his bed and cracked the fingers of both hands. Each finger twice, expertly, once at the knuckle, then at the joint closest to the nail. He could also crack his toes — each toe just once, though — but he did not feel like it right now. Don't crack your fingers, they used to tell him, your hands will become fat and ugly. For a while then he had cracked his knuckles more fervently than ever, hoping they would swell into fists the size of a face. Such fists would be useful to scare someone off in a fight. But the hands had remained quite normal. (Mistry 1987, p. 40)

In the following section, odds ratios as proxies for effect size are shown for data from the *TIC* database. In children, joint-cracking had an overlap with trichotillomania (OR 3), skin-picking (OR 1.7), nail-biting (OR 2.8), awake bruxism (OR 2.8), rocking (OR 2.5), nose-picking (OR 2.3), spitting (OR 2.3), contrary urges (OR 2.3) and SIB (OR 1.7). There was no significant overlap with bruxism in sleep, smelling, coprophenomena, lip-licking, social skill deficits, anger control problems or anxiety disorder. In adults, the significant relationships were with spitting (OR 7.6), skin-picking (OR 4.1) and OCD (OR 3.3).

S<small>KIN-PICKING</small>

With the advent of the DSM-5, excoriation (skin-picking) is now a bona fide disorder, the criteria for which include "repeated attempts to decrease or stop skin picking". Skin-picking can be quite damaging both physically and socially. In the *TIC* database, the following correlations were found between excoriation disorder and other BFRBs in children: trichotillomania (OR 5.5, 52% of those with trichotillomania have had skin-picking), awake bruxism (OR 4.2), smelling (OR 3.4), nail-biting (OR 3.2), nose-picking (OR 2.3), rocking (OR 2.6), SIB (OR 4.0, 50% of skin-pickers were rated as self-injurious), joint-cracking (OR 2.3), contrary urges (OR 2.0), and weak social skills (OR 2.4). In adults, associations were with trichotillomania (OR 8.8), SIB (OR 5.5), nail-biting (OR 4.3), and rocking (OR 2.6).

N<small>OSE-PICKING</small> (R<small>HINOTILLEXOMANIA</small>)

Spitting has a robust association with nose picking (OR 4.8), contrary urges (OR 4.2) and rocking (OR 3.0).

H<small>EAD-BANGING/SELF-HITTING</small>

Head-banging and self-hitting was associated with ADHD (OR 2.2), OCD (OR 2.1), and the following with odds ratios of around 2: mood disorder, anxiety disorder, conduct disorder/ODD, sleep problems, stuttering, social skill deficits, nail-biting, skin-picking, smelling and contrary urges. Much stronger associations were with SIB (OR 9), coprophenomena (OR 3.2), rocking (OR 3.8) and spitting (OR 3.5).

L<small>IP-LICKING</small>

Lip-licking occurred in 8% of patients with TS-only in the *TIC* database. Significant associations were with ADHD (OR 1.9), anxiety disorders (OR 1.8), SIB (OR 2.1), nose-picking (OR 1.9), smelling things (OR 1.8), rocking (OR 2.0) and (not surprisingly) contrary urges (OR 2.1).

R<small>EPETITIVE MOTOR BEHAVIORS AND COMORBIDITY</small>

In the *TIC* database a significant positive correlation was found between number of RMBs and comorbidity score (n=685 children) of 0.28 (Spearman's rho), p<0.01, df = 682, and Pearson correlation 0.313, p<0.01. TS-only children had a history of 1.3 RMBs; this mean number increases gradually with increasing comorbidity score to 4.6 RMBs with a comorbidity score of 5. Looking at those with 3 or more RMBs compared with none, the proportion is about double for anger control problems, sleep problems, coprophenomena and social skill deficits, with even higher rates for SIB. These findings may merit further research.

D<small>EVELOPMENT OF 'NEW' REPETITIVE MOTOR BEHAVIORS</small>

A stereotyped pattern can arise irregularly during development (indeed in adult life) and one may not be fully aware that it is helping with concentration (and may persist due to automatic reinforcement). For example, most of us are aware that our need for intense concentration may be fostered by closing our eyes or looking up at the ceiling, perhaps to reduce surrounding irrelevant stimuli. This is so common that others watching this may think nothing of it, and never ask for an explanation.

CAN A RESPONSE TO A SENSORY TRIGGER BECOME A REPETITIVE MOTOR BEHAVIOR?
The answer is probably yes. For example, allergies producing an itchy nose can lead to repetitive nose-rubbing and in some individuals can become a 'habit' when the trigger is gone and later seem to be an RMB.

CAN A REPETITIVE BEHAVIOR SWITCH CATEGORIES?
Can a ritual become practised so often that it loses its cognitive component and becomes an RMB or a tic? This is unclear, but probably so. A repetitive pattern may replace another. Or a repetitive behavior only later may come to be considered a tic because it was the first repetitive pattern, before what were later recognized as tics.

WHAT HAPPENS TO A REPETITIVE MOTOR BEHAVIOR WHEN THE PERSON HAS A TIC UPSURGE?
We do not know, as this appears to have never been published. The question should be amenable to research.

Self-injurious behavior

> SIBs are a frequent contributor to concern and impairment. Although their causes are poorly understood, there are complex relationships between SIBs and comorbid disorders and other behavior patterns, many possibly related to weak self-regulation. Because of behavioral heterogeneity and unclear category boundaries, this section should be considered in conjunction with those on SMD, RMBs and ASD.

It is difficult to define SIB unless there is obvious tissue damage. Tics themselves can be self-injurious, sometimes because of the need to get the extreme position of the tic just right (e.g. rotating joints), or the feeling of connecting with an object just right. If the object is a person, there may be social effects. This may be seen with arm or leg abduction. A child who had an irresistible urge to abduct his knee into the person sitting next to him was able to describe how the urge began with the perception of the other's body in his visual field. This may dictate a different seating position in the classroom.

Examples of SIB in persons with Tourette syndrome include knee-knocking, head or face hitting, lip or cheek chewing, ankle-twisting, skin-rubbing, eye-rubbing and -poking, jaw punching, and temporomandibular joint popping. Unusual urges can result in unusual behaviors. The role of Tourette syndrome in these is often unclear, because as will be seen below, comorbidity is an important factor. SIB is uncommon in TS-only.

Sometimes there is disagreement or doubt whether an SIB pattern is – or is not – a tic. Of course there is no way to be absolutely sure, but one may get a good enough description of the pattern's development over time to conclude that it is a tic. Merely being a pattern among several tics doesn't prove 'guilt by association'. On occasion we may conclude that it is 'tic-like', but without a very good description of evolution of the pattern and what accompanies it internally we simply will not know. For treatment, with all its uncertainties, it may not matter at this point in our knowledge.

Practice point

Sometimes a repetitive pattern, because it occurs among several tics, is assumed to be a tic. This may not seem to matter, but if the tics are treated, for example pharmaco-logically, the clinician may wrongly expect the SIB pattern to respond as the tics do. 'Guilt by association' shouldn't be assumed.

NON-TIC PATTERNS

More detailed information may be found in the section on RMBs. Nail-biting is the most common pattern, but often causes only cosmetic changes. Lip-licking may cause thickened, cracked, reddened and painful lips during the winter months (but usually not as much at other times). Cold air may be very dry, and the dryness of forced-air house heating (with-out a humidifier) may also contribute to excessive drying of the lips and other mucous mem-branes. The self-injurious act itself may need to be combined with other factors (e.g. pre-dispositions, infection) for injury to occur. Fungal or bacterial secondary infections may supervene. Pigmentary changes may develop in some. Irritation of the lips can cause skin irregularities and result in picking, triggering other patterns. It is important to realize that lip-licking, like many other RMBs, may be more complex than as it first appears or is described. It may be associated with a mouth-opening tic that causes skin cracking, which triggers more licking. Once lip-licking causes discomfort or unsightliness, parents may try to manage it and unwittingly cause more of a problem. Many parents believe that more is better, so that lip balm containing antibiotics or other chemicals, or 'natural' products con-taining beeswax are better, when dermatologists advise that these can be sensitizing or cause pain. They strongly recommend very frequent application of the simplest lip balm (with the least extra ingredients) to restore moisturization, unless infection or other complications ensue.

Mathews et al. (2004) examined the relationship between SIB and other behavioral fea-tures. They found that mild to moderate SIB was associated with OCD, while severe SIB was more closely related to affect or impulse dysregulation, episodic rages and risk-taking behaviors. Overall, 29% of patients had SIB, 4% severe. Their findings led to the sugges-tion that mild/moderate and severe SIB may be different phenomena.

Eisenhauer and Woody (1987) described two cases of persons with Tourette syndrome who mutilated themselves, one a child who had eye-poking urges and loosened several teeth when under severe family-based stress, the other an adult who had gouged his eyes and by age 12 had blinded himself. Later he had a cervical disc subluxation with spinal cord dam-age due to violent neck-twisting tics. The authors recommended that physical examination include checking for physical signs of self-mutilation as well as asking the patient and family about urges to self-mutilate. An example of what can happen when such recommendations are not followed and an SIB history is not realized to reflect a risk of serious damage is that of 'Joshua' in Chapters 7 and 17.

In the following example, damage was wrongly assumed to be due to SIB in Tourette syndrome.

Case example

'Neil' was 18 when first seen, and had a history of not only severe tics but also significant social relationship difficulties. He was living by himself in a subsidized apartment, on a disability pension. He had been poking his eyes for a long time, causing retinal detachments. Heroic ophthalmologic treatment had saved some vision in one eye, but the surgeons wanted him to stop the poking before all vision was lost. After a number of contacts he came in with a white cane. Why would he do that, when usually people going blind delay such learning? That was the puzzle. The reason turned out to be that he expected to be completely blind. Why? Because he wanted to be! No one had considered that possibility.

Comment: We all assume that no one would want to be blind. However, this young man was so tortured by his lack of success with women that he couldn't tolerate seeing them. His autistic limitations not only accounted for some of his sexual failures, but also his failure to tell any of his physicians of the fact or reasons for his unusual motivation.

In another instance, a young child developed early self-injurious tics.

Case example

'Lisa', 5 years old, was doing well in school and socially. Then motor tics started, which involved flinging her arms out, which sometimes seemed to accidentally hit things and hurt her hands. Later she smacked herself in the face, which resulted in bruising and occasional nose-bleeds. Vocal tics started (sniffing and inspiratory noises). Under stress causing anxiety these tics worsened.

Comment: This is a not uncommon history of gradual development of SIB.

In the *TIC* database (Freeman et al. 2000), SIB is much more common in children with TS+ (15.3%) than in those with TS-only (4.2%, p<0.001, OR 3.6). In terms of comorbidity scores, among children with two comorbid disorders 15% had reports of SIB, and at a score level of five disorders, 41%. Coprophenomena occur in children at a rate of 30% if they have SIB, 9% if they do not. In adults, comparable figures are 36% versus 14% if they do not. These are highly statistically significant findings and also have clinical significance. For TS-only cases, significantly higher rates of SIB are found only in females (8.2% vs 2.8%),

TABLE 12.6
Self-injurious behavior in children (*TIC* data, n=5247)

	Without coprolalia (n=4531)		With coprolalia (n=666)		*p*	Odds ratio
	n	*%*	*n*	*%*		
Female sex	747	16.3	122	18.2	ns	—
Medication for tics (ever)	2094	46.2	377	56.5	<0.001	1.5
Pre-/perinatal problems	770	18.8	143	23.4	0.008	1.3
ADHD	2638	57.6	456	68.0	<0.001	1.6
OCD	751	16.4	199	29.7	0.019	2.1
SLD	1032	22.6	196	29.3	<0.001	1.4
Mood disorder	465	10.2	123	18.3	<0.001	2.0
Anxiety disorder	650	14.2	180	26.8	<0.001	2.2
Sleep disorder (now)	190	29.4	734	17.3	<0.001	4.4
Anger (now)	1134	25.5	302	47.3	<0.001	2.0
Trichotillomania	77	1.7	53	7.9	<0.001	5.0
Social skill deficits (now)	671	14.7	167	24.9	<0.001	1.9
Coprophenomena (ever)	400	8.7	199	29.7	<0.001	4.4

Excluded: intellectual disability, ASD and psychosis.
ADHD, attention-deficit–hyperactivity disorder; OCD, obsessive–compulsive disorder; SLD, specific learning disability; ns, non-significant.

and in those with severe tics (26.3% vs 9.8% for mild), anger control problems (9.3% vs 3.5%) and social skill problems (12.8% vs 3.7%), with significantly lower rates in children (3.4% vs 7.1% in adults, probably because of the longer years with the symptom). It may be that some of these associations are linked, i.e. SIB, coprophenomena, sleep problems, anger control and social skill deficits may be manifestations of weak self-regulation.

Also in the *TIC* database, SIB was reported in 39% of adults with intellectual disability as against 23% of those without, and in 26% of children with intellectual disability versus 13% of those without (OR 2.3); and likewise, SIB was reported in 21% versus 13% of children and 35% versus 24% of adults with and without ASD. Other results are displayed in Table 12.6.

> **Practice point**
> When SIB is associated with coprophenomena, sleep problems, anger control problems and social skill deficits, those symptoms may be manifestations of weak self-regulation. This combination is likely to cause significant difficulties in clinical management.

NOSE-PICKING

Nose-picking (rhinotillexomania) was studied in a survey by Andrade and Srihari (2001). They reported that 17% of surveyed adolescents thought this was a serious problem for themselves; 25% had caused nosebleeds and 4.5% ate the results of their picking. In the *TIC* database there was no significant association with trichotillomania.

SKIN-PICKING

Excoriation (skin-picking) disorder is related to trichotillomania. In the *TIC* database, 19% of those with Tourette syndrome were reported to have skin-picked (141 of 742). In a quarter this was intermittent; 81% of the 141 were still picking at the time seen. It was judged to be self-injurious in half. Mean onset in children was 6.9 years (SD 3.6y). Of those who picked at their skin, 14% also had a history of trichotillomania and 52% of nail-biting. Skin-picking children were almost six times as likely as others to have pulled their hair out, and for adults this was even higher (almost nine times) (see also Chapter 10).

SELF-CUTTING

Self-cutting is a form of non-suicidal self-injury in most cases (Wilkinson and Goodyer 2011, Ougrin et al. 2012). It is thought to serve as a way of reducing distressing feelings or signalling emotional need to others. It is often wrongly assumed to reflect suicidal intent. At least 7% to 14% of adolescents are reported to have engaged in self-injury at least once. In the *TIC* database, self-cutting was reported in 7% of 91 female children with Tourette syndrome, and 1% of 486 male children (OR 5.3, p<0.005); and in three of 26 female adults and 9% of 68 male adults. It was associated with higher comorbidity scores in both sexes: 3.2 vs 1.8 in male children, and 2.6 vs 1.4 in female children.

MISCELLANEOUS TICS

Miscellaneous tics of many kinds can do damage. Fusco et al. (2006) presented the case of a 13-year-old boy who had OCD in addition to a pattern of sitting down on his heels abruptly and rapidly getting up again, repeated many times a day. This resulted in stress fractures of both peroneal bones. Stress fractures present with pain that is much worse during exercise. In this case the bones healed well due to spontaneous reduction in the causative tic. Calvo et al. (1995) described a clavicular fracture in a 26-year-old woman who developed another fracture of a similar kind on the contralateral side; after many studies the cause was finally attributed to a 'nervous tic' consisting of circumduction of her shoulder ('shoulder rolls'); she started with the second clavicle when immobilized for treatment of the first. Because of the risk of a neoplastic cause, overtreatment is a potential problem if the causative move-ment is not reported or observed. Moon et al. (1998) reported the case of an 11-year-old girl with left shoulder pain due to a non-displaced fracture of the acromion. After healing took place, she developed a rib fracture. Further questioning of the parents revealed a frequent shoulder-shrug with other components, exacerbated by stress, but "surprisingly she had not exhibited this unusual behavior during any of her previous clinic visits" (p. 405). Other reports of SIBs are available, e.g. Krauss and Jankovic (1996), Dobbs and Berger (2003), Lin et al. (2007), Isaacs et al. (2010), Ko et al. (2013). These reports illustrate the potential diversity of orthopedic damage that can sometimes be caused by frequent tics and how easy it is to initially miss the causative factor.

UNINTENDED SELF-INJURIOUS TICS

Some other tic situations can lead to injuries. Margo (2002) described two men with

Tourette syndrome who failed to tell the physician who was examining their eyes that they had Tourette syndrome, resulting in unintended laceration, hemorrhage or corneal abrasion. In one of these cases the occasion for the visit to the emergency room was a fight that was probably the result of misinterpretation of the tics. Lim (2004) reported a 25-year-old man who had eye-blinking, blepharospasm, jabbing his fingers into his eyes and punching himself in the periorbital area. Ophthalmologic examination revealed multiple injuries to both eyes, including retinal tears requiring surgery. Mashor et al. (2011) described keratoconus (progressive thinning and steepening of the cornea), likely to have been at least partly caused by eye-rubbing in three patients with Tourette syndrome. Each rubbed predominantly one eye, and the damage was identified only in that eye.

Leksell and Edvardson (2005) described a 4-year-old girl who had such severe grinding of her teeth (bruxism) that she loosened a primary canine and then removed it. A behavioral approach was used to diminish the SIB.

TREATMENT

Treatment of SIB is often unsatisfactory and depends upon identification of the causative factors in the associated neurodevelopmental or other pathology. Thus there is no single therapeutic medical or behavioral approach. A functional analysis of the symptom is generally regarded as advisable.

Speech and language disorders

> Speech and language problems are common in tic disorders but there is little settled knowledge about the mechanisms by which this occurs. Some severe stutterers with secondary abnormal movements made in an effort to force the blocked sound probably have patterns indistinguishable from tics, or may have a tic disorder. Specific language impairment or language disorder (in DSM-5) and social (pragmatic) communication disorder may also overlap with tic disorders and merit specialist evaluation in their own right, but relationships with tic disorders have not been well investigated. This is an area ripe for further research.

It is surprising that so little research has been devoted to speech and language problems in tic disorders, given the historically predominant interest in coprolalia, palilalia (repetition of a word or phrase) and echolalia (involuntary repetition of part of another's utterance). Features of speech and language in some persons with Tourette syndrome also include blocking, emphasis upon certain sounds (e.g. |k| or |s|) or syllables, change in speech intensity, repetitions, prolongations, false starts, accents, blockages, and reversals of yes/no (Van Borsel and Vanryckeghem 2000). Reports on speech and language in persons with tics are few and the results contradictory (Mulligan et al. 2003, Van Borsel et al. 2004, Legg et al. 2005, Thirumalai et al. 2007, Burd et al. 2008).

Children with speech problems frequently have associated motor problems (Visscher et al. 2007). This is another area of complex comorbidity. It would not be at all surprising if they also had a higher than expected rate of ADHD and tics.

STUTTERING

Stuttering (in DSM-5 termed 'childhood-onset fluency disorder') is common in children generally: 9% at age 3 years (Reilly et al. 2009), though other estimates have been as low as 4% and as high as 31%. Age at onset is between 2 and 6 (mean 5) years, with a male excess. The rate of spontaneous recovery is high. Persistent stuttering can be socially and vocationally impairing. But is what we sometimes encounter in Tourette syndrome stuttering or cluttering? Cluttering involves interjections of whole words or phrases. It might be that both stutterers and persons with Tourette syndrome have factors impairing stability of the speech fluency system (Ludlow et al. 1982, De Nil et al. 2005).

In the *TIC* database (Freeman et al. 2000), 'stuttering' was almost twice as common in persons with TS+ (6.8%) as in TS-only (3.7%, p<0.001, OR 1.8), and interestingly it was almost twice as common in those with coprolalia as in those without. In the Pauls et al. (1993) genetic study, stuttering occurred in 15% and other speech problems in 9% of patients, with no increase in their first-degree relatives, leading to the conclusion that there was no genetic relationship between tics and stuttering.

> **Practice point**
> Dysfluencies are more common in TS+ and in persons manifesting coprophenomena.

SPECIFIC LANGUAGE IMPAIRMENT

Specific language impairment (SLI) is a developmental disorder characterized by language impairments in individuals who have normal nonverbal ability, neurologic status and hearing (St Clair et al. 2011), with a prevalence estimated at 7%. Children with SLI have increased rates of emotional, behavioral and ADHD symptoms and impaired social adaptation, with an increased risk of psychiatric disorder in adult life (Clegg et al. 2005, Snowling et al. 2006, Yew and O'Kearney 2012). About one-third also qualify for DCD (Flapper and Schoemaker 2013). Those with SLI+DCD showed impairment in autonomy and social functioning. Although no study of SLI in tic disorders was found, the category overlaps indicate that many children with Tourette syndrome, for example, may have an SLI and merit evaluation.

In DSM-5 the equivalent diagnosis is *language disorder*, which is defined as a persistent difficulty in the acquisition and use of language across modalities at a level substantially below expectation for age, with onset during the developmental period, and not attributable to hearing or other sensory impairment, motor dysfunction or other medical condition, or better explained by intellectual disability or global developmental delay.

The other associated diagnosis in DSM-5 is *social (pragmatic) communication disorder*, defined as having (1) deficits in social usage, impairment in register-switching (changing communication to adapt to context), difficulty following rules of conversation and story-telling, and difficulties in making inferences (usage of nonliteral meanings); (2) functional limitations; and (3) onset in the early developmental period; and (4) not being attributable to another medical condition or better explained by ASD, intellectual disability or global delay.

Even though speech and language pathologists may not be very familiar with some of the peculiar speech patterns of those with tics, it may still be useful to have an assessment.

Sexually inappropriate behavior

> Sexually inappropriate behavior is associated with SIB and comorbidity in both children and adults, but absolute rates are low. It may be linked to weak self-regulation and control, as seen in other potentially disruptive behavior patterns. Treatment options are behavioral or pharmacological, but have not been well demonstrated to be effective.

In the *TIC* database (Freeman et al. 2000), reports of inappropriate sexual behavior are strongly associated with comorbidity. It was reported more commonly in TS+ (5.3%) than in TS-only (1.4%, p<0.001, OR 3.5), but the absolute proportion was still very low. The varieties of behavior can be very extensive: open masturbation, hands down the pants, sexual touching, pelvic thrusting, certain noises, and humping (sexual rubbing against another person or object, this occurring even in very small children).

Sexually inappropriate behavior is also associated with SIB in children (10% accompanying SIB vs 4% without, p<0.001, OR 2.6) and for adults (7% vs 2%, p<0.001, OR 3.5). (Some of the hazards of assuming sexual abuse as a causative factor have been considered in Chapter 3.)

Rödöö and Hennberg (2013) followed, to age 8 years, 19 Swedish girls who had had reported onset of infantile masturbation at a mean of 10.4 months and whose episodes of masturbation occurred from a few times a week to 50 a day. Twelve stopped at a mean age of 66 months. Although no patient was reported to have tics, these findings indicate that the presence of masturbation may involve developmental and other factors, so that it should not automatically be assumed to be a 'sexually inappropriate behavior' associated with a persistent tic disorder.

Sexually inappropriate behaviors may be associated with coprophenomena and social skill deficits, and may be intermittent rather than persistent.

> **Case examples**
> *'Michelle', 13, started tics at age 7 with eye-blinking and facial grimacing, but what was more a cause of concern was that she sometimes licked a finger and inserted it into her vagina in public. She also had shoulder-shrugging and mouth-opening. At age 9 sniffing began, and the tics waxed and waned. At 11 snorting began, followed by expletives. Her school did a count of her coprolalia, and on one day the estimate for*

"Fuck!" was over 1000 times. She was described as moody, irritable and oversensitive. Haloperidol improved the symptoms but caused too much sedation, so she could attend school only part-time. A trial of tetrabenazine was unsuccessful. Pimozide, 4mg/d was more successful. At interview she was cooperative but restless, with obvious motor and vocal tics. She told immediately about her touching herself, not realizing it could be part of Tourette syndrome; she had told her girlfriends about it so they wouldn't think she was masturbating. Later there was a parental complaint that she was behaving provocatively with boys. She was placed in a foster home and contact was lost.

Comment: Was there a relationship between her unusual 'tic' and her inappropriate sexual behavior? This was unclear.

'Frank', age 17, was a foster child seen over 20 years ago because of sexually inappropriate behavior since age 12. This consisted largely of agreeing to engage in any sexual acts that were available or that he had an urge to do. He had Tourette syndrome and ADHD with impulsivity, but also a history of preterm birth, maternal rejection, and a series of foster homes and institutional placements that resulted in attachment disorder and sexual abuse. He had been placed in care by age 2, but periodic involvement of his birth father delayed adoption for several years. Notably he showed a foot fetish by age 4. At age 5 psychological testing indicated average cognitive potential. The diagnosis of TS+ADHD was made only at age 16. It appeared that tics had been interpreted as attention-seeking behavior at times in the past. Pimozide improved his tics, but not his impulsive sexual behavior.

Comment: In the midst of such a mixed history and chaotic patterns of behavior, tics were not recognized. At what age they began and whether they and the ADHD added significantly to the clinical picture could not be determined.

Is not known how likely sexually inappropriate behaviors are to respond to behavioral or pharmacological methods of treatment. Some behaviors are quite socially embarrassing and may impair quality of life.

Practice point

In persons manifesting inappropriate sexual behavior other types of inadequate impulse control require investigation.

It may be pertinent here to point out that very little is known about how tics affect 'normal' or appropriate sexual behavior. One would think that this would be a fascinating area to investigate, but there is relatively little research on this subject, apart from some reports that tics improve after orgasm (Robertson et al. 1988, Robertson 1990, Jankovic 2001, Janik et al. 2014).

Contrary urges

> Urges to do what you are warned not to do (and know you should not do) can cause social problems and physical injury. Prevalence has been found to be almost 9%, most likely to occur in those with OCD, and with a higher comorbidity score and number of RMBs. This symptom can be considered part of a disorder of impulse control. (The name 'contrary urges' is purely descriptive and not used elsewhere.)

What are here termed 'contrary urges' are quite specific. They are not part of general oppositional behavior. These individuals have an overwhelming urge to do what specifically they were told not to do, *just because* they've been told that, and it 'sticks' in their mind and won't let go. Common examples are "Don't touch that, it's hot (or sharp)!" and then they touch it and may even sustain some injury. A more serious example is around the time of an eclipse of the sun, when people are warned not to stare at the phenomenon because it may cause permanent retinal damage. But they have to do it, and so must sometimes be restrained physically.

> I've always had to touch things. Sometimes I touch things I'm forbidden to touch... I stepped outside a store at a mall holding a dress with a plastic security tag attached to it, knowing an alarm would go off, mortified at the thought of being mistaken for a shoplifter but unable to resist bringing it — and me — over the invisible line... Sometimes I touch things that cause me pain, for the same reason: because my brain sends me a firm message to do so. I have often burned the tips of my fingers by touching stove burners (much in the same way I look directly at the sun until all I see is a hot white light, even though I know this is asking for permanent eye damage in the form of burned retinas). (Wilensky 1999, pp. 92–4)

In the *TIC* database (Freeman et al. 2000) there are original data on 52 children with this symptom, out of a total of 594 (8.7%). Most impressive is this pattern's relationship to comorbidity. The rate of such urges is much higher in TS+ than in those with TS-only. The average child with contrary urges has a comorbidity score of 2.48, whereas in children without contrary urges the average comorbidity score is 1.67 ($p<0.001$). Similarly, for (presumably non-tic) RMBs the average number is 4.7 vs 1.9 ($p<0.001$); the major differences among the disorders are strongest with OCD (OR 5.6), and somewhat less robust with anxiety and ADHD. Among the symptoms, spitting, a history of SIB, trichotillomania, nose-picking, rocking, smelling things, awake bruxism and coprophenomena are most strongly associated. This suggests that contrary urges are part of a spectrum of impulse control disorder symptoms and/or related to OCD. There are insufficient patients with contrary urges (n=51) to make statistical comparisons, but the trends may be of interest: the strongest associations with urges (in declining order of strength) are spitting, rocking, OCD, smelling, awake bruxism, coprophenomena and trichotillomania.

Sensory over-responsivity/sensory processing disorder/misophonia

> Sensory over-responsivity (SOR) is important and can be a significant feature of neuro-developmental disorders, including tic disorders, OCD and ASD, or may merit its own diagnostic category. Unfortunately, despite some evidence of its independence, it was not accepted for DSM-5. There is a strong clinical impression that occupational therapy assessment is valuable in exploring SOR, but that evidence in favor of sensory integration therapy is not yet well enough established to be highly recommended. Families may become accustomed to accommodate their member with SOR and not report it in the clinical evaluation unless it is asked about. There is evidence that persons with tic disorders are more likely to have high sensitivity to endogenous or exogenous sensation.
>
> Misophonia is the unofficial term for strong negative reactions (often quite specific) to sounds. It can be a minor personal peculiarity or impairing when it leads to physical and social avoidances. It is not rare. Reactions may involve the limbic and autonomic systems.

There has been anecdotal evidence for a long time about sensory peculiarities in the field of occupational therapy, but only recently has early evidence for treatment effects become available, and it is still in contention (American Academy of Pediatrics 2012).

In the *TIC* database (Freeman et al. 2000) differences in the tactile mode are most frequent, perhaps related to premonitory sensations in Tourette syndrome.

CLINICAL APPEARANCE

Many examples can be provided but only a few are mentioned here. In the *tactile mode*, annoying sensations that persist (or that children cannot ignore) are seams in socks, tags in new clothing, tightness around the waist (belts) or neck (turtle-neck sweaters), textures of materials, and tightness of shoes. Parents may describe going shopping for clothing or shoes for their child, finally picking some that seem acceptable, only to have them rejected forcefully when first put on at home. Children may refuse to go to school, because they believe that the unpleasant feeling will last all day. In the *auditory mode* specific types of sounds (e.g. vacuum cleaners, fireworks) may evoke unpleasant reactions; sometimes the over-responsivity diminishes or abates with further development. In the *olfactory mode*, there may be general sensitivity or reactions to specific kinds of smells, perhaps leading to disgust, gagging or even vomiting. Strong reactions to tastes and textures of food are common in young children, whose gustatory system has not yet fully reached its adult status and causes parental concern. This often changes with further development. There may also be unusually strong negative reactions to bright lights, heights, vestibular sensations affecting playground equipment, rides, elevators and escalators, hyperactive gag reflex and startle, and so on, or sometimes the opposite (an unusual attraction to the same stimuli). These characteristics may become the basis for phobic avoidances or habits.

It seems obvious that children with strong sensory dysfunction will live different lives, as will their families. Several publications have explored this field (e.g. Miller 2006, Carter et al. 2011). There is some evidence that children with significant sensory differences tend to engage in more ritualistic behavior (Dar et al. 2012).

EVIDENCE LIMITATIONS

There are no generally accepted clinical standards, and the reactions are matters of degree, life situation and context. They may not be reported because the sensitivity has reduced over time or the family has accommodated to them.

Is there enough evidence for a sensory integration or processing disorder diagnostic category, or are unusual sensory differences just manifestations of various disorders or symptoms? This question has been approached by Reynolds and Lane (2008), Carter et al. (2011), Keuler et al. (2011) and Van Hulle et al. (2012). They studied sensory over-responsivity in its relationship to psychopathology and found that the former exists independently of recognized diagnoses but also in association with them. This was contentious during the run-up to DSM-5; the result was that the category has not been included in DSM-5, even as a research category.

Sensory peculiarities appear to be especially common among persons with ASD (Baranek et al. 2007, Ben-Sasson et al. 2013), but there appears to be no good evidence of efficacy in favor of sensory integration therapy for it (Lang et al. 2012). The prevalence of SOR among persons with tic disorders is probably higher than in those without, but has not been adequately studied, beyond the report of Belluscio et al. (2011). Nevertheless, sensitivities may be clinically important! For the most recent review, including the important symptom of excessive evaluation of one's own behavior, see Houghton et al. (2014).

Practice point

Asking about sensitivities (past or present) that have caused concern or avoidances, in tactile, auditory, olfactory, vestibular, visual and temperature modes should be part of a complete history if a competent occupational therapy assessment has not been done. Even when not especially revealing it can be a good way to learn about your patient and sometimes family members as well.

MISOPHONIA

Misophonia is the name of an uncommon disorder where the person cannot tolerate specific sounds (Stansfield 1992, Coelho et al. 2007, Hadjipavlou et al. 2008, Asha'ari et al. 2010, Schwartz et al. 2011, Johnson et al. 2013, Wu et al. 2014) owing to extreme over-responsivity. Little is known about it, but most people are familiar with one example: intolerance to chalkboard-scratching, which is very individually specific and apparently does not remit with advancing age (no studies were available on this point). Other well-known examples are intolerance of the sounds of chewing, swallowing, slurping, sneezing, nose-blowing, breathing, silverware touching teeth or plates, and scratching or rubbing something made of styrofoam against something else. These intolerances may persist in unchanged form or may spread or worsen (perhaps because of the development of hypervigilance) and cause significant impairment. In many cases the intolerance is more severe in association with sounds made by the parents, especially the mother or a sibling.

Practice point

For reasons not well understood, hyper-responsivity to specific sounds made by the mother are more common than those made by others.

Onset of misophonia is often in mid- to late childhood, and other family members may also be affected. It is of interest that the range of triggers may expand, and can include *seeing* the sound-producing activity, or *imagining* the activity, and the child may even *mimic* the sound trigger, which can sometimes weaken the unpleasant effect. For example, in someone exquisitely sensitive to chalkboard scratching, one has only to raise one's hand and mimic the action, without explanation, to cause a reaction (often described as "a chill down my spine"). Neal and Cavanna (2012) described a 52-year-old man with Tourette syndrome whose misophonia developed before his tics.

The etiology is speculative, but in the still quite limited audiology literature it is said that the problem is not in the auditory tracts but may lie in the connections to the limbic and autonomic systems. Hyperacusis (generalized lowered loudness discomfort level associated with abnormal annoyance with sounds) is reported to occur in many children, and of those, half of a randomly selected sample also had tinnitus (Coelho et al. 2007) of which many parents were unaware.

The only experimental research was in an important paper by Edelstein et al. (2013). The patients interviewed reported that the worst trigger sounds were chewing, eating and crunching sounds, followed by lip-smacking, pen-clicking and clock-ticking. Reactions included a range of negative feelings and thoughts. These included intense anxiety, panic, anger, extreme irritation and even rage. Physical reactions included feelings of pressure in the chest, arms, head or entire body as well as tightened muscles, sweating, difficulty breathing and increase in heart rate (all reactions of autonomic arousal). The symptoms did not fit with any conventional diagnostic category. Skin conductance responses indicated that auditory stimuli were more aversive than visual stimuli, and stronger in misophonic individuals than in a comparison group. The suggestion from the experiments was that reactions of misophonic indivuals are exaggerated normal reactions. The findings were consistent with the proposed diagnostic criteria of Schröder et al. (2013).

Johnson et al. (2013) make a strong point that the reactions of a person with misophonia are often modified by familiarity (less assertive or aggressive with strangers than with family) and there is typically considerable family accommodation.

Wu et al. (2014) assessed 483 undergraduate students through self-report measures and found that almost 20% reported misophonic symptoms. There were associations with other modalities, impairment, and moderate associations with anxiety, depressive and OCD-like symptoms. Anger outbursts were related to significant anxiety levels.

In the *TIC* database (Freeman et al. 2000), 30% of children were reported to have or to have had auditory hypersensitivity, not always reported unless asked about directly. Common triggers, especially in young children, are fireworks, popping of balloons, vacuum cleaners, leaf-blowers, chainsaws, sirens, foghorns, blenders, lawn mowers and sonic booms. These sensitivities can lead to avoidances and affect family life. The association of auditory sensitivity was strongest with anxiety disorder (OR 6.6) and OCD (OR 3.8); of those reported as having auditory sensitivity, 73% had an anxiety disorder and 48% had OCD, whereas the association with ADHD was non-significant. [These results dovetail well with those of the Wu et al. (2014) study.]

A common misophonic reaction is to joint-cracking. Clinically, we often observe that one family member is repelled by the sounds and sometimes also the look of their child doing this. They like the popular myth that joint-cracking will lead to arthritis later (a common misunderstanding in our culture) and feel supported by that belief in trying to scare their child out of the 'habit', but correcting the myth does not change the negative reaction. If said in front of the child, a common (hopefully temporary) response of the child is to perform it more forcefully in the mother's presence (as if to make up for her efforts to suppress it). This can sometimes cause a negative feeling about the clinician.

We have encountered patients with TS+ who cannot tolerate their mother making specific sounds (typically consonantal like |k| or |p|) in her speech, placing a demand upon her to select words of similar meaning without the offending sounds, or to avoid the combination of certain words with nonverbal communication of specific feelings.

Case examples

'Anthony' was assessed when he was 12. He had been diagnosed with Tourette syndrome and ADHD and had a long history of exquisite sensitivity to bumps caused by rolling over pine cones when in his baby carriage and later on a bicycle; the event triggered a rage reaction. This quite severe sensitivity was hard to believe, so I began to ask him about "pi--" and that was as far as I got, because he instantly leapt towards me, shrieking "I'm going to kill you!" and then within a few seconds apologized. It is hard to convey how sudden and shocking this reaction was! His mother had not exaggerated. In this case it seemed that the early tactile reaction spread to the word. (The father also had misophonia.)

'Dale' was 14, diagnosed with Tourette syndrome, ADHD and OCD. Among his many symptoms were that he could not tolerate |p| or |k| sounds or speech with wet lips, especially with his parents. When it was encountered he reacted with anger and might hit them, expressing remorse later.

Comment: Aggressive reactions are not typical, but have been reported in some cases by Edelstein et al. (2013) and Schröder et al. (2013).

'Jay' was 12 years old with Tourette syndrome that included fairly loud vocal tics. His

younger brother had ASD and was exquisitely sensitive to an increase in Jay's vocals, resulting in a deterioration of his behavior. This became a powerful family-based reason for treating Jay's tics with medication.

These examples of unusually specific and extreme reactions to a trigger, presently and unofficially termed misophonia, are presented because (1) persons with Tourette syndrome and/or OCD may manifest them; (2) they may have siblings who react this way to one or more of their tics; and (3) they are likely to be misunderstood as reacting this way purely because of some dysfunctional family relationship. With regard to tics or repetitive motor behaviors as triggers for misophonia, the following are listed in the literature: throat-clearing, coughing, gulping, sniffing, tapping, eye-blinking and joint-cracking. Note that phonophobia (a fear of all or any loud sounds) is classifiable as a form of 'specific phobia, other' in DSM-5. Thus, misophonia has as yet no clear place in the DSM classification.

Neuroimaging studies have not been reported as yet, but should not be methodologically difficult. Fine-tuning of brain reactions to sensation should not be surprising, and lesser extremes than discussed here are common. There are rare cases of seizures being triggered by music in a specific key, but not if a half-tone higher or lower, or by one specific person's voice.

Treatment is not well established, but systematic desensitization by pairing with positive sounds appears to be efficacious according to Jastreboff and Jastreboff (2003).

Other physical symptom patterns

Headaches are common in children and there is some evidence that headaches in general and migraine in particular are more common in tic disorders than in those without. The clinical course is variable. New tics of the head, neck and shoulders can cause pain and aggravate headaches in those susceptible to them, an indication for careful exploration before starting systemic medication for tics. Enuresis, encopresis and persistent 'cough' can have multiple causes related to tics that may be misunderstood and lead to requests for unnecessary specialist referral and extensive tests.

HEADACHE/MIGRAINE

Kwak et al. (2003) have reported that migraine is more common in Tourette syndrome (25%), four times the population prevalence. Previously Barabas et al. (1984) reported a figure of 26.6%. Many authors accept that a substantial increase is associated with Tourette syndrome. Ghosh et al. (2012) interviewed 109 patients with Tourette syndrome at or under the age of 21 and found headaches in 55%, with migraines four times more common than in the general population, and tension-type headaches more than five times as common. Migraine in children and adolescents now has a first-line evidence-based treatment of CBT and amitriptyline (Powers et al. 2013).

A good review of the field of pediatric headache is by Hershey (2010). Tension-type headaches are very common generally (5% to 15%) while migraine in various studies ranges from 2% to 5%. Forty per cent to 50% of children reported having at least one headache a week. The criteria to establish migraine as a diagnosis are not entirely satisfactory. In the transition from late adolescence to adulthood the prevalence of migraine increases significantly (Wang et al. 2009, Hershey 2010). Some of these children resolve their chronic daily headaches that were considered tension-type, some do not, and many of those who continue to have headaches were later diagnosed with episodic migraine. Thus the course is quite variable.

Since some children with tics have powerful, frequent and sudden movements of their head, neck and/or shoulders, local pain and headaches may be reported and thought to be tic-related. This is not uncommon in children with new head-shaking tics. Occasionally headache is complained of after a new drug (such as methylphenidate) is started.

PAIN

It is not uncommon for persons with tics to complain of pain due to a new tic, intensification of an existing tic, an accidental encounter with an object in the performance of a tic, or a self-injurious tic. The complaints are most often voiced to the mother during the vulnerable time after the child is in bed. It is the source of problems brought to specialist or primary care clinicians, and can exert pressure to medicate (which may, however, merit caution and temporizing).

Before a decision to medicate the tics, one should examine the area expressing the pain, determine the nature of the complaint and the change in the tic situation that seems to have been the origin of the suffering, and gain some idea of whether the family can support conservative measures rather than systemic medication (at least temporarily). If you start with medication, you could be in for a long and complex course that may be unnecessary. How much complaining can the parent(s) tolerate? Do they realize that sore muscles from tics can be the result of over-exercise that can occur with any new activity? This is usually the point at which common pain-relieving measures should be discussed and instituted for muscle aches, such as massage, local heat, mild analgesics and reassurance, with an agreement to report back on results. If these are not successful, more robust methods may be required, including medication or even (rarely) botulinum toxin therapy.

> **Practice point**
> The development of pain that appears to be related to tics should be cause to assess the situation carefully, and if it results from a frequent new tic, advise conventional and conservative measures before instituting medication for tics.

ENURESIS AND ENCOPRESIS

In years past many common 'special symptoms' were rather loosely lumped together, possibly because of presumed psychogenic explanations. Although there is more than one type of enuresis (developmental, regressive, nocturnal, diurnal; Kiddoo 2012), there seems to be little evidence of any close relationship between this category and tics. The same may be said for encopresis. Perusing a 'Google Scholar' search for enuresis and tics, most of the references to books and journal articles date from 50 to 100 years ago. However, happy to say, a comprehensive handbook on both enuresis and encopresis was produced by von Gontard and Nevéus in 2006. There is some evidence that in children with the inattentive type of ADHD (where enuresis is common) enuresis may reflect a disorder of arousal (Elia et al. 2009).

What may be of more current importance, though, is how tics may cause or trigger enuretic or encopretic-seeming behavior.

Case example

'Cathy' was 5 when she developed severe tics with coprolalia and echolalia. She had a history of some recurrent bladder infections and started having abdominal tics with a Valsalva maneuver. She engaged in scratching of the perianal area but no infection or parasite was found. She began to insert her finger into her anus and said she always felt as if she had a full rectum and would have to defecate, sometimes passed some stool and had an accident in school. She had several months-long tic-free periods. Finally on examination she was found to have an internal hemorrhoid; when this was treated her symptoms gradually subsided. When followed up at age 11 she was doing well on low-dosage medication with occasional coprolalia but no recurrence of the problem with bowel movements.

__Comment:__ It was not clear which came first: the hemorrhoid or the repetitive Valsalva maneuver producing stool expulsion, but treatment was able to reverse an increasingly complex symptom development.

A very recent phenomenon, a 'sign of the times', should be noted here. Children and adolescents who are heavily involved in video gaming, especially those who are competitive with others online, may be penalized by the software timing if they take a break to go to the toilet, because they may lose their hard-won place. As a consequence we are seeing some children and adolescents who have urinary incontinence because they will not take a break, or wait too long, especially if their tics involve abdominal contractions or they have urological problems.

Practice point

Interference with ordinary habits may have a simple cause (or a phobic avoidance) that only requires sensible questioning before specialist referral and tests are considered.

COUGH

Cough is a common symptom with many potential causes, already mentioned in Chapters 2 and 3 (Irwin et al. 2006). Here is but one example.

Case example

'Amir' was 13, an only child of an Asian family, regarded as precious, important and bright by his extended family. Schooling had been split between two countries. He was so shy and anxious that he barely spoke and had great difficulty making friends. After a mild upper respiratory illness he developed a persistent 'cough' associated with normal findings: bronchoscopy, pulmonary function studies, radiography and computerized tomography. The symptom did not occur in sleep. Unfortunately for the family, all assessments showed mild intellectual disability, even when tested in his native language. The parents did not accept this. The 'cough' had an unusual quality, a biphasic expiratory noise. He said he had a strange feeling of too much saliva in the back of his throat. His parents denied any other tics, but occasional eye-blinking and facial grimacing were observed. The parents insisted that the otolaryngologist had not spent enough time with him to find the organic cause of his 'cough'. "There must be something there." An 'organic' cause was not confirmed on a brief hospital admission for observation (during which the parents refused to leave his bedside) and he was discharged against medical advice.

Comment: Although a respiratory tic was suspected, the situation may have been complicated by the parents sponsoring extended family members to immigrate and their fear that the process might be jeopardized if their son was found to have a chronic 'mental' condition. In this instance powerful family and cultural forces seemed to be at work, obscuring the clinical picture and truncating the completion of an agreed-upon diagnostic process.

REFERENCES

Allen RP, Singer HS, Brown JE, Salam MM (1992) Sleep disorders in Tourette syndrome: a primary or unrelated problem? *Pediatr Neurol* 8: 275–80. doi: 1-s2.0-0887899492903656.

American Academy of Pediatrics Section on Complementary and Integrative Medicine and Council on Children with Disabilities (2012) Policy Statement. Sensory integration therapies for children with developmental and behavioral disorders. *Pediatrics* 129: 1186–9 doi; 10.1542/peds.2012-0876.

Andrade C, Srihari BS (2001) A preliminary survey of rhinotillexis in an adolescent sample. *J Clin Psychiatry* 62: 426–31.

Asha'ari ZA, Zain NM, Razali A (2010) Phonophobia and hyperacusis: practical points from a case report. *Malaysian J Med Sci* 17: 49–51.

Bachara GH, Phelan WJ (1980) Rhythmic movement in deaf children. *Percept Motor Skills* 50: 933–4.

Barabas G, Matthews WS, Ferrari M (1984) Tourette's syndrome and migraine. *Arch Neurol* 41: 871–2. doi: 10.1001/archneur.1984.04050190077018.

Baranek GT, Boyd BA, Poe MD, et al. (2007) Hyperresponsive sensory patterns in young children with autism, developmental delay, and typical development. *Am J Ment Retard* 112: 233–45.

Bate KS, Malouff JM, Thorstcinsson ET, Bhullar N (2011) The efficacy of habit reversal therapy for tics, habit disorders, and stuttering: a meta-analytic review. *Clin Psychol Rev* 31: 865–71. doi: 10.1016/j.cpr.2011.03.013.

Baum KT, Desai A, Field J, et al. (2014) Sleep restriction worsens mood and emotion regulation in adolescents. *J Child Psychol Psychiatry* 55: 180–90. doi: 10.1111/jcpp.12125.

Belluscio BA, Jin L, Watters V, et al. (2011) Sensory sensitivity to external stimuli in Tourette syndrome patients. *Mov Disord* 26: 2538–43. doi: 10.1002/mds.23977.

Ben-Sasson A, Soto TW, Martínez-Pedraza F, Carter AS (2013) Early sensory over-responsivity in toddlers with autism spectrum disorders as a predictor of family impairment and parenting stress. *J Child Psychol Psychiatry* 54: 846–53. doi: 10.1111/jcpp.12035.

Borda T, Feinstein BA, Neziroglu F, et al. (2013) Are children with obsessive–compulsive disorder at risk for problematic peer relationships? *J Obsess-Compuls Relat Disord* 2: 359–65. doi: 10.1016/j.jocrd.2013.06.006.

Budman C (2006) Treatment of aggression in Tourette syndrome. *Adv Neurol* 99: 222–6.

Budman C, Coffey BJ, Shechter R, et al. (2008) Aripiprazole in children and adolescents with Tourette disorder with and without explosive outbursts. *J Child Adolesc Psychopharmacol* 18: 509–15. doi: 10.1089/cap.2007.061.

Budman CL, Rockmore L, Stokes J, Sossin M (2003) Clinical phenomenology of episodic rage in children with Tourette syndrome. *J Psychosom Res* 55: 59–65. doi: 10.1016/S0022-3999(02)00584-6.

Burd L, Christensen T, Kerbeshian J (2008) Speech, language, and communication in Tourette's syndrome. *Ann Rev Appl Linguistics* 28: 170–90. doi: 10.1017/S026719050808001X.

Calvo E, Fernández-Yruegas D, Alvarez L, et al. (1995) Bilateral stress fracture of the clavicle. *Skeletal Radiol* 24: 613–6.

Carlson GA, Potegal M, Margulies D, et al. (2009) Rages – what are they and who has them? *J Child Adolesc Psychopharmacol* 19: 281–8. doi: 10.1089/cap.2008.0108.

Carter AS, O'Donnell DA, Schultz RT, et al. (2000) Social and emotional adjustment in children affected with Gilles de la Tourette's syndrome: associations with ADHD and family functioning. *J Child Psychol Psychiatry* 41: 215–23. doi: 10.1111/1469-7610.00602.

Carter AS, Ben-Sasson A, Briggs-Gowan MJ (2011) Sensory over-responsivity, psychopathology, and family impairment in school-aged children. *J Am Acad Child Adolesc Psychiatry* 50: 1210–9. doi: 10.1016/j.jaac.2011.09.010.

Chen K, Budman CL, Herrera LD, et al. (2013) Prevalence and clinical correlates of explosive outbursts in Tourette syndrome. *Psychiatry Res* 205: 269–75. doi: 10.1016/j.psychres.2012.09.029.

Chervin RD, Archbold KH, Dillon JE, et al. (2002) Associations between symptoms of inattention, hyperactivity, restless legs, and periodic leg movements. *Sleep* 25: 213–8.

Clegg J, Hollis C, Mawhood L, Rutter M (2005) Developmental language disorders — a follow-up in later adult life. Cognitive, language and psychosocial outcomes. *J Child Psychol Psychiatry* 46: 128–49. doi: 10.1111/j.1469-7610.2004.00342.x.

Coelho CB, Sanchez TG, Tyler RS (2007) Hyperacusis, sound annoyance, and loudness hypersensitivity in children. *Prog Brain Res* 166: 169–78.

Dar R, Kahn DT, Carneli R (2012) The relationship between sensory processing, childhood rituals and obsessive–compulsive symptoms. *J Behav Ther Exper Psychiatry* 43: 679–84. doi: 10.1016/j.jbtep.2011.09.008.

De Laat A, Macaluso GM (2002) Sleep bruxism as a motor disorder. *Mov Disord* 19 Suppl 2: S67–9. doi: 10.1002/mds.10064.

De Nil LF, Sasisekaran J, Van Lieshout PHHM, Sandor P (2005) Speech disfluencies in individuals with Tourette syndrome. *J Psychosom Res* 58: 97–102. doi: 10.1016/j.jpsychores.2004.06.002.

Dobbs M, Berger JR (2003) Cervical myelopathy secondary to violent tics of Tourette's syndrome. *Neurology* 60: 1862–3. doi: 10.1212/01.WNL.0000064285.98285.CF.

Eddy CM, Cavanna AE (2013) 'It's a curse!': coprolalia in Tourette syndrome. *Eur J Neurol* 20: 1467–70. doi: 10.1111/ene.12207.

Edelstein M, Brang D, Rouw R, Ramachandran VS (2013) Misophonia: physiological investigations and case descriptions. *Front Hum Neurosci* 7: 296. doi: 10.3389/fnhum.2013.00296.

Egermark I, Carlsson GE, Magnusson T (2001) A 20-year longitudinal study of subjective symptoms of temporomandibular disorders from childhood to adulthood. *Acta Odont Scand* 59: 40–8. doi: 10.1080/000163501300035788.

Eisenhauer GL, Woody RC (1987) Self-mutilation and Tourette's disorder. *J Child Neurol* 2: 265–7. doi: 10.1177/088307388700200405.

Elia J, Takeda T, Deberardinis R, et al. (2009) Nocturnal enuresis: a suggestive endophenotype marker for a subgroup of inattentive attention-deficit/hyperactivity disorder. *J Pediatr* 155: 239–44. doi: 10.1016/j.jpeds.2009.02.031.

Ellison JM, Stanziani P (1993) SSRI-associated nocturnal bruxism in four patients. *J Clin Psychiatry* 54: 432–4.

Flapper BCT, Schoemaker MM (2013) Developmental coordination disorder in children with specific language impairment: co-morbidity and impact on quality of life. *Res Dev Disabil* 34: 756–63. doi: 10.1016/j.ridd.2012.10.014.

Freeman RD (2007) Tic disorders and ADHD: answers from a world-wide clinical dataset on Tourette syndrome. Tourette Syndrome International Database Consortium. *Eur Child Adolesc Psychiatry* 16 (Suppl 1): 15–23. doi: 10.1007/s00787-007-1003-7.

Freeman RD, Fast DK, Burd L, et al. (2000) An international perspective on Tourette syndrome: selected findings from 3500 individuals in 22 countries. *Dev Med Child Neurol* 42: 436–7. doi: 10.1111/j.1469-8749.2000.tb00346.x.

Freeman RD, Zinner SH, Müller-Vahl KR, et al. (2009) Coprophenomena in Tourette syndrome. *Dev Med Child Neurol* 51: 218–27. doi: 10.1111/j.1469-8749.2008.03135.x.

Fusco C, Bertani G, Caricati G, Della Giustina E (2006) Stress fracture of the peroneal bone secondary to a complex tic. *Brain Dev* 28: 52–4. doi: 10.1016/j.braindev.2005.03.009.

Ghanizadeh A (2008) Association of nail biting and psychiatric disorders in children and their parents in a psychiatrically referred sample of children. *Child Adolesc Psychiatry Ment Health* 2: 13.

Ghosh D, Rajan PV, Dad D, et al. (2012) Headache in children with Tourette syndrome. *J Pediatr* 161: 303–7. doi: 10.1016/j.jpeds.2012.01.072.

Gingras JL, Gaultney JF, Picchietti DL (2011) Pediatric periodic limb movement disorder: sleep symptom and polysomnographic correlates compared to obstructive sleep apnea. *J Clin Sleep Med* 7: 603–9.

Grant J, Stein D, Woods D, Keuthen NJ, eds (2012) *Trichotillomania, Skin-Picking, and Other Body-Focused Repetitive Behaviors*. Arlington, VA: American Psychiatric Publishing.

Gruber R, Carrey N, Weiss SK, et al. (2014) Position statement on pediatric sleep for psychiatrists. *J Can Acad Child Adolesc Psychiatry* 23: 174–95.

Hadjipavlou G, Baer S, Lau A, Howard A (2008) Selective sound intolerance and emotional distress: what every clinician should hear. *Psychosom Med* 70: 739–40.

Hanisch C, Hautmann C, Plück J, et al. (2014) The Prevention Program for Externalizing Problem Behavior (PEP) improves child behavior by reducing negative parenting: analysis of mediating processes in a randomized controlled trial. *J Child Psychol Psychiatry* 55: 473–84. doi: 10.1111/jcpp.12177.

Hershey AD (2010) Recent developments in pediatric headache. *Curr Opin Neurol* 23: 249–53. doi: 10.1097/WCO.0b013e3283391888.

Hoban TF (2004) Sleep and its disorders in children. *Semin Neurol* 24: 327–40. doi: 10.1055/s-2004-835062.

Houghton DC, Capriotti MR, Conelea CA, Woods DW (2014) Sensory phenomena in Tourette syndrome: their role in symptom formation and treatment. *Curr Dev Disord Rep* (online Aug 23) doi: 10.1007/s40474-014-0026-2.

Irwin RS, Glomb WB, Chang AB (2006) Habit cough, tic cough, and psychogenic cough in adult and pediatric populations: ACCP evidence-based clinical practice guidelines. *Chest* 129: 174S–179S.

Isaacs JD, Adams M, Lees AJ (2010) Noncompressive myelopathy associated with violent axial tics of Tourette syndrome. *Neurology* 74: 697–8.

Janik P, Milanowski L, Szejko N (2014) [Psychogenic tics: clinical characteristics and prevalence.] *Psychiatr Pol* 48: 835–45 (in Polish).

Jankovic J (2001) Tourette's syndrome. *N Engl J Med* 345: 1184–92. doi: 10.1056/NEJMra010032.

Jastreboff PJ, Jastreboff MM (2003) Tinnitus retraining therapy for patients with tinnitus and decreased sound tolerance. *Otolaryngol Clin* 36: 321–36.

Johnson KP, Giannotti F, Cortesi F (2009) Sleep patterns in autism spectrum disorders. *Child Adolesc Psychiatr Clin N Am* 18: 917–28.

Johnson PL, Webber TA, Wu MS, et al. (2013) When selective audiovisual stimuli become unbearable: a case series on pediatric misophonia. *Neuropsychiatry* 3: 569–75.

Keuler MM, Schmidt NI, Van Hulle CA, et al. (2011) Sensory overresponsivity: prenatal risk factors and temperamental contributions. *J Dev Behav Pediatr* 32: 533–41.

Kiddoo DA (2012) Nocturnal enuresis. *CMAJ* 184: 908–11. doi: 10.1503/cmaj.111652.

Kim KL, Reynolds KCV, Alfano CA (2012) Social impairment in children with obsessive–compulsive disorder: do comorbid problems of inattention and hyperactivity matter? *J Obsess-Compuls Relat Disord* 1: 228–33. doi: 10.1016/j.jocrd.2012.06.005.

Ko DY, Kim SJK, Chae JH, et al. (2013) Cervical spondylotic myelopathy caused by violent motor tics in a child with Tourette syndrome. *Childs Nerv Syst* 29: 317–21. doi: 10.1007/s00381-012-1939-x.

Kotagal S, Silber MH (2004) Childhood-onset restless legs syndrome. *Ann Neurol* 56: 803–7.

Krauss JK, Jankovic J (1996) Severe motor tics causing cervical myelopathy in Tourette's syndrome. *Mov Disord* 11: 563–6. doi: 10.1002/mds.870110512.

Kurlan R, Daragjati C, Como PG, et al. (1996) Nonobscene complex socially inappropriate behavior in Tourette's syndrome. *J Neuropsychiatr Clin Neurosci* 8: 311–7.

Kushner HI (1995) Medical fictions: the case of the cursing marquise and the (re)construction of Gilles de la Tourette's syndrome. *Bull Hist Med* 69: 224–54.

Kwak C, Dat Vuong K, Jankovic J (2003) Migraine headache in patients with Tourette syndrome. *Arch Neurol* 62: 1595–8. doi: 10.1001/archneur.60.11.1595.

Lang R, O'Reilly M, Healy O, et al. (2012) Sensory integration therapy for autism spectrum disorders: a systematic review. *Res Aut Spect Disord* 6: 1004–18.

Legg C, Penn C, Temlett J, Sonnenberg B (2005) Language skills of adolescents with Tourette syndrome. *Clin Ling Phonetics* 19: 15–33. doi: 10.1080/02699200410001665270.

Leksell E, Edvardson S (2005) A case of Tourette syndrome presenting with oral self-injurious behaviour. *Int J Paediatr Dentistry* 15: 370–4. doi: 10.1111/j.1365-263X.2005.00652.x.

Lespérance P, Djerroud N, Diaz Anzaldua A, et al. (2004) Restless legs in Tourette syndrome. *Mov Disord* 19: 1084–7. doi: 10.1002/mds.20100.

Lewin AB, Murphy TK, Storch EA, et al. (2012) A phenomenological investigation of women with Tourette or other chronic tic disorders. *Compr Psychiatry* 53: 525–34. doi: 10.1016/j.comppsych.2011.07.004.

Lim S (2004) Self-induced bilateral retinal detachment in Tourette syndrome. *Arch Ophthalmol* 122: 930–1.

Lin J-J, Wang H-S, Wong M-C, et al. (2007) Tourette's syndrome with cervical disc herniation. *Brain Dev* 29: 61–3.

Lobbezoo F, Ahlberg J, Glaros AG, et al. (2013) Bruxism defined and graded: an international consensus. *J Oral Rehabil* 40: 2–4. doi: 10.1111/joor.12011.

Ludlow CL, Polinsky RJ, Caine ED, et al. (1982) Language and speech abnormalities in Tourette syndrome. *Adv Neurol* 35: 351–61.

Manfredini D, Lobbezoo F (2010) Relationship between bruxism and temporomandibular disorders: a systematic review of literature from 1998 to 2008. *Oral Surg Oral Path Oral Radiol Endodontol* 109: e26–50. doi: 10.1016/j.tripleo.2010.02.013.

Manfredini D, Landi N, Fantoni F, et al. (2005) Anxiety symptoms in clinically diagnosed bruxers. *J Oral Rehabil* 32: 584–8. doi: 10.1111/j.1365-2842.2005.01462.x.

Margo CE (2002) Tourette syndrome and iatrogenic eye injury. *Am J Ophthalmol* 134: 784–5.

Mashor RS, Kumar NL, Ritenour RJ, Rootman DS (2011) Keratoconus caused by eye rubbing in patients with Tourette syndrome. *Can J Ophthalmol* 46: 83–6. doi: 10.3129/i10-072.

Mathews CA, Waller J, Glidden DV, et al. (2004) Self injurious behavior in Tourette syndrome: correlates with impulsivity and impulse control. *J Neurol Neurosurg Psychiatry* 75: 1149–55.

McGough JJ (2014) Chronic non-episodic irritability in childhood: current and future challenges. *Am J Psychiatry* 171: 607–10 (editorial). doi: 10.1176/appi.ajp.2014.14030385.

McGuire JF, Kugler BB, Park JM, et al. (2012) Evidence-based assessment of compulsive skin picking, chronic tic disorders and trichotillomania in children. *Child Psychiatry Hum Dev* 43: 855–83.

Micheli F, Fernandez Pardal M, Gatto M, et al. (1993) Bruxism secondary to chronic antidopaminergic drug exposure. *Clin Neuropharmacol* 16: 315–23.

Miller LJ (2006) *Sensational Kids: Hope and Help for Children with Sensory Processing Disorder.* New York: Penguin.

Mindell JA, Owens JA (2010) *A Clinical Guide to Pediatric Sleep: Diagnosis and Management of Sleep Problems, 2nd edn.* Philadelphia: Wolters Kluwer/Lippincott Williams & Wilkins.

Mistry R (1987) *Tales from Firozsha Baag.* Toronto: McLelland & Stewart.

Moon BS, Price CT, Campbell JB (1998) Upper extremity and rib stress fractures in a child. *Skeletal Radiol* 27: 403–5.

Müller-Vahl K (2010) *Tourette-Syndrom und andere Tic-Erkrankungen in Kindes- und Erwachsenenalter.* Berlin: Medizinisch Wissenschaftliche Verlagsgesellschaft.

Mulligan HF, Anderson TJ, Jones RD, et al. (2003) Tics and developmental stuttering. *Parkinsonism Relat Disord* 9: 281–9. doi: 10.1016/S1353-8020(03)00002-6.

Neal M, Cavanna AE (2012) Selective sound sensitivity syndrome (misophonia) and Tourette syndrome. *J Neurol Neurosurg Psychiatry* 83: e1 (abstract). doi: 10.1136/jnnp-2012-303538.20.

Ohayon MM, O'Hara R, Vitiello MV (2012) Epidemiology of restless legs syndrome: a synthesis of the literature. *Sleep Med Rev* 16: 283–95. doi: 10.1016/j.smrv.2011.05.002.

Ougrin D, Tranah T, Leigh E, et al. (2012) Self-harm in adolescents. *J Child Psychol Psychiatry* 53: 337–50. doi: 10.1111/j.1469-7610.2012.02525.x.

Owens JA, Mindell JA (2005) *Taking Charge of Your Child's Sleep.* New York: Marlowe/Avalon.

Pauls D, Leckman J, Cohen D (1993) Familial relationship between Gilles de la Tourette syndrome, attention deficit disorder, learning disability, speech disorders, and stuttering. *J Am Acad Child Adolesc Psychiatry* 32: 1044–50. doi: 10.1097/00004583-199309000-00025.

Petit D, Touchette E, Tremblay RE, et al. (2007) Dyssomnias and parasomnias in early childhood. *Pediatrics* 119: e1016–25. doi: 10.1542/peds.2006-2132.

Picchietti D, Allen RP, Walters AS, et al. (2007) Restless legs syndrome: prevalence and impact in children and adolescents – the Peds REST Study. *Pediatrics* 120: 253–66. doi: 10.1542/peds.2006-2767.

Picchietti DL, England SJ, Walters AS, et al. (1998) Periodic limb movement disorder and restless legs syndrome in children with attention-deficit hyperactivity disorder. *J Child Neurol* 13: 588–94. doi: 10.1177/088307389801301202.

Picchietti DL, Bruni O, de Weerd A, et al. (2013) Pediatric restless legs syndrome diagnostic criteria: an update by the International Restless Legs Syndrome Study Group. *Sleep Med* 14: 1253–9. doi: 10.1016/j.sleep.2013.08.778.

Picchietti MA, Picchietti DL (2010) Advances in pediatric restless legs syndrome: iron, genetics, diagnosis and treatment. *Sleep Med* 11: 643–51. doi: 10.1016/j.sleep.2009.11.014.

Powers SW, Kashikar-Zuck SM, Allen JR, et al. (2013) Cognitive behavioral therapy plus amitriptyline for chronic migraine in children and adolescents: a randomized clinical trial. *JAMA* 310: 2622–30.

Pullen SJ, Wall CA, Angstman ER, et al. (2011) Psychiatric comorbidity in children and adolescents with restless legs syndrome: a retrospective study. *J Clin Sleep Med* 7: 587–96. doi: 10.5664/jcsm.1456.

Rapp JT, Vollmer TR (2005a) Stereotypy I: a review of behavioral assessment and treatment. *Res Dev Disabil* 26: 527–47. doi: 10.1016/j.ridd.2004.11.005. doi: 10.1016/j.ridd.2004.11.006.

Rapp JT, Vollmer TR (2005b) Stereotypy II: a review of neurobiological interpretations and suggestions for an integration with behavioral methods. *Res Dev Disabil* 26: 548–64.

Reynolds S, Lane SJ (2008) Diagnostic validity of sensory over-responsivity: a review of the literature and case reports. *J Autism Dev Disord* 38: 516–29.

Robertson MM (1990) Gilles de la Tourette's syndrome. *Eur J Nucl Med* 16: 843–5.

Robertson MM, Trimble MR, Lees AJ (1988) The psychopathology of the Gilles de la Tourette syndrome. A phenomenological analysis. *Brit J Psychiatry* 12: 383–90.

Rödöö P, Hellberg D (2013) Girls who masturbate in early infancy: diagnostics, natural course and a long-term follow-up. *Acta Paediatr* 102: 762–6. doi: 10.1111/apa.12231.

Roy AK, Klein RG, Angelosante A, et al. (2013) Clinical features of young children referred for impairing temper outbursts. *J Child Adolesc Psychopharmacol* 23: 588–96. doi: 10.1089/cap.2013.0005.

Roy AK, Lopes V, Klein RG (2014) Disruptive mood dysregulation disorder: a new diagnostic approach to chronic irritability in youth. *Am J Psychiatry* 171: 918–24. doi: 10.1176/appi.ajp.2014.13101301.

Schröder A, Vulink N, Denys D (2013) Misophonia: diagnostic criteria for a new psychiatric disorder. *PLoS ONE* e54706. doi: 10.1371/journal.pone.0054706.

Schwartz P, Leyendecker J, Conlon M (2011) Hyperacusis and misophonia: the lesser-known siblings of tinnitus. *Minn Med* 94: 42–3.

Snorrason I, Woods DW (2014) Nail picking disorder (onychotillomania): a case report. *J Anx Disord* 28: 211–4. doi: 10.1016/j.janxdis.2013.10.004.

Snowling MJ, Bishop DVM, Stothard SE, et al. (2006) Psychosocial outcomes at 15 years of children with a preschool history of speech-language impairment. *J Child Psychol Psychiatry* 47: 759–65. doi: 10.1111/j.1469-7610.2006.01631.x.

Snyder G, Friman PC (2012) Habitual stereotypic movements: a descriptive analysis of four common types. In: Grant JE, Stein DJ, Woods DW, Keuthen NJ, eds. *Trichotillomania, Skin Picking, & Other Body-focused Repetitive Behaviors.* Arlington, VA: American Psychiatric Publishing, pp. 43–64.

St Clair MC, Pickles A, Durkin K, Conti-Ramsden G (2011) A longitudinal study of behavioral, emotional and social difficulties in individuals with a history of specific language impairment (SLI). *J Commun Disord* 44: 186–99.

Stansfield SA (1992) Noise, noise sensitivity and psychiatric disorder: epidemiological and psychophysiological studies. *Psychol Med Mongr Suppl* 22: 1–44.

Stein MA, Weiss M, Hlavaty L (2012) ADHD treatments, sleep, and sleep problems: complex associations. *Neurotherapeutics* 9: 509–17.

Storch EA, Milsom V, Lack CW, et al. (2009) Sleep-related problems in youth with Tourette's syndrome and chronic tic disorder. *Child Adolesc Ment Health* 14: 97–103.

Sukhodolsky DG, Scahill L (2012) *Cognitive–Behavioral Therapy for Anger and Aggression in Children.* New York: Guilford Press.

Sukhodolsky DG, Vitulano LA, Carroll DH, et al. (2009) Randomized trial of anger control training for adolescents with Tourette's syndrome and disruptive behavior. *J Am Acad Child Adolesc Psychiatry* 48: 413–21. doi: 10.1097/CHI.0b013e3181985050.

Thirumalai S, Gray-Holland S, Shah NS (2007) Are we overlooking Tourette syndrome in children with persistent developmental stuttering? *J Pediatr Neurol* 5: 111–5.

Trichotillomania Learning Center (2011) *Expert Consensus Treatment Guidelines for Trichotillomania, Skin Picking and Other Body-Focused Repetitive Behaviors* (available online at www.trich.org).

Van Borsel J, Vanryckeghem M (2000) Dysfluency and phonic tics in Tourette syndrome: a case report. *J Commun Disord* 33: 227–39. doi: 10.1016/S0021-9924(00)00020-4.

Van Borsel J, Goethals L, Vanryckeghem M (2004) Dysfluency in Tourette syndrome: observational study in three cases. *Folia Phoniatr Logop* 56: 358–66. doi: 10.1159/000081083.

Van Hulle CA, Schmidt NL, Goldsmith HH (2012) Is sensory over-responsivity distinguishable from childhood behavior problems? A phenotypic and genetic analysis. *J Child Psychol Psychiatry* 53: 64–72. doi: 10.1111/1469-7610.2011.02467.x.

Visscher C, Houwen S, Scherder EJA, et al. (2007) Motor profile of children with developmental speech and language disorders. *Pediatrics* 120: e158–63. doi: 10.1542/peds.2006-2462.

Voderholzer U, Muller N, Haag C, et al. (1997) Periodic limb movements during sleep are a frequent finding in patients with Gilles de la Tourette's syndrome. *J Neurol* 244: 521–6. doi: 10.1007/s004150050136.

von Gontard A, Nevéus T (2006) *Management of Disorders of Bladder and Bowel Control in Childhood. Clinics in Developmental Medicine no. 170.* London: Mac Keith Press.

Wang S-J, Fuh J-L, Lu S-R (2009) Chronic daily headache in adolescents: an 8-year follow-up study. *Neurology* 73: 416–22. doi: 10.1212/WNL.0b013e3181ae2377.

Wilensky AS (1999) *Passing for Normal: a Memoir of Compulsion.* New York: Broadway Books.

Wilkinson P, Goodyer I (2011) Non-suicidal self-injury. *Eur Child Adolesc Psychiatry* 20: 103–8. doi: 10.1007/s00787-010-0156-y.

Wise M (2001) Citalopram-induced bruxism. *Br J Psychiatry* 178: 182. doi: 10.1192/bjp.178.2.182-a.

Wong MW, Williamson BD, Qiu W, et al. (2014) Growing pains and periodic limb movements of sleep in children. *J Paediatr Child Health* 50: 455–60. doi: 10.1111/jpc.12493.

Worbe Y, Mallet L, Golmard J-L, et al. (2010) Repetitive behaviours in patients with Gilles de la Tourette syndrome: tics, compulsions, or both? *PLoS ONE* 5: e12959. doi: 10.1371/journal.pone.0012959.

Wu MS, Lewin AB, Murphy TK, Storch EA (2014) Misophonia: incidence, phenomenology, and clinical correlates in an undergraduate student sample. *J Clin Psychol*, epub 17 April 2014. doi: 10.1002/jclp.22098.

Yew SGK, O'Kearney R (2012) Emotional and behavioural outcomes later in childhood and adolescence for children with specific language impairments: meta-analyses of controlled prospective studies. *J Child Psychol Psychiatry* 54: 516–24. doi: 10.1111/jcpp.12009.

Yilmaz K, Kilincaslan A, Aydin N, Kor D (2011) Prevalence and correlates of restless legs syndrome in adolescents. *Dev Med Child Neurol* 53: 40–7. doi: 10.1111/j.1469-8749.2010.03796.x.

Yoon SY, Jain U, Shapiro C (2012) Sleep in attention-deficit/hyperactivity disorder in children and adults: past, present and future. *Sleep Med Rev* 16: 371–88. doi: 10.1016/j.smrv.2011.07.001.

Yüce M, Karabekiroğlu K, Say GN, et al. (2013) Buspirone in the treatment of atomoxetine-induced bruxism. *J Child Adolesc Psychopharmacol* 23: 634–5. doi: 10.1089/cap.2013.0087.

13
TICS IN OTHER MEDICAL CONDITIONS

This chapter provides examples of some medical conditions in which tics can also occur. Their inclusion here is based upon experience and a sometimes unrecognized potential for misunderstanding. It is recognized that there could be additional examples, with no obvious limit.

Epilepsy

> The many kinds of movements and changed behaviors accompanying seizures or other paroxysmal events may sometimes be confused with tics, and tics may sometimes be triggered or aggravated by anticonvulsant medication. Medication for tics may sometimes alter the seizure threshold of vulnerable individuals. There is also an increased incidence of seizures in persons with ADHD, who are more likely to have tics.

Paroxysmal events are often misdiagnosed (Uldall et al. 2006). Half the children referred to a tertiary epilepsy center were discharged with a diagnosis of nonepileptic seizures. Of those referred with no doubts about the diagnosis, 35% turned out to not have epilepsy. Children or adults with tonic tics, often described as 'freezing', may be thought to have seizures or catatonia. In addition, paroxysmal episodes may be neither (DiMario 2006). Tics may sometimes be triggered or aggravated by anticonvulsants, or even appear after long-term treatment with risperidone in children with ASD (Feroz-Nainar and Roy 2006).

Choreoacanthocytosis (a rare autosomal recessive disorder) can present in adult life with seizures and tics and be misdiagnosed as Tourette syndrome (Al-Asmi et al. 2005).

There are a large number of types, mechanisms and combinations of paroxysmal events, and accurate diagnosis may be difficult (Plioplys et al. 2007b). Collaboration with a pediatrician or neurologist familiar with seizures may be necessary.

Rizzo et al. (2010) have described the comorbid pattern of Tourette syndrome with ADHD and epilepsy, and Cohen et al. (2013) determined the general population prevalence of epilepsy in Israel as 0.5% and of ADHD as 12.6%; more than a quarter of the children with epilepsy were also diagnosed with ADHD, and children with ADHD had twice the risk of seizures.

Musiek et al. (2010) have summarized the literature on tics provoked (or probably caused) by the anticonvulsant lamotrigine, and presented two new cases. These tics did not fully remit after discontinuation of the drug. Sotero de Menezes et al. (2000) presented five pediatric cases, and others have presented still more (e.g. Lombroso 1999). Carbamazepine can also trigger transient tics (Robertson et al. 1993).

Many other paroxysmal symptoms or disorders may be confused with epilepsy and these include certain kinds of tics and other repetitive motor behaviors. Careful workup by an epilepsy specialist may be necessary, including video–EEG study (Watemberg et al. 2005).

Functional or 'psychogenic' non-epileptic seizures also occur, as well described by Plioplys et al. (2007a) and Schachter and LaFrance (2010).

Visual impairment

> Stereotypies are almost universal in children with the early onset of significant visual impairment and are often a concern of parents and schools. They may serve to regulate arousal. In childhood their form, with the exception of eye-pressing and -poking, may represent spontaneous patterns unmodified by cultural influences. Blindness in many of the children may be associated with complicated medical/genetic etiologies, making stereotyped patterns of movement more likely. Tics are much more difficult than usual to diagnose in the midst of these other stereotypic behaviors. In early life, stereotypies typically are quite stable and do not change their pattern frequently, unlike the tics of Tourette syndrome. Clinically this may or may not matter, depending upon their type, intrusiveness and severity. Stereotypies may persist but become private after social awareness is fully developed (which would not be typical of tics).

Children with early-onset significant visual impairment typically develop stereotypies in early life, originally termed 'blind mannerisms' or just 'blindisms' for short. These are broadly similar to stereotypies in non-visually impaired individuals with the exception of eye-poking and -pressing, which can be intense and persistent and may result in distortion of the growth of the orbit (Jan et al. 1983, 1994). The prevalence of stereotypies is positively correlated with the severity of the visual impairment and inversely with the age at onset.

> **Practice point**
> Stereotypies are almost universal in early-onset visual impairment. They are positively correlated with the severity of the visual impairment and inversely with the age at onset.

The nature of stereotypies was discovered to roughly indicate the mechanism of the visual impairment: children who eye-press or -poke have intact optic tracts and usually have retinal or other ocular disease as the source of their visual impairment (Jan et al. 1977). They press to stimulate the visual (occipital) cortex (so a causative factor seems to be sensory deprivation). Children with optic nerve hypoplasia do not engage in this behavior.

In this case, defining a stereotypy as 'non-functional' or 'purposeless' is obviously incorrect. No one seems to have thought about asking blind people about their subjective experiences in doing — or suppressing — their stereotypy, so that assertions that they have no premonitory sensations are dubious at best. What differentiates their other stereotypies from tics? This is not a simple question in the presence of both, as well as when there are other repetitive motor behaviors that may not be either. This is probably not the only mechanism: stereotypies may function as self-regulation when arousal is too low or too high (Jan et al. 1977, McHugh and Lieberman 2003, Molloy and Rowe 2011). There may be a distorting effect of sensory processing dysfunction in these children, which it would be prudent to take into account (Gal and Dyck 2009).

Tics tend to be rapid, isolated and non-rhythmic, whereas stereotypies are often rhythmic, usually slower and may be more prolonged. Stereotypies tend to be non-vocal, although sounds may sometimes accompany them. Children with cortical visual impairment may have normal eyes but may have stereotypies associated with other patterns associated with the causative factors (Freeman 2010), and assumptions about the natural history of tics may no longer apply. For example, in an uncommon condition known as oculomotor apraxia lateral eye movements may be difficult or impossible to make, so that head-turning is compensatory and may appear to be tic-like. Compensatory head-shaking may be confused with spasmus nutans (Jan et al. 1990), an uncommon condition of nystagmus with anomalous head position and head-nodding or titubation. In one published case it was confused with Tourette syndrome (Bray 1990). Newer imaging techniques might in the future be able to identify correlations of which we are presently unaware.

> **Practice point**
> Some persons with normal eyes have cortical visual impairment. They may make unusual compensatory head or other movements that can be confused with tics.

Stereotypies in blind children usually persist into adolescence, and in adult life may become private in those with good social awareness, but usually do not completely cease. This conclusion is from the only follow-up study of a total population of legally blind children into adult life (Freeman et al. 1991). Whether tics in blind children follow the same course of improvement with age as in sighted children is unknown and may be complicated by the complex and changing etiologies of the visual impairment. This could be a fruitful area for longitudinal research.

Both stereotypies and tics in visually impaired children tend to be very aversive to parents because they make the children seem even more different from others, and may be associated in the public's mind with intellectual disability or ASD. Much like children with stereotypic movement disorder, the patients don't complain about their movement patterns — others do (McHugh and Lieberman 2003). Occasionally persons with visual impairment may become resentful that they are expected to change their behavior based upon the reactions of sighted people.

> **Practice point**
>
> Visually impaired persons with stereotypies ordinarily do not complain about their movements, others do, but they may become concerned once they become aware of how the movements affect sighted people.

The following four vignettes illustrate some of the complexities encountered in assessing repetitive stereotyped behavior in people with a visual impairment. In some ways they are extreme cases (because of when and why they were seen) and are not meant to be representative of the average person with visual impairment.

> **Case examples**
>
> *'Lorraine' was 15 when assessed 45 years ago, and as was common at that time, was totally blind from retinopathy of prematurity, associated with early (but not continuing) seizures and normal intelligence. She was seen specifically because of bad 'gestures' or 'habits' that had become seriously problematic for her mother and her church associates, who regarded them as literally sinful. These consisted of throwing her head back, stiffening her arms and pursing her lips that all became more obvious about age 12. She had been spanked when these occurred in states of apparent boredom. (No eye-pressing was noted, though it would not have been surprising.) She was noted in the interviews to rock, grunt and throat-clear, but tics had not been entertained as a possibility. She was almost completely under her mother's domination, constantly criticizing herself in her mother's manner. Her mother periodically observed her in school and tried to stay in the assessment interviews by pretending to leave the room. Lorraine confessed that sometimes she engaged in her behaviour 'on purpose' because it felt good, but she knew it was sinful.*
>
> ***Comment:*** *This situation illustrates the complexity of several intertwined patterns, with difficulty in differential diagnosis. When work towards some individuation of Lorraine moved forward, her mother terminated treatment. It is the common opinion that tics are not enjoyable. Lorraine's confession is therefore more compatible with stereotypies, and it can be wondered whether they were one of her only 'individual' outlets. But at least some of the movements seemed characteristic of tics, which in this case may have had an unusal role to play in relation to her mother.*
>
> *'Sam' was 13 when initially seen, blind from birth for reasons never fully determined, and of low average tested intelligence. He was left on his own much of the time when he was not in school, and his eyes were deep-set from pressing. The presenting complaint was of mannerisms: eye-blinking, -pressing and -poking, facial grimacing, rocking, lip-biting, shoulder-shaking, leg-shaking, finger-twisting, bruxism, ear-pulling, noises with his lips on his teeth, sniffing, joint-cracking, throat-clearing, snorting, 'jaw-jerking', tongue-clicking and rapid fluttering movements of his hands. These were very embarrassing to his mother and his teachers, partly because he also often*

expressed unusual ideas, some of which took a concrete religious form. Contact with him was sporadic because he lived far away. Seen again at age 24 he claimed that spirits were making him cough and that his noises had 'special significance'. He spent time typing endless but disorganized stories about a fictitious person who deserved to be killed and about how he himself would obtain power. No placement for work experience was possible because of his odd behaviour and activities: when left alone he rode elevators up and down for long periods, often singing to himself. Tourette syndrome was considered as a possibility by his mother, but in the midst of his complex problems was not judged of the greatest importance, and was never officially diagnosed (although he fulfilled criteria).

Comment: This individual story, also from over 30 years ago, brings in factors of social isolation, stereotypies, body-focused repetitive motor patterns (bruxism, joint-cracking), tics, atypical development and finally, delusional thinking. The difficult question was: were his abnormal movements tics, stereotypies often seen in early-onset blindness and sometimes in psychosis, or some mixture?

'Jeremy' was 10 when seen on a home and school visit because of multiple unusual movements. He had a history of mild athetoid cerebral palsy and visual impairment, retaining some light perception. He had eye-pressing, rocking, head-shaking and interrupted speech. What was of interest was that while he had athetoid movements, he also had stereotypies, multiple tics, and the secondary manifestations of stuttering. Vigorous head-shaking was observed to occur only when he was trying to talk, not at other times.

At age 10 'Hugh' was seen in consultation in what was then a school for students with visual impairment. He was born preterm with retinopathy of prematurity and had no useful vision but at least average intelligence. He showed eye-pressing and many other stereotypies that bothered the parents and school. Efforts were made to suppress them, to no avail. He was seen for treatment later from age 16 intermittently through age 24, when he was living on his own. His movements included eye-winking, noises, some rocking, facial grimacing, and patterns of lightning-like sexual touching of men that he initially claimed were accidental.

Comment: The touching turned out to be deliberate with a compulsive element, but could have been considered (under other circumstances) to be a complex tic. That some of the movements were tic-like was considered only after many years of contact, because of other movements, noises, and the complexities of his behavior.

Hearing impairment

Stereotypies are not more common in persons with hearing disorders than in those without. Some repetitive behaviors of deaf individuals may seem strange to the un-initiated but may be adaptive for them. Tics may occur, and in signing deaf persons may be the medium for copropraxia. Differentiation of stereotypies from tics and other repetitive behaviors may require consultation with a clinician with special experience and skill.

A serious error has crept into the scientific literature that should be corrected. A paper was published by Murdoch (1996) about stereotyped behavior in sensory disability (emphasizing hearing loss with or without vision loss). The majority of children (79%) had additional disabilities, and in that subgroup the rate of stereotypy was 35%. The research, undertaken in three residential schools found that deaf children without other disabilities do not show stereotyped behaviour at a significantly higher rate than children with typical development: "For the sample studied, it is clear that deaf and hard of hearing students without additional disabilities do not show behaviors likely to be interpreted as stereotyped. Students with disabilities in addition to hearing loss are significantly more likely to show such behaviors" (p. 385).

To add to this point, in a review of patient records from the past 40 years many blind children were seen with stereotyped behavior, but none with hearing impairment unless they also had ASD, intellectual disability or visual impairment. (As a consultant psychiatrist to programs for both hearing and visual impairment, I have seen about equal numbers of each.)

Many studies of stereotypic behavior over the years have mentioned deaf persons, but almost all are about persons with additional disabilities, most often intellectual disability, ASD or visual impairment, and therefore are not evidence of stereotypic behavior in hearing-impaired persons as such. In many of the residential programs in which studies were carried out, the categorization methods of additional disabilities were arguably inadequate.

It is therefore proposed here that clinicians and researchers stop making statements about stereotypy in individuals with sensory impairments that include hearing impairment unless new and properly obtained evidence is brought forward.

Hearing-impaired children can, like anyone, have tics and other stereotyped behaviors (Bachara and Phelan 1980). Dalgaard et al. (2001) presented a 10-year-old boy with tics who developed signing coprolalia. Children who are quite deaf may engage in behavior that seems strange to unfamiliar hearing persons, but may be functional for them (modified by cultural differences): touching or tapping complete strangers to get attention, making seemingly inarticulate and poorly modulated sounds when the public may think of them as actually 'deaf and dumb' or 'deaf–mute' (which are misleading and offensive outmoded terms). Deaf persons who have some residual bone conduction may grind their teeth (bruxism) to produce some input to their auditory cortex. Those with partial hearing losses (which may be worse on one side) may show postural or positional differences. These patterns may at times create confusion as to the differential diagnosis. In signing deaf persons who do have Tourette syndrome, copropraxic tics may be expressed in sign language, as one might expect (Rickards 2001). Consultation with a clinician expert in both repetitive behaviors (including tics) and deafness may occasionally be required.

Case example

'Brandon' is now 18. There is no family history of tics. In addition to profound congenital sensorineural deafness, he has mild cerebral palsy, ASD, OCD, ADHD, SLD and mild cortical visual impairment. He also has Tourette syndrome, with loud vocal tics, head-shaking and throat-clearing. His eye contact is abnormal, making it difficult for him to track what he should be seeing from a sign language interpreter. Several years ago he developed absence seizures and was found to have an abnormal but non-diagnostic EEG, and recently had several major convulsions. He also has had a chronic sleep disorder and sudden aggressive behavior when frustrated. His management at home has been very stressful for the family. He attended a school for the deaf and lived in a dormitory setting where his behavioral problems presented frequent challenges. His tics have not usually been the most important of his diagnoses or symptoms, and have not been treated. Their nature and role was explained to the school staff on a visit there.

Comment: *Tourette syndrome in this boy probably represents one facet of a complex neurodevelopmental disorder.*

Cerebral palsy

Cerebral palsy is a broad term for movement and posture disorders having their onset in utero or in infancy and caused by damage to the brain, often associated with many kinds of deficits in other areas of function. Abnormalities of movement (athetosis, chorea, spasticity) may make identification of tics and stereotyped behaviors problematic. Difficulty in modulating movement may be mirrored in weak emotional control that can be wrongly assumed to be due to a concurrent tic disorder. Children with cerebral palsy have a much higher rate of behavioral problems than those with typical development. Already impaired quality of life can be further affected by the presence of significant tics, which can aggravate difficult motor coordination.

In one definition, the term 'cerebral palsy'

> … describes a group of permanent disorders of the development of movement and posture, causing activity limitation, that are attributed to non-progressive disturbances that occurred in the developing fetal or infant brain. The motor disorders of cerebral palsy are often accompanied by disturbances of sensation, perception, cognition, communication, and behaviour, by epilepsy, and by secondary musculoskeletal problems. (Rosenbaum et al. 2006, p. 9)

This is a descriptive, not etiologic, definition. Although the etiologic factors are non-progressive, the functional consequences tend to be progressive, and may accelerate in adult life (somewhat like post-polio syndrome). The presence of significant tics may complicate problems of motor coordination and emotional control, both for the patient and for those trying to understand his or her skills and disability.

197

A splendid book that covers the field from birth to old age has been written by Rosenbaum and Rosenbloom (2012), and is equally informative for clinicians and interested lay persons. It is unusual because it includes an explanation of the nature and limitations of evidence and how it is derived, the value of which has applicability far beyond cerebral palsy.

Children with cerebral palsy are known to have high rates of behavioral and emotional problems (Parkes et al. 2008), approximately 25% versus 10% in those without (Novak et al. 2012). A parenting intervention has been shown to reduce these problems (Whittingham et al. 2014). How tics interact with these problems is not well known at this time.

Case examples

'Cameron' was seen first at age 7 because of tics and aggressive behavior. He was born preterm and suffered a brain hemorrhage leading to what was then termed mild spastic hemiplegia. There was a family history of tics. He had many kinds of tics along with ADHD, explosive temper associated with very low frustration tolerance and long-standing sleep disorder. Some complex tics had initially been suspected to be seizures. There were additionally several SIBs (nail-picking and lip-biting), obsessive–compulsive behaviors, and very poor emotional regulation. Medication trials were minimally effective. Years later as a teenager he was failing all subjects in school and manifesting challenging and sometimes violent behavior.

Comment: Abnormal movements of various kinds in cerebral palsy can be confused with — or co-exist with — tics.

'Julia' was 6 when first seen because of perfectionistic trends and stereotyped movements. Her prenatal history was marked by a cerebral hemorrhage; hydrocephalus and cerebral palsy were diagnosed later. Her main problems seemed to be perfectionistic and also repetitive behaviors, frustration intolerance, difficulty making decisions, sleeping problems, anxiety and ADHD features. Psychological testing revealed many scattered strengths and weaknesses. At her first interview she jumped, bounced, and displayed rapid hand mannerisms and eye-rolling. She was thought to have some tics and stereotypic movement patterns along with her motor deficits, and obsessive–compulsive features. Her sleep initiation difficulty responded to melatonin. There was a family history of obsessive–compulsive symptoms. Seen again several years later she had developed specific quite severe fears, further OCD symptoms, anxiety and depression.

Comment: Brain damage, and genetic and environmental factors probably combined to produce a complex clinical picture that included movement, cognitive and emotional disorders.

Tics in persons with various forms of brain damage are not at all uncommon, but can be difficult to distinguish from movement disorders that are part of what we call cerebral palsy and/or a variety of other movements that can include the patterns in Table 13.1. If the movements are impairing, treatment may depend upon the understanding of their nature.

TABLE 13.1
Abnormal movements to consider in cerebral palsy (in addition to neurological symptoms)

Movement type	Characteristics	Typical associations
Stereotypy	May be self-injurious; hard to distinguish from other patterns	Early-onset visual impairment, intellectual disability, ASD
Stereotypic movement disorder	Occur in excitement, fantasy, sometimes self-regulation	May have a familial pattern (inquire)
Speech dysfluency	Occur when trying to speak, not otherwise	Stuttering, oral–motor dyspraxia
Tics	Rapid, non-rhythmic, partially suppressible	Positive family history, changeable and variable (especially in childhood)
OCD/OCB	Ritualistic features	May have anxiety
'Habits' or RMBs	Uncertain, but may occur out of full awareness	Common also in typical development

ASD, autism spectrum disorder; OCD/OCB, obsessive–compulsive disorder/obsessive–compulsive behavior; RMB, repetitive motor behavior.

Fetal alcohol syndrome (FAS)

> Exposure to alcohol in utero is now known to frequently cause multiple developmental problems that may be permanent and limit life's accomplishments. When a tic disorder is added there is a chance that its symptoms and functional effects may be misunderstood.

Although in the not too distant past the UK government concluded that FAS was not a significant problem, we now know that it is (Preece and Riley 2011, Autti-Rämö 2013). O'Leary et al. (2013) expressed the opinion that in Western Australia at least 3.8% of cases of intellectual disability could be avoided by preventing maternal alcohol use (1.3% in non-Aboriginal and 15.6% in Aboriginal children), and that one-third of children diagnosed with FAS had intellectual disability. Fernández Mayoralas et al. (2010) reported that nine of 138 adopted children (7%) were diagnosed with FAS and Tourette syndrome.

Persons with FAS may have tics to add to their often lifelong woes resulting from psychopathology (Steinhausen et al. 1993, Streissguth et al. 2004, Davis et al. 2011). The frequent burden of poor self-regulation, compromised cognitive functioning including attentional problems and failure to learn from social consequences may then have the additional complication of easy-to-misunderstand tics and comorbid disorders.

The 4-Digit Diagnostic Code, developed at the University of Washington, defines diagnoses of FAS, partial FAS and alcohol-related neurodevelopmental disorder (Astley 2004). The difficulty has been that the consequences of alcohol exposure are variable and complex, and that many of the children to whom the criteria are applied have lived through atypical experiences. Many of them qualify for ADHD (Fryer et al. 2007), but their pattern of attentional difficulties is still contested (Lane et al. 2014).

In DSM-5, FAS is classified as a "condition for further study" with the title "neuro-behavioral disorder associated with prenatal alcohol exposure" and the following proposed criteria: more than minimal exposure to alcohol during gestation; impaired neurocognitive functioning manifested by one or more of impairment in global intellectual performance, executive functioning, learning, memory and visuospatial reasoning, and impaired self-reg-ulation (mood or behavioral or attention deficit and impulse control); impaired adaptive functioning; and onset in childhood. (This allows for diagnosis whether facial dysmorphology is manifested or not.)

Case example

'Amber', a 9-year-old girl, was diagnosed with Tourette syndrome, partial FAS, ADHD, OCD, anxiety and sleep disorder. She had been removed from her mother who had been (and still was) an alcoholic, was placed with relatives, and again removed and placed into a foster home because of abuse. Observed were an expiratory tic ("Heh!"), head-shaking, lip-pursing, knee-knocking, tongue-thrusting, face-hitting, self-biting, throat-clearing, sniffing hands and fingers, repeating words, grunting, abdom-inal contractions, eye-rolling, coughing, grimacing, shoulder-shrugging, flapping and full-body tics. She also engaged in suicidal talk, ripping her clothes, bedtime rituals, gorging on food, sensory sensitivities and aggression. She tended to misread others' facial expressions and intentions. She had episodes of visual and auditory hallucina-tions, and was on multiple medications. On physical examination she met three of the four criteria for FAS, namely distinctive facial features, documented exposure to alco-hol during gestation and static encephalopathy, but not documented growth failure.

*   **Comment:** Amber had experienced the disrupted background that is all too com-mon in persons with FAS, but also the early onset of multiple and complex tics, along with comorbid ADHD, OCD, mood and anxiety features, dysregulation of appetite and sleep as well as sensory over-responsivity, weak self-regulation, learning problems and odd misperceptions.*

Neuromuscular disorders

Tics can co-occur in any disease, disorder or syndrome, or in conjunction with any other symptom. Whether the tics are noticed or reported will depend upon their im-portance relative to other concerns. Little is likely to be known about whether their natural history is any different than in those without the co-occurring condition. If the diagnosis of a tic disorder is made it will be important to explain its level of impor-tance and to alert families to the possibility of tics being misunderstood, especially in the presence of other conditions.

To illustrate how unexpected it can be to find tics in combination with some rare other disorders, here are examples of two *females* with Duchenne-type muscular dystrophy (in itself rare, and occurring when there is severely skewed X-inactivation) in whom tics were only incidentally identified. In rare cases, a female carrier of the mutation can have a progressive course similar to that of males (Leyser et al. 2013).

Case examples

'Sandra' was 11 and in a wheelchair when seen long ago for oppositional and rigid behavior. She was on steroid treatment like many with muscular dystrophy. For difficult behavior she had been on an SSRI and a second-generation antipsychotic. She had some compulsive hand-washing, SLD, anxiety and sensory over-responsivity, with impaired executive functions and self-regulation. On an extended home visit eye-blinking with blepharospasm and facial grimacing were observed. Her mother acknowledged that these had been present for some years, but neither she nor previous clinicians or anyone at the specialty clinic had ever mentioned or noted them. She was given a new diagnosis of chronic motor tic disorder (DSM-IV-TR).

'Mary' was 7 when seen twice long ago. She presented with sensory over-responsivity and distractibility. There was a family history of mild obsessive–compulsive symptoms. In the interview, eye-blinking, eye-winking and facial grimacing were observed on both visits. Her mother acknowledged that she had had these patterns for a few years, but no clinicians had ever mentioned them (or noted them in the record). As with Sandra, she was diagnosed with chronic motor tic disorder.

What is important here is that in the multiplicity of concerns about these girls' increasing disability, non-impairing tics were apparently not considered important, and though at least some of the specialty clinic's staff were familiar with tics, no mention was ever made of them. This shows the importance of context and meaning.

Case example

'Fred' was 12 when first seen for behavioral issues and school learning concerns. He had a rare congenital condition, amyoplasia, a non-progressive muscle disorder. He also had borderline intellectual functioning on psychological testing. Not noted in his medical chart, he also had chronic motor tics. When retested several years later his intellectual functioning was found to be in the mild range of intellectual disability. When followed up in his early 20s his tics were not a problem, but his participation in activities was minimal and he had no friends.

*   **Comment:** This young man's evolution of tic symptoms seems to have been typical and apparently was unaffected by his muscle disorder.*

There seems to be a tendency to ignore non-impairing tics when persons have other significant health conditions. This is not to imply that more than is necessary should be made of them, but if at some point the tics change, increase, or are misunderstood by someone involved, their nature and earlier history may need appropriate consideration.

Neurofibromatosis type 1 (NF-1)

> NF-1 is fairly common, with a variable clinical course, risk of further tumors and related physical impairment. Associated neurodevelopmental disorders may be seen, along with weak self-regulation and social skills, ADHD in 30% to 50%, and tics. Management is complex.

Much attention has been paid to cognitive profiles in NF-1 (Levine et al. 2006). Overall, there is a tendency toward a slightly lower tested IQ, with common (but not universal) deficits in reading, mathematics, spelling, visual perception, language, social skills and memory (Lehtonen et al. 2013). About 30% to 50% of patients qualify for a diagnosis of ADHD (Huijbregts et al. 2010, Isenberg et al. 2013). The frequency of symptoms of ASD is also elevated, as high as 15% to 30% (Garg et al. 2013, Walsh et al. 2013).

Pride et al. (2013) examined social skills in adults with NF-1 and found that deficits continue into adult life in about half, more so in males. It is clinically important that adults showed reduced awareness of their deficits. This might be attributable to the high rate of ADHD with its accompanying weak emotional regulation and reduced ability to process social information. (Tics were not mentioned in that report.)

Tics can occur in NF-1. Cosentino and Torres (2000) presented the case of an 11-year-old boy with NF-1 and Tourette syndrome, in whom magnetic resonance imaging showed bilateral pallidal hyperintensities. The three boys described below all had learning problems, multiple tics qualifying them for a diagnosis of Tourette syndrome, deteriorating school achievement, and comorbid disorders. In addition, although they were reluctant to discuss the subject, they were aware of the threat of further disability from NF-1 lurking in the background. NF-1, which is not rare, can be associated with both tics and other neurodevelopmental disorders.

> ### Case examples
> *'Kyle' was 17 when he presented with parental complaints of poor socialization, easy angering, worries, irritability, tics and compulsions. He had developed concerns and rituals about germs that necessarily involved his family, excessive checking, and repeated reassurance-seeking. The significance of these he denied. School work had declined and teachers described him as not interested in social relationships. Tics had started about 10 years before, and the variety had increased. His NF-1 was closely monitored but was not very progressive or impairing; however, the family had been affected by the prognostic information they had been given. Kyle refused to describe his obsessions, and when offered the opportunity to return for further assessment and counseling, he declined.*

'Chris' was 13 when first seen. He lived far away from the medical center. He had a history of recurrent episodes of depressed, slowed-down mood (about every few months for a few weeks), circumscribed interest patterns, and fears about health and dying. Motor and vocal tics began at age 6 and became quite varied and noticeable. Psychological testing showed a mixed pattern, with non-verbal learning disability and a high degree of distractibility. He did not have many friends or age-appropriate social skills. The diagnoses were Tourette syndrome, ADHD and SLD. The family was lost to follow-up.

'Shawn' was seen at age 10 for an increasingly bad temper, verbal abuse of his mother (but not others), worsening tics with swearing, insomnia and resistance to completing school work (but with good behavior there). He was very anxious about illness and germs and constantly asked for reassurance. He also had a history of self-injurious lip-licking, eye-rubbing, and atypical sensory processing in more than one modality. There was a family history of tics, aggressive behavior, learning problems and other chronic health problems. Psychological testing showed average Full-Scale IQ but visuospatial weaknesses and very weak mathematical and writing skills. Fine motor coordination was weak. In the interview he would say very little about himself, as was also true at home. He met criteria for Tourette syndrome, OCD, generalized anxiety disorder and DCD. He declined to be seen again, despite increasing anxiety.

Comment: *Shawn's anxiety may have been aroused partly because of the important role of illness and injury in his family. He was becoming aware of how different he was from his peer group.*

There seems to be a tendency to ignore non-impairing tics when persons have other significant health conditions. This is not to imply that more than is necessary should be made of them, but if at some point the tics change, increase, or are misunderstood by someone involved, their nature and earlier history may need appropriate consideration.

Gastroesophageal reflux disorder (GERD)

The diagnosis of GERD is not simple, since correlations between symptoms and pathology are highly variable and still controversial among gastroenterologists (Blanco et al. 2012). Many symptoms involving the larynx, nasopharynx, ears and lungs have been attributed to this commonly invoked condition. Children with sniffing, coughing, snorting, throat-clearing and respiratory tics have had them attributed to the extra-esophageal manifestations of GERD, and in some cases have had unnecessary endoscopy. Of course GERD could also aggravate or trigger tics, so sometimes a course of treatment for GERD is recommended initially, even when the diagnosis of tics is considered likely. It is helpful if gastroenterologists are aware of the similarity of some putative GERD symptoms to tics and possible combinations of GERD symptoms and tics.

Wilson disease

> Wilson disease is a rare progressive metabolic error that is treatable. It can manifest with movement disorders that can be confused with tics as well as with other movement disorders and neuropsychiatric symptoms. The average specialist will never see a case, but to miss the diagnosis is tragic.

Wilson disease is a rare autosomal recessive disorder of copper metabolism, caused by mutations on chromosome 13, but is treatable (Bandmann 2013). Its presentation is hugely variable. The occurrence is rare (1:30,000) so that it can easily be missed. Failure to excrete sufficient extra copper eventually leads to systemic copper poisoning with progressive liver damage and toxic accumulation in brain and other tissues. Presentation is neurologic in about 40%, the rest with liver disease or psychiatric symptoms, including change in personality, mood, impulsivity, antisocial behavior and school work. Symptoms can start as early as 4 years or as late as 50 or older (Pfeiffer 2007, Lorincz 2010). Diagnosis requires a 24-hour urine copper determination. Treatment is by careful use of zinc, D-penicillamine, trientine, or sometimes liver transplantation, but is not always satisfactory (Fox 2013, Rana et al. 2013).

Clearly one should not miss this important diagnosis. In practice many neurologists confronted by a movement disorder will do a screening test for Wilson disease, but given its rarity, other physicians may wait to test only if some other symptoms point the way.

> **Case example**
> *Many years ago a school-age boy was treated as having a child psychiatric behavior problem with some abnormal movements thought to be tics, but the therapist did not suspect a progressive neurologic disorder, even when the child developed difficulty feeding himself. His symptoms were thought to possibly represent childhood schizophrenia. By the time Wilson disease was diagnosed he was physically incapacitated. Treatment eventually improved his neurologic disorder, but he was left with persisting impulsivity and callous disregard for the feelings of others. His sister was tested and found to have presymptomatic Wilson disease and treatment thereby spared her a repetition of her brother's disability.*

Additional examples

BRAIN TUMORS

Peterson et al. (1996) described patients in whom tics appeared in the course of progressive and inoperable brain tumors. In two there was a family history of tics and in the other there were obsessive–compulsive manifestations. A 'genetic diathesis' was invoked, rather than an assumption that the tumor was the sole cause of the tics. It is of interest, though, that in one case the very significant tics and OCD, starting at age 4–5 years, improved around ages 16–17, and were mild in early adult life. Thus the presence of an extensive tumor that could not be removed did not prevent the typical mid-adolescent improvement that we see with tics and Tourette syndrome.

CHARGE SYNDROME

CHARGE (*c*oloboma, *h*eart, *a*tresia of the choanae, *r*etardation of growth and development, *g*enitourinary and *e*ar anomalies and hearing loss) has only been recognized as a syndrome since 2004; before that it was considered an 'association' of characteristics. A gene affecting many patients was found in that year. Children with the syndrome have serious problems in early life, among them behavior disturbance, and yes, they can have tics and OCD-like features, which can be confused with other patterns (Hartshorne et al. 2011). Three case examples are provided here to demonstrate the huge range of variation.

Case examples

'Max' was 11 and was in a foster home. His functioning level was very low and he had little communication. He engaged in SIBs when upset or frustrated. His behavior had become more irritable in the past year, with periods of crying. The team wondered whether he was in pain (nothing specific was found) or depressed. In addition, he had jerking movements that some suspected might be brief seizures. Assuming that environmental changes might be a factor, telephone interviews were held with all those involved with him in the school. It turned out that there had been many changes that were beyond staff control (a huge increase in the number of students in the school and consequent changes in the space that Max had become used to) and differences in goals among staff. When Max was seen, he obviously had multiple motor tics, not seizures.

Comment: This child represents a fairly common pattern for those with developmental delay and very limited communication: apparently small changes in their environment can cause increased stress and therefore behavioral change. Among all the other atypical patterns, tics can easily be missed or misinterpreted.

'Arnold' was 12 when first seen and had had marked gross and fine motor delay, a moderately severe hearing loss, hypogonadism and a renal anomaly. In addition, there were sleep problems, ADHD, repetitive motor patterns (including head-banging) and low Performance IQ (but not in the intellectual disability range). His tics consisted of excessive eye-blinking with blepharospasm, facial grimacing, head and neck tics, and screeching. He also showed contamination fears. He was friendly and sociable, but very self-critical. At age 15 his behavior had improved and tics had decreased. At age 25 he had made steady gains and was fully employed and functioning remarkably well.

Comment: This is a success story, radically different from 'Max', and indicates the wide range of outcomes for CHARGE syndrome.

'Barbara' was 6 when first seen for speech dysfluency, combined soon afterwards with head and body movements, followed by skin-picking after the tics subsided. Assesment included mild global developmental delay, ADHD, possible OCD-like behaviors and the plethora of congenital anomalies often seen: tracheoesophageal fistula, reflux, hearing loss, hypoplasia of the cerebellar vermis, chewing, feeding and sleeping problems, hypotonia and ataxia, visual impairment with colobomata, ptosis, fascination with part-objects, and easy frustration. Spitting was present for a while. Her movements were diagnosed as tics, but did not return, and many of her ASD-like patterns partially resolved with further development.

Comment: Her tics appeared to be transient, and it is interesting that they appeared around the time when severe skin-picking and spitting were also present. Improvement in overall functioning was evident, but she was only followed for 2 years before contact was lost.*

CHROMOSOMAL DISORDERS

Many varieties of chromosomal disorders might involve tics, but so far none has been found to have a specific relationship to tics.

Case example

'Russell' was 12 when seen for unusual movements and increasingly unacceptable behavior. He had been found to have both Down and Klinefelter syndromes (karyotype 48, XXY, +21), an unlikely combination estimated at that time to occur only once in over 350,000 births. A younger brother with a normal karyotype had tics. For years Russell had eye-blinking and facial grimacing, and then around age 11 frequent head-nodding appeared. He also showed some obsessive–compulsive rituals and preoccupations as well as tactile, auditory and vestibular over-responsivity. Academic functioning was 3 years behind age expectations. A diagnosis was made of chronic motor tic disorder (DSM-IV-TR).

Comment: This is another example of how tics can occur in any condition, and in this instance were probably related to a familial pattern.*

A recent review of sex chromosome aneuploidies by Hong and Reiss (2014) suggested a neurocognitive pattern for the XYY syndrome among the increased rates of neurological and psychiatric disorders in Turner, Klinefelter and XYY syndromes. (Tics were not mentioned.)

Case example

'Jordan' was 7 when first seen for his multiple tics, but it quickly became apparent that he had many other peculiarities of behavior and development. At that time his 47,XYY karyotype was not known to reflect a behavioral phenotype. In brief, Jordan had many

learning problems, ADHD, impulsivity, DCD, a well above average number of RMBs (some self-injurious), extreme SOR in the tactile mode causing turmoil each morning in order to get him dressed for school, sensitivity to sounds and specific visual patterns, OCD-like rituals, pica, self-touching involving hands down pants then smelling and licking fingers and touching eyelashes that caused negative social reactions from peers, and much more. He was assessed for ASD but did not meet criteria. Medications to modify the SOR did not help.

Comment: Surprisingly, substantial improvement occurred after an exorcism was performed.

CLEFT PALATE

Cleft lip and palate typically require one or more surgical procedures, and may have other congenital abnormalities, making generalizations about their liability to psychopathology questionable. Many genetic syndromes are associated with orofacial clefts, particularly the 22q11 deletion syndrome, which is associated with a high rate of ADHD, ASD and intellectual disability (Niklasson et al. 2009). Outcomes are highly variable according to the relatively few studies. Demir et al. (2011) found that social anxiety disorder and major depression were significantly more frequent than in comparison children. (None of these studies reported patients with tics.) In patients with tics, the changed oral/facial sensations may be triggers for new tics, or self-consciousness about speech or facial appearance may be aggravated by the tics.

Case example

'Austin' had to have several surgical procedures, but eventually had a good result. He did well academically and socially. Tics (with a family history of tics) began around age 8 with loud coprolalia, but he also had echolalia. What was unusual about the coprolalia was that the words had to be repeated three times. Around age 13 he started to chew an ulcer in his cheek and claimed he could not stop it; dental work may have triggered this tic. Shortly thereafter he started medication which seemed to help, but he tapered it off at age 18 when his tics were less troublesome.

Comment: Despite moderately severe tics that included self-injury and coprolalia, Austin was able to cope with them throughout secondary school; complex dental reconstructive surgery may have been a tic-provoking factor.

FRAGILE X SYNDROME

Fragile X is the most common genetic cause of inherited intellectual disability and the most common single-gene cause of ASD (Kidd et al. 2014). Movement disorders, such as hand-flapping (Hagerman and Hagerman 2002), are also said to be common. Reports of tic frequency vary from 16% to 45%, but a figure of around 6% as reported from the Fragile X

Clinical and Research Consortium (reviewed by Kidd et al. 2014) is more likely. Hagerman and Hagerman (2002) observed that coprolalia seemed to be most common where the patient was living in a situation in which swearing was common, therefore imitation was assumed to be a factor. An important point is that parent reports may confuse tics with stereotypies, and it should be noted that this difficulty probably affects the determination of tic prevalence in other genetic conditions as well. Both movement patterns may be suppressed during a clinician's interview.

SOTOS SYNDROME

Sotos syndrome is caused by a mutation in the *NSD1* gene, a relatively rare autosomal dominant disorder (usually sporadic), also known as cerebral gigantism, that is marked by early accelerated growth, expressive language delay, specific learning disabilities, and often mild intellectual disability. It may be associated with ADHD, irritability, stereotypies, seizures, cardiac anomalies and aggressive behavior. A few patients have similar characteristics without the mutation, known as a 'phenocopy'. However, patients with the mutation were found to be less affected than those without (de Boer et al. 2006).

Case example

'Oliver' was diagnosed with the Sotos mutation. He was 13 when seen for SIB and sleep difficulty. He picked his skin to the point of scarring and bit his nails till they bled. His teachers wanted him assessed for seizures because he 'twitched' when he walked and also showed 'shaking' of his hands and head. On testing he showed mild intellectual disability and additional specific learning problems. It took him about 2 hours to fall asleep at night, and as a consequence he was sleepy in school. His noticeable movements that caused concern were tics, not seizures.

*   **Comment:** This boy did not show the irritability, aggression and anxiety frequently mentioned in the Sotos syndrome literature, where tics are not mentioned.*

SPASTIC PARAPARESIS

Hereditary spastic paraplegia is a slowly progressive lower-limb-predominant disorder of corticospinal motor neurons, now thought to be caused by one of four mutations in BICD2, a protein that interacts with the motor complex critical to motor neuron development and maintenance (Oates et al. 2013).

Case study

'Harvey' was first seen at age 10. He had spastic paraparesis with associated chronic pain. At age 8 tics had started, including tongue-thrusting, noises, urges to touch people and objects, and 'giving the finger' (copropraxia). His teacher reported short attention span and distractibility, homework was a battle, and ADHD was diagnosed.

He became very self-conscious about people teasing him because of his gait. Sensory over-responsivity was also present. Coprolalia developed, but later subsided. OCD features developed and he appeared depressed. Psychological testing indicated above-average intelligence. At age 12 spitting started, and a year later tongue-biting, then contrary urges. At age 14 vocal tics were loud enough to cause complaints by neighbors, and at 17 school work was affected by ADHD and OCD, as well as continuing depression, but he was not ready for counseling or psychotherapy. Medication was tried, with limited success and frequent side-effects. At age 20 his tics were minimal, but OCD persisted. He had briefly attended university, but left because if not interested he could not pay adequate attention in class. Only then did he express more interest in exploring his feelings about his disability and his life.

*   **Comment:** *This is an example of Tourette syndrome with a co-occurring significant neurological disorder (and chronic pain) with four additional comorbidities. The tics were present throughout, with severe symptoms (coprophenomena, spitting, touching, self-injurious tongue-biting) that were transient, associated with persisting ADHD, OCD, anxiety and mood disorder, and suboptimal response to numerous medications. Note that tics caused trouble only intermittently, eventually remitted, and were not usually the most important problem.*

THYROID DISEASE

There is little useful information available on tics and thyroid disease. What there is suggests that tics (especially eye-blinking tics) are common or related to either hyperthyroidism or hypothyroidism, more the former, where an increase in anxiety might plausibly increase the likelihood of tics (Bagheri et al. 1999). There seem to be no data showing that tics (not just any movement disorder) are more frequent in thyroid disease, nor the utility of screening persons with tics for thyroid dysfunction. Another difficulty is that there is great confusion on the internet about the distinction between eyelid tics, myokymia and blepharospasm, even on sites claiming to represent eye specialists (e.g. www.eyedoctorguide.com). Readers need to be aware that confusing and misleading information on this topic is readily available to anyone with an internet connection.

Case example

'Burt', a 15-year-old boy, had onset of anxiety and tics around age 3, but was not diagnosed with Tourette syndrome until age 13. He developed an unusual pattern of making himself retch and vomit to relieve anxiety. His mood was labile, he had low energy and had difficulty falling asleep. Family history was positive for thyroid disease, anxiety and depression. Eventually Hashimoto thyroiditis was diagnosed and he was started on levothyroxine (a synthetic thyroid hormone), but anxiety with some obsessive–compulsive features remained a problem. Severe head-shaking developed and may have provoked headaches (also described as a symptom of this type of thyroiditis,

along with anxiety and depression). Later he was tested and a diagnosis of SLD was made.

Comment: This is an example of some symptoms of Tourette syndrome overlapping with those of another disorder. Retching and vomiting are also a pattern occasionally reported in Tourette syndrome (Rickards and Robertson 1997), and the relief of anxiety bears a possible relationship to bulimia. Such a complex picture may be clarified over time only by collaboration between pediatrician, endocrinologist, the movement disorder clinician, and possibly others.

TRAUMATIC BRAIN INJURY (TBI)

Recent years have seen greatly increased awareness of the consequences of mild traumatic brain injury, especially in contact sports. The outcome is highly variable (Ranjan et al. 2011, Forsyth and Kirkham 2012). Max et al. (2012) performed a follow-up study and found that personality change and affective disorders (new psychiatric disorders) were much more common in the TBI group than in comparison children (who had orthopedic injury). The review of the outcomes by Li and Liu (2013) concluded that about 50% of the time TBI is followed by behavioral problems and disorders. Krauss and Jankovic (1997) presented the cases of three adults who developed multifocal motor and vocal tics following craniocerebral trauma in motor vehicle accidents, with a latency of 1 day to a few weeks. The important question is: if tics appear or seem to worsen after TBI, is TBI the sufficient or additive cause of the tics? This question can arise in cases of litigation and compensation, where the interpretation of pre-existing tics or other repetitive behaviors may be crucial to the outcome.

Case examples

'Ben' was 8 when first seen. He was injured in a hockey game but did not become unconscious. He had had tics (throat-clearing) before the injury, but afterwards developed more eye-blinking, head-shaking, kissing noises, humming, rubbing his nose and repeatedly saying inappropriate words. His teacher reported that he couldn't focus as well as before. He fulfilled criteria for Tourette syndrome, with a fairly typical onset age, and MRI was normal. Other than the changes reported by the school, there was nothing in the clinical sequence or pattern to prove (or disprove) cause-and-effect. There were no adequate pre-accident baseline data.

Comment: Weaker focus is not unusual when there is a significant increase in tics. In this instance a connection to brain injury was dubious.

'Beverly' was 8 when she suffered a skull fracture in a playground accident. CT showed brain swelling during 4 days of hospitalization while unconscious. There was no family history of tics nor any known indication of tics prior to the injury. Post-accident physical and imaging findings were all normal, but some skills seemed to have declined; she had notably less energy, and became irritable and occasionally aggressive, as well

as light- and sound-sensitive. Multiple tics developed: eye-blinking, head-shaking and noises. Psychological testing revealed a weakness in verbal concepts and both short- and long-term memory deficits. She no longer liked reading.

Comment: *She was felt to have clear neurologically based learning and behavior problems secondary to her TBI, and given a diagnosis of 'tic disorder not otherwise specified' (DSM-IV-TR). The role of the head injury in causing tics was unclear, given her age at onset, but was an attractive speculation.*

REFERENCES

Al-Asmi A, Jansen AC, Badhwar A, et al. (2005) Familial temporal lobe epilepsy as a presenting feature of choreoacanthocytosis. *Epilepsia* 46: 1256–63. doi: 10.1111/j.1528-1167.2005.65804.x.

Astley SJ (2004) *Diagnostic Guide for Fetal Alcohol Spectrum Disorder: the 4-Digit Diagnostic Code.* Seattle, WA: University of Washington.

Autti-Rämö I (2013) Heavy alcohol consumption and motherhood — a negative match. *Dev Med Child Neurol* 55: 205–6. doi: 10.1111/dmcn.12048.

Bachara GH, Phelan WJ (1980) Rhythmic movement in deaf children. *Percept Motor Skills* 50: 933–4.

Bagheri MM, Kerbeshian J, Burd L (1999) Recognition and management of Tourette's syndrome and tic disorders. *Am Fam Physician* 59: 2263–72.

Bandmann O (2013) Wilson disease. In: Burn DJ, ed. *Oxford Textbook of Movement Disorders, 2nd edn.* Oxford: Oxford University Press, pp. 241–6.

Blanco FC, Davenport KP, Kane TD (2012) Pediatric gastroesophageal reflux disease. *Surg Clin N Am* 92: 541–58. doi: 10.1016/j.suc.2012.03.009.

Bray PF (1990) Can maternal alcoholism cause spasmus nutans in offspring? *N Engl J Med* 322: 554. doi: 10.1056/NEJM199002223220815.

Cohen R, Senecky Y, Shuper A, et al. (2013) Prevalence of epilepsy and attention-deficit hyperactivity (ADHD) disorder: a population-based study. *J Child Neurol* 28: 120–3. doi: 10.1177/0883073812440327.

Cosentino C, Torres L (2000) Tourette's syndrome and neurofibromatosis type 1. *Pediatr Neurol* 22: 420–1. doi: 10.1016/S0887-8994(00)00124-7.

Davis K, Desrocher M, Moore T (2011) Fetal alcohol spectrum disorder: a review of neurodevelopmental findings and interventions. *J Dev Phys Disabil* 23: 143–67. doi: 10.1007/s10882-010-9204-2.

de Boer L, Röder I, Wit JM (2006) Psychosocial, cognitive, and motor functioning in patients with suspected Sotos syndrome: a comparison with and without *NSD1* gene alterations. *Dev Med Child Neurol* 48: 582–8. doi: 10.1111/j.1469-8749.2006.tb01319.x.

Demir T, Karacetin G, Baghaki S, Aydin Y (2011) Psychiatric assessment of children with nonsyndromic cleft lip and palate. *Gen Hosp Psychiatry* 33: 594–603. doi: 10.1016/j.genhosppsych.2011.06.006.

DiMario FJ Jr (2006) Paroxysmal nonepileptic events of childhood. *Semin Pediatr Neurol* 13: 208–21. doi: 10.1016/j.spen.2006.09.002.

Fernández-Mayoralas DM, Fernández-Jaén A, Muñoz-Jareño N, et al. (2010) Fetal alcohol syndrome, Tourette syndrome, and hyperactivity in nine adopted children. *Pediatr Neurol* 43: 110–6. doi: 10.1016/j.pediatrneurol.2010.03.008.

Feroz-Nainar C, Roy M (2006) Risperidone and late onset tics. *Autism* 10: 302–7.

Forsyth R, Kirkham F (2012) Predicting outcome after childhood brain injury. *CMAJ* 184: 1257–64.

Fox S (2013) Treating neurological Wilson's disease; the expert opinion is not good enough. *Can J Neurol Sci* 40: 445 (editorial).

Freeman RD (2010) Psychiatric considerations in cortical visual impairment. In: Dutton GN, Bax M, eds. *Visual Impairment in Children Due to Damage to the Brain. Clinics in Developmental Medicine no. 186.* London: Mac Keith Press, pp. 174–80.

Freeman RD, Goetz E, Richards DP, Groenveld M (1991) Defiers of negative prediction: results of a 14-year follow-up study. *J Vis Impair Blind* 85: 365–70.

Fryer SL, McGee CL, Matt GE, et al. (2007) Evaluation of psychopathological conditions in children with heavy alcohol exposure. *Pediatrics* 119: 733–40. doi: 10.1542/peds.2006-1606.

Gal E, Dyck MJ (2009) Stereotyped movements among children who are visually impaired. *J Vis Impair Blind* 103: 754–65.

Garg S, Lehtonen A, Huson SM, et al. (2013) Autism and other psychiatric comorbidity in neurofibromatosis type 1: evidence from a population-based study. *Dev Med Child Neurol* 55: 139–45. doi: 10.1111/dmcn.12043.

Hagerman RJ, Hagerman PJ, eds (2002) *Fragile X Syndrome: Diagnosis, Treatment, and Research, 3rd edn.* Baltimore: Johns Hopkins University Press.

Hartshorne TS, Hefner MA, Davenport SLH, Thelin JW, eds (2011) *CHARGE Syndrome.* San Diego: Plural Publishing.

Hong DS, Reiss AL (2014) Cognitive and neurological aspects of sex chromosome aneuploidies. *Lancet Neurol* 13: 306–18. doi: 10.1016.S1474-4422(13)70302-8.

Huijbregts S, Swaab H, de Sonneville L (2010) Cognitive and motor control in neurofibromatosis type 1: influence of maturation and hyperactivity–inattention. *Dev Neuropsychol* 35: 737–51. doi: 10.1080/87565641.2010.508670.

Isenberg JC, Templer A, Gao F, et al. (2013) Attention skills in children with neurofibromatosis type I. *J Child Neurol* 28: 45–9. doi: 10.1177/0883073812439435.

Jan JE, Freeman RD, Scott EP (1977) *Visual Impairment in Children and Adolescents.* New York: Grune & Stratton.

Jan JE, Freeman RD, McCormick AQ, et al. (1983) Eye-pressing by visually-impaired children. *Dev Med Child Neurol* 25: 755–62. doi: 10.1111/j.1469-8749.1983.tb13844.x.

Jan JE, Groenveld M, Connolly MB (1990) Head shaking by visually impaired children: a voluntary neuro-visual adaptation which could be confused with spasmus nutans. *Dev Med Child Neurol* 32: 1061–6. doi: 10.1111/j.1469-8749.1990.tb08524.x.

Jan JE, Good WV, Freeman RD, Espezel H (1994) Eye-poking. *Dev Med Child Neurol* 36: 321–5. doi: 10.1111/j.1469-8749.1994.tb11852.x.

Kidd SA, Lachiewicz A, Barbouth D, et al. (2014) Fragile X syndrome: a review of associated medical problems. *Pediatrics* 134 (online October 6). doi: 10.1542/peds.2013-4301.

Krauss JK, Jankovic J (1997) Tics secondary to craniocerebral trauma. *Mov Disord* 12: 776–82. doi: 10.1002/mds.870120527.

Lane KA, Stewart J, Fernandes T, et al. (2014) Complexities in understanding attentional functioning among children with fetal alcohol spectrum disorder. *Front Hum Neurosci* 8: 119. doi: 10.3389/fnhum.2014.00119.

Lehtonen A, Howie E, Trump D, Huson SM (2013) Behaviour in children with neurofibromatosis type 1: cognition, executive function, attention, emotion, and social competence. *Dev Med Child Neurol* 55: 111–25. doi: 10.1111/j.1469-8749.2012.04399.x.

Levine TM, Materek A, Abel J, et al. (2006) Cognitive profile of neurofibromatosis type 1. *Semin Pediatr Neurol* 13: 8–20. doi: 10.1016/j.spen.2006.01.006.

Leyser M, Marques FJP, Elias MAC, et al. (2013) Classic mainfestations of Duchenne dystrophy in a young female patient: a case report. *Eur J Paediatr Neurol* 17: 212–8. doi: 10.1016/j.ejpn.2012.08.002.

Li L, Liu J (2013) The effect of pediatric traumatic brain injury on behavioral outcomes: a systematic review. *Dev Med Child Neurol* 55: 37–45. doi: 10.1111/j.1469-8749.2012.04414.x.

Lombroso CT (1999) Lamotrigine-induced tourettism. *Neurology* 52: 1191–4.

Lorincz MT (2010) Neurologic Wilson's disease. *Ann NY Acad Sci* 1184: 173–87.

Max JE, Wilde EA, Bigler ED, et al. (2012) Psychiatric disorders after pediatric traumatic brain injury: a prospective, longitudinal, controlled study. *J Neuropsychiatry Clin Neurosci* 24: 427–36. doi: 10.1176/appi.neuropsych.12060149.

Molloy A, Rowe FJ (2011) Manneristic behaviors of visually impaired children. *Strabismus* 19: 77–84.

Murdoch H (1996) Stereotyped behaviors in deaf and hard of hearing children. *Am Ann Deaf* 141: 379–86.

Musiek ES, Anderson CT, Dahodwala NA, Pollard JR (2010) Facial tic associated with lamotrigine in adults. *Mov Disord* 25: 1512–3. doi: 10.1002/mds.23120.

Niklasson L, Rasmussen P, Óskarsdóttir, Gillberg C (2009) Autism, ADHD, mental retardation and behavior problems in 100 individuals with 22q11 deletion syndrome. *Res Dev Disabil* 30: 763–73. doi: 10.1016/j.ridd.2008.10.007.

Novak I, Hines M, Goldsmith S, Barclay R (2012) Clinical prognostic messages from a systematic review on cerebral palsy. *Pediatrics* 130: e1285–e1312. doi: 10.1542/peds.2012-0924.

Oates EC, Rossor AM, Hafezparast M, et al. (2013) Mutations in BICD2 cause dominant congenital spinal muscular atrophy and hereditary spastic paraplegia. *Am J Hum Genet* 92: 965–73. doi: 10.1016/j.ajhg.2013.04.018.

O'Leary C, Leonard H, Bourke J, et al. (2013) Intellectual disability: population-based estimates of the proportion attributable to maternal alcohol use disorder during pregnanacy. *Dev Med Child Neurol* 55: 271–7. doi: 10.1111/dmcn.12029.

Parkes J, White-Koning M, Dickenson HO, et al. (2008) Psychological problems in children with cerebral palsy: a cross-sectional European study. *J Child Psychol Psychiatry* 49: 405–13. doi: 10.1111/j.1469-7610.2007.01845.x.

Peterson BS, Bronen RA, Duncan CC (1996) Three cases of symptom change in Tourette's syndrome and obsessive–compulsive disorder associated with pediatric cerebral malignancies. *J Neurol Neurosurg Psychiatry* 61: 497–505.

Pfeiffer RF (2007) Wilson's disease. *Semin Neurol* 27: 123–32. doi: 10.1055/s-2007-971173.

Plioplys S, Asato MR, Bursch B, et al. (2007a) Multidisciplinary management of pediatric nonepileptic seizures. *J Am Acad Child Adolesc Psychiatry* 46: 1491–5. doi: 10.1097/chi.0b013e31814dab98.

Plioplys S, Dunn DW, Caplan R (2007b) 10-year research update review: psychiatric problems in children with epilepsy. *J Am Acad Child Adolesc Psychiatry* 46: 1389–1402. doi: 10.1097/chi.0b013e31815597fc.

Preece PM, Riley EP (2011) *Alcohol, Drugs and Medication in Pregnancy: The Long-term Outcome for the Child. Clinics in Developmental Medicine no. 188.* London: Mac Keith Press.

Pride NA, Crawford H, Payne JM, North KN (2013) Social functioning in adults with neurofibromatosis type 1. *Res Dev Disabil* 34: 3393–9. doi: 10.1016/j.ridd.2013.07.011.

Rana AQ, Avan A, Aftab A, et al. (2013) A viewpoint about the treatment of Wilson's disease. *Can J Neurol Sci* 40: 612–14.

Ranjan N, Nair KP, Romanoski C, et al. (2011) Tics after traumatic brain injury. *Brain Inj* 25: 629–3.

Rickards H (2001) Signing coprolalia and attempts to disguise in a man with prelingual deafness. *Mov Disord* 16: 790–1. doi: 10.1002/mds.1158.

Rickards H, Robertson MM (1997) Vomiting and retching in Gilles de la Tourette syndrome: a report of ten cases and a review of the literature. *Mov Disord* 12: 531–5. doi: 10.1002/mds.870120409.

Rizzo R, Gulisano M, Calì PV, Curatolo P (2010) ADHD and epilepsy in children with Tourette syndrome: a triple comorbidity? *Acta Paediatr* 99: 1894–96. doi: 10.1111/j.1651-2227-2010.01951.x.

Robertson PL, Garofalo EA, Silverstein FS, Komarynski MA (1993) Carbamazepine-induced tics. *Epilepsia* 34: 965–8.

Rosenbaum P, Paneth N, Leviton A, et al. (2006) A report: the definition and classification of cerebral palsy. *Dev Med Child Neurol* 49 Suppl 109: 8–14.

Rosenbaum PL, Rosenbloom L (2012) *Cerebral Palsy: from Diagnosis to Adult Life.* London: Mac Keith Press.

Schachter SC, LaFrance WC Jr, eds (2010) *Gates and Rowan's Nonepileptic Seizures, 3rd edn.* Cambridge/New York: Cambridge University Press.

Sotero de Menezes MA, Rho JM, Murphy P, Cheyette S (2000) Lamotrigine-induced tic disorder: report of five pediatric cases. *Epilepsia* 41: 862–7.

Steinhausen HC, Willms J, Spohr H-L (1993) Long-term psychopathological and cognitive outcome of children with fetal alcohol syndrome. *J Am Acad Child Adolesc Psychiatry* 32: 990–4. doi: 10.1097/00004583-199309000-00016.

Streissguth AP, Bookstein FL, Barr HM, et al. (2004) Risk factors for adverse life outcomes in fetal alcohol syndrome and fetal alcohol effects. *Dev Behav Pediatrics* 25: 228–38.

Uldall P, Alving J, Hansen LK, et al. (2006) The misdiagnosis of epilepsy in children admitted to a tertiary epilepsy centre with paroxysmal events. *Arch Dis Child* 91: 219–21. doi: 10.1136/adc.2004.064477.

Walsh KS, Vélez JI, Kardel PG, et al. (2013) Symptomatology of autism spectrum disorder in a population with neurofibromatosis type 1. *Dev Med Child Neurol* 55: 131–8. doi: 10.1111/dmcn.12038.

Watemberg N, Tziperman B, Dabby R, et al. (2005) Adding video recording increases the diagnostic yield of routine electroencephalograms in children with frequent paroxysmal events. *Epilepsia* 46: 716–9.

Whittingham K, Sanders M, McKinlay L, Boyd RN (2014) Interventions to reduce behavioral problems in children with cerebral palsy: an RCT. *Pediatrics* 133: e1249–e1257. doi: 10.1542/peds.2013-3620.

14
NEUROPSYCHOLOGY

> Patients with Tourette syndrome combined with other neurodevelopmental disorders are likely to show problems in memory and executive functioning, although studies on TS-only cases suggest that there are no pathognomonic abnormalities. Problems with working memory and processing speed are frequent psychological assessment findings in ADHD, and OCD typically can add problems of rumination, obsessional doubting, perfectionism and compulsions. Tics themselves can affect performance, so the combined factors are many. Whatever the deficits in learning or performance, competent psychological assessment is usually valuable and may be essential to individualized educational planning.

Despite papers suggesting otherwise, statements on the internet and the beliefs of some educators, the preponderance of evidence is that there are no universal psychological problems with intelligence, memory, or executive function in TS-only, although in practice such problems are common because of the frequency of comorbid disorders. Thorough discussions of this area have been contributed by Eddy et al. (2009), Rasmussen et al. (2009) and Sukhodolsky et al. (2010). Comorbid ADHD often implicates working memory impairment, and many studies have provided mixed results, probably because of inadequate or uncertain exclusion of comorbid disorders. The presence of OCD features may affect cognition because of rumination or obsessional, intrusive thoughts, and waxing–waning tic severity is another possibly confounding factor. Rasmussen et al. (2009), however, did not find differences in their patients with TS+OCD.

A somewhat contrary opinion was presented by Como (2001) that, despite methodological flaws in previous studies, there was some evidence for learning problems specifically in math and written language, and for cognitive deficits in visuomotor integration, fine motor skill and executive dysfunction. The latter functions may not be assessed in a school psychologist's psychoeducational evaluation. Como also pointed out that intellectual ability is normally distributed in Tourette syndrome. Channon et al. (2003) compared TS-only, TS+ADHD and TS+OCD on executive functioning, learning and memory, and found only one domain affected (inhibition and strategy generation).

One needs to be aware of other pitfalls in psychologists' interpretations of a child's behavior during an assessment (and psychologists often have the most time observing a child):
- Tics may be missed entirely because they are misinterpreted as 'nervousness' due to frustration or anxiety associated with the test situation.

- Increases in tics during a session may be interpreted as solely due to stress or fatigue, when the time of day may also be important.
- RMBs may be assumed to be tics, may increase under 'stress' like tics can, and then the 'tics' may be said to interfere with performance.

Case example

'Brad', a very bright boy with Tourette syndrome and ADHD, performed largely in the gifted range educationally, with no tested areas of weakness. RMBs specifically interpreted as motor tics included hands in mouth, finger-picking, sucking and biting fingers, scratching, and picking at teeth, all of which were said to affect his focus.

*   **Comment:** In the context of a very helpful assessment by an otherwise competent neuropsychologist, one can see that many RMBs were definitively classified as tics with little or no justification for this. This brings to mind the warning not to assume that "If you have tics, all other repetitive behaviors are also tics." Having said that, it is also true that at times the dividing line between tics and other patterns of behavior can be far from clear or agreed-upon.*

Here we can again see the phenomenon of 'diagnostic overshadowing'. What is often attributed to Tourette syndrome may be related to Tourette syndrome comorbidity. Books and materials developed for teaching children with TS+ADHD may be very useful, but not necessarily because the children have tics (Dornbush and Pruitt 2008, Packer and Pruitt 2010).

REFERENCES

Channon S, Pratt P, Robertson MM (2003) Executive function, memory, and learning in Tourette's syndrome. *Neuropsychology* 17: 247–54. doi: 10.1037/0894-4105.17.2.247.

Como P (2001) Neuropsychological function in Tourette's syndrome. *Adv Neurol* 85: 103–11.

Dornbush MP, Pruitt SK (2008) *Tigers, Too: Executive Functions/Speed of Processing/Memory.* Atlanta, GA: Parkaire Press.

Eddy CM, Rizzo R, Cavanna AE (2009) Neuropsychological aspects of Tourette syndrome: a review. *J Psychosom Res* 67: 503–13. doi: 10.1016/j.jpsychores.2009.08.001.

Packer LE, Pruitt SK (2010) *Challenging Kids, Challenged Teachers: Teaching Students with Tourette's, Bipolar Disorder, Executive Dysfunction, OCD, ADHD, and More.* Bethesda, MD: Woodbine House.

Rasmussen C, Soleimani M, Carroll A, Hodlevskyy O (2009) Neuropsychological functioning in children with Tourette syndrome (TS). *J Can Acad Child Adolesc Psychiatry* 18: 307–15.

Sukhodolsky DG, Landeros-Weisenberger A, Scahill L, et al. (2010) Neuropsychological functioning in children with Tourette syndrome with and without attention-deficit/hyperactivity disorder. *J Am Acad Child Adolesc Psychiatry* 49: 1155–64. doi: 10.1016/j.jaac.2010.08.008.

15
INTERVENTIONS AND TREATMENT

Slow progress has been made in choices of treatment, both within medication and in behavioral approaches. The first and most important question is whether treatment is needed, and whether the preliminary steps have been taken. Those steps involve 'psychoeducation' and a delineation of the context in which tics occur. Specific treatment decisions aren't simple, and usually are not inherent in the diagnosis. Vocal tics are more likely than motor tics to cause problems in school. If antipsychotic medication is to be used, weight gain and metabolic changes are significant hazards, requiring baseline laboratory tests and close monitoring. Caution is needed switching from brand-name to generic psychotropic medications.

A major dilemma in conceptualization affects both clinician and patient thinking: how to interpret behavioral problems that go beyond 'core' tics. Are they 'part of Tourette syndrome', sometimes referred to vaguely as 'full-blown Tourette syndrome'? Studies have shown that persons with chronic tic disorders are more likely than those with typical development to display emotional and behavioral difficulties, as well as what we call comorbidity. If caution is not applied, this can provide a possibly pseudo-explanatory short-cut that can bypass helpful therapeutic efforts or lead to a therapeutic dead end. In this chapter a brief summary of current concerns is provided, but anyone using pharmacologic or behavioral interventions should read the most recent reviews.

Intervention implies help, but not necessarily medication. What is that help? — to learn or discover what would make your 'new' life with tics livable. Often this could mean taking better charge of the meanings others assign to your tics and therefore feeling less victimized thereby. Also, to acquire information about the disorders that have been diagnosed, and develop a simple explanation in plain language. This won't be perfect, especially with strangers, but even then skills can improve. With children this includes parents and other important family members.

Fundamental to psychoeducation is to demystify the meaning of Tourette syndrome as contrasted with 'tic disorder'. Then the usual course of persistent tic disorders in childhood needs to be grasped so as to minimize a strong negative reaction to every tic change or increase. If this is not accomplished there is a risk of overmedication. It can be helpful to share successes in managing awkward situations that the child has with parents and therapist. (Humor should not be omitted from otherwise serious situations.) This is also one function of a good support group. A study by Olufs et al. (2013) showed that adults learning about Tourette syndrome acquired more knowledge when there was self-disclosure rather than the usual talk with audiovisual enhancement.

"Provision of a diagnostic label alone appears insufficient" (Nussey et al. 2013, p. 617). These authors performed a review of the evidence of the helpfulness of education, and specifically with comorbid ADHD. Information was helpful, for children, parents and teachers. Psychoeducation needs to include help for parents (with supervision by a clinician experienced in behavioral approaches) to collect evidence of environmental factors influencing tic frequency and severity, and to modify those when identified (Bennett et al. 2013). This is a change from the traditional content. Important changes in evidence-based advice have been very well summarized in their paper and should be required reading. The following is a brief summary of the changes in current clinical recommendations and how they differ from previous ones (and from most of those on the internet).

- Becoming more aware of tics (rather than ignoring them)
- Realizing that individuals can learn to manage their tics (rather than seeing them as uncontrollable)
- Providing social reward for successful management of the tics
- Using behavioral strategies rather than assuming that these are ineffective
- Learning to control tics through focused attention and competing responses to break the reinforcement cycle, and that the urges will fade away (rather than assuming that suppression will cause a rebound or worsen premonitory urges)
- Coming to the understanding that new tics don't develop from behavioral strategies
- Realizing that tics can wax and wane and therefore be influenced by inner and outer environmental factors, that need to be identified as part of management.

Who needs treatment?

Treatment implies something specific. But what is usually needed isn't specific treatment, but more likely counseling, ecological management (sometimes), support and advocacy. For dramatic symptoms or complaints, reassurance may be appropriate and necessary, but can be hard to achieve when a premonitory sensation strongly suggests a physical problem, the source of which hasn't been located. Reassurance that does not take account of symptoms that change or of the level of parental anxiety often fails or makes things worse. When the diagnosis is made, parents may then move on to what seems the logical next step: "What do we do, then?" They need to learn that usually there is nothing curative to 'do' right away. This, however, has its own problems for them, because it recommends tolerating the passivity of what could well be their child's unpredictable symptom storms. Parents who have a strong need to 'know' and thereby feel competent or who themselves have obsessive–compulsive traits may have special difficulty without something to do. What there is to do in the absence of a specific treatment, however, is to provide psychoeducation and to put into practice those "little things that truly make a difference" (Ryan and Leventhal 2012), such as developing better treatment motivation, building better liaison with parents, other important family members and teachers, and (sometimes) ensuring treatment of significant disorders in family members.

The conceptual trap of a behavior problem seen as 'part of Tourette syndrome'
Treatment decisions aren't simple, and usually are not inherent in the diagnosis or diagnoses. Parents, patients — and all too often clinicians — may attribute the development or presence of behavioral problems to the tic disorder itself. This may seem to reduce uncomfortable uncertainty, but can be dangerous. How? It is true that studies of persons with chronic tic disorders (even without comorbidity) show that as a group they have more emotional and behavioral problems than those without, but that provides much too easy a way out of deeper thinking, and can be a trap. Those findings do not justify the conclusion that the problem in a particular individual is part of Tourette syndrome. Do persons without tics sometimes have the same problems? Probably yes; maybe often. Boundaries around our disorder categories are not sharp and are known to overlap. If this is granted, it seems that the same thoughtfulness that we apply to those persons without tics should be applied to those with tics. The rarely (if ever) defined phrase 'full-blown Tourette syndrome' is best retired.

What treatments are appropriate?
In almost all cases (assuming that the diagnosis of Tourette syndrome is correct), the provision or enhancement of understanding is the first priority for tics (sometimes termed 'psychoeducation'), and often the only intervention needed. What is it that patients or their parents want? From both research and clinical experience, an explanation of the symptoms and what is feared to lie behind them; reassurance about symptom course, fluctuations in the future, risk of teasing or bullying; and of course an abolition of the tics and other problems, if possible. Secondly, any situation or comorbid disorder that may be triggering tics or contributing to their exacerbation or overall impairment should be modified. While patients and their families rarely ask for it explicitly, they may value, and benefit from, sharing the story of their experience of the disorder and how it is affecting their lives (Frank 2002).

These goals depend for their continuing success upon clinician accessibility. One initial assessment session that goes well is rarely found to be sufficient. People go away, talk about the session, and generate new questions or a need for clarification.

If treatment is needed, then one has a choice of medication or a behavioral approach (or both).

Interventions for tics
You can have thousands of extra eye-blinks a day without much social impairment, but spit five times or touch inappropriately and everything changes. Blinking is with both eyes; winking is with only one, but socially it can be much more impairing because it is a social signal that is being misapplied.

Resorting to medication immediately, except when there is severe impairment, is not a good idea. Withholding that treatment isn't to assert that suffering is good for the soul, but so that the ways, areas and meanings of suffering are understood and that strengths in the individual, family, school and community are developed to maximize tolerance of symptoms. Since tics can't be cured by medications, and tend to improve in and after adolescence, moving too quickly to medication may bypass tolerance processes and not build whatever mastery can be achieved. Each upsurge may then be the occasion for medication increases, and medication usage exposes the patient to short- and long-term risks (Sandor and Carroll 2012) against which the clinical need must be weighed.

Recently help has become available through the publication of European (Müller-Vahl et al. 2011; Roessner et al. 2011a,b; Verdellen et al. 2011) and Canadian evidence-based treatment guidelines (Pringsheim et al. 2012, Steeves et al. 2012) covering pharmacotherapy, behavioral therapy, deep brain stimulation, and transcranial magnetic stimulation. The European guidelines also cover assessment (Cath et al. 2011). Clinicians considering treatment of tics would be well advised to read these guidelines. The editorial accompanying the Canadian guidelines (Sandor and Carroll 2012) is a model of the appropriate approach to treatment. American practice parameters have just been published (Murphy et al. 2013; a short critique of a few points is presented in Appendix 4). Since different medications are available in different countries, there are differences in the three publications; all have useful ideas and are worth careful attention.

The recently validated behavioral treatment known as CBIT (Comprehensive Behavioral Intervention for Tics) should also be carefully considered (Meidinger et al. 2005; Woods et al. 2009, 2011; Capriotti et al. 2014b) and is discussed in more detail below.

Tics that seem to require urgent treatment

There are some tics that present to clinicians as an intolerable situation, crying out for something effective to minimize them. These are often very loud, frequent, piercing vocal tics that are disturbing to everyone but especially in a classroom, or self-injurious tics. In school they may result in exclusion from the classroom, sitting in a hallway or the principal's office, frequent calls to the home to come and pick up the child, staying at home for prolonged periods, even home-schooling. When other parents start to call the principal and register complaints, tics cannot be ignored. A decision to medicate the child appears necessary and rapid. However, not so fast! Some of these situations require a closer look. While that closer look is evolving, the offending tic may subside. One should look at what factors in the child's life may be exacerbating the premonitory urges or triggering the tics, the sensitivities and expectations of the teacher, characteristics of the classroom or class, and adequacy of classroom supports. The level of tolerance may not be as rigidly low as initially thought. Supportive contact with the school may have salutary effects even without commencing effective medication.

Case example

'Garth' was only 8 years old when his vocal tics underwent a large increase that could not be ignored by his classmates or teacher. The school asked the mother to take him home on about half the school days, placing stress on her job. Search for triggers

---

produced the terminal illness of a much-loved grandmother. Exploration of the school situation showed that the teacher had a well-known sensitivity to sound and a need for a quiet, well-ordered atmosphere in her class; classmates' voices had to be raised to overcome the effect of the frequent vocal tics. The teacher had no prior experience with tics and wasn't sure whether the vocal tics were really involuntary or might be at least partially deliberate.

Comment: A meeting to work out strategies to reduce stress and improve understanding obviated the necessity for medication.

In situations where a quick response is necessary, there is a difference among classes of medication. If a child cannot attend school and the parents are not able or willing to take the responsibility of home-schooling, the most rapidly effective drug is necessary. The safest drugs unfortunately require longer to evaluate effects and the results may be less robust. They are likely to have some side-effects. These first-line drugs are clonidine and guanfacine, but their benefit is likely to be limited to mild or moderate cases. The quickest and most dependable response, especially with more severe symptoms is with antipsychotic (neuroleptic) drugs (second line), which have the strongest evidence base: 'first generation' antipsychotics (FGAs) such as haloperidol, pimozide, and fluphenazine; substituted benzamides such as tiapride (Eggers et al. 1988), sulpiride (Robertson et al. 1990), and amisulpride; and 'second generation' antipsychotics (SGAs) such as risperidone and ziprasidone. A newer drug in a special category is aripiprazole (Masi et al. 2012, Rizzo et al. 2012, Wenzel et al. 2012). A different drug with relatively rapid onset is tetrabenazine (Kenney et al. 2007, Chen et al. 2012), which has a weaker evidence base and is therefore considered third line.

There are others with little current evidence base, such as topiramate, and still more have been advocated or are being investigated currently.

It used to be assumed that SGAs have fewer side-effects and long-term effects (are more tolerable) that FGAs. This may not be so, and it appears that efficacy is equivalent for the two groups (Kompoliti et al. 2010).

Two examples indicate the complexity of the decision to employ medication.

Case examples

'Frances' was an overweight 18-year-old when seen again for consideration of medication because of an upsurge of tics before an important imminent job interview. Careful interviewing revealed that her tolerance for her tics was low: she was very self-conscious about her vocal tics in particular and assumed that people would reject her. She also had some obsessive–compulsive symptoms and a delayed sleep phase disorder. After reaching a better understanding and clarifying some misunderstandings, medication seemed unnecessary. However, within a short time she had a more severe upsurge that was so impairing that medication had to be reconsidered and finally became necessary.

At age 14 'Ivan' was referred to obtain recommendations for medication. He was sad about his tics because he hated them and they led to teasing; he was starting to withdraw from his peer group. The teasing was partly due to his moving into a new social group in a different school, but he never explained his tics to the class, instead making a different and sometimes far-fetched excuse for each different tic (of many). Questioning revealed that he was not much bothered by his tics when alone or when he was with accepting adults. He was hyper-aware of the possibility that out of his view peers who had noticed his tics were making fun of him.

Comment: The question arose: should he be medicated because of his sensitivity, or would it be more appropriate to attempt to modify his social context and improve his explanation of his tics?

Considerations in using medication for tics

- Children who are suffering with pain or other distress may want medication immediately, whereas many parents (especially in developed countries) are likely to have misgivings and be much more cautious, more so the younger the child.
- You cannot count on tic observation in the office to fully assess the need for medication or any other intervention.
- If medication is tried, careful monitoring is required, especially at first, including (for some drugs) blood tests or electrocardiography (Maayan and Correll 2011, Ronsley et al. 2012).
- Significant comorbid disorders often need to be treated first (especially ADHD and OCD).
- Clinicians who are not familiar with the use of medications for tics should read recent reviews and if at all possible consult with a local or regional specialist.
- Starting at too high a dosage for the patient may lead to early adverse effects such as dystonic reactions, which, while not directly harmful, can turn the patient and family against medication in general. The 'start low, go slow' rule is a good one.
- The waxing–waning course of tics often confuses the need for continuing medication. Many parents and patients are unaware that despite effective treatment in lessening overall tic severity, tic upsurges will continue to occur. This point should be an integral part of psychoeducation.
- Polypharmacy is common, especially when there is significant comorbidity. Drug interactions must be considered, and risks may increase if more than one drug in the same category is used.
- Tapering dosage can be tricky because of timing and situational factors. (Is the time appropriate? What if worse symptoms emerge just at this time?)
- After a time on medication the patient or family may feel that it is not helping. Rather than have an older child or adolescent stop suddenly on his or her own (and perhaps suffer rebound symptoms), it is better to engage in a planned tapering with monitoring of changes. The result may be a significant recrudescence of target symptoms showing that there was indeed a treatment effect, to which people had become accustomed.

• Switching from brand-name to generic medications or between generics. Generic medications do not undergo the same approval process as required of original medications. Clinical deterioration and decreased tolerability may occur with generic substitution, but this is not well-known to many clinicians. A review of reports by Desmarais et al. (2011) showed some such problems with anticonvulsants, antidepressants, anxiolytics and antipsychotics such as risperidone. The authors recommend individual consideration and close monitoring during a transition. A further point can be made: the equivalence standards allow for deviations from one generic to another (e.g. when a pharmacy switches suppliers) that may cause significant therapeutic effects for some patients.

General tips for the use of medication
There are a number of pitfalls for the unwary, as follows.

(1) *People who can't take pills.* Not many drugs are available in liquid or similar vehicles. If they are, their taste may be a problem, especially individuals with ASD or sensory sensitivities. Others may fear choking. Always ask whether your patient can take pills — even with adults. Some compounding pharmacists can prepare a suspension from pills at extra cost.

(2) *Sustained-release preparations.* Parents who break up or grind up pills in this category may not realize that the desired sustained effect is lost by so doing. In addition, the more acute increase in blood level of the drug may produce significant side-effects.

(3) *Monitoring.* It is not a good idea to start a new medication just before you go away, leaving the responsibility for coverage to a colleague who does not know the patient. It is standard practice to monitor closely at the start of a new medication, or after dosage changes. The patient or family needs to know how to contact you in case of difficulty. Few situations are more frustrating than being unable to reach the prescribing physician when there is a problem.

(4) *Baseline electrocardiogram.* This is a consideration (but not officially a standard of care in North America), before using a stimulant for ADHD or pimozide or ziprasidone for tics (Lombroso and Scahill 2008). The latter medications can lengthen the QTc or make the person vulnerable to further lengthening when certain other drugs are used simultaneously.

Case example
'Jeff' had obvious Tourette syndrome symptoms and significant ADHD. He was planning to engage in competitive sports and to undergo a trial of stimulant medication. A baseline ECG was obtained and found to be quite abnormal. Further testing revealed hypertrophic cardiomyopathy, and the affected autosomal dominant gene was identified. Investigation of immediate family members showed that his brother and father also had the condition and had had episodes that were misdiagnosed as exercise-

---

induced asthma and panic attacks respectively. Two other extended family members were found to carry the same gene but were unaffected (incomplete penetrance).

Comment: Originally thought to be rare, hypertrophic cardiomyopathy is now known to be "a relatively common cardiomyopathy with variable and an often benign, or at least manageable, clinical course" (Jacoby et al. 2013, p. 132).

(5) *Metabolic syndrome (MetS)*. The recent increase in Type 2 diabetes mellitus in children and adolescents has received worldwide attention (Groner et al. 2006, Sellers et al. 2008, Varda and Gregoric 2009). Diagnosis may not be made for years because of delayed symptom appearance. Increased diabetic and cardiovascular risk with the use of SGAs and the likelihood that changes can be induced rapidly and possibly permanently are cause for considerable worry (Correll et al. 2009, Panagiotopoulos et al. 2009, Varley and McClellan 2009, Maayan and Correll 2011). Metabolic syndrome is a collection of risk factors, the definition of which has not yet reached universal agreement. Despite attempts by several organizations to develop guidelines for research and practice, there is still no general agreement on all aspects and therefore studies are not always comparable. There is evidence that lifestyle monotherapy can be successful in about half of cases (Wittmeier et al. 2012). However, in a recent editorial, the summary statement was:

> Increased adiposity during childhood has a significant impact on cardiometabolic health and, perhaps most alarmingly, is highly predictive of obesity during adulthood along with a broad range of adverse health effects that are independent of adult body mass index. Clinicians and public health professionals have an acute need for effective interventions to mitigate these factors. (Crume and Harrod 2013, p. 697)

Many clinicians are still not taking account of the metabolic risks (Panagiotopoulos et al. 2009, Morrato et al. 2010). Evidence-based guidelines for monitoring safety have recently been published (Pringsheim et al. 2011), and guidelines for management of metabolic complications are now also available (Ho et al. 2011). The institution of a Metabolic Monitoring Training Program in British Columbia showed that monitoring can be improved, and that the rate of prescribing SGAs can be substantially reduced (Ronsley et al. 2012). An excellent review of the entire situation was presented by Panagiotopoulos et al. (2010). There is now evidence that discontinuation of risperidone, even after years of usage, may reverse excessive weight gain and cardiometabolic parameters (Calarge et al. 2014).

Usage of SGAs has increased, especially in North America (Patten et al. 2012), for disruptive behavior disorders (ADHD and conduct disorder) and ASD. FGAs are still used in Europe and other countries, but SGA usage has increased there as well. It is disconcerting, then, to find out that there is very weak placebo-controlled evidence for efficacy of risperidone (the most prescribed drug) in adolescents with average intelligence, and virtually none for FGAs (Pringsheim and Gorman 2012). A very helpful synthesis of current research by Dent et al. (2012) provides a ranking of potential weight gain for most of the psychotropic drugs. It also shows how inadequate current knowledge is. With regard to antipsychotic medication for tics, the following ranking was concluded, in descending order of risk: olanzapine, quetiapine, risperidone, amisulpride, aripiprazole, haloperidol, fluphenazine and ziprasidone. (Note that there is insufficient comparative evidence to rank pimozide, sulpride, tiapride or tetrabenazine.) Children and adolescents who are already overweight before commencing medication are at higher risk. The study by Kompoliti et al. (2010) reported that although children receiving antipsychotic drugs were significantly more likely to experience weight gain than those not taking those drugs, in this regard there was no difference between FGAs and SGAs.

(6) *Constipation.* Chronic constipation in children has been reported to occur in about 7%, associated with lack of exercise, avoidance of using the school toilet, low consumption of fruits and vegetables, high levels of milk products, family history of constipation, and some medications (including antipsychotics).

(7) *Using drugs intermittently for upsurges may be less effective in influencing the course than continuous treatment.* A study of this question, using pimozide in a pilot study on a small group (Tourette Syndrome Study Group 1999) showed a beneficial long-term effect, but it has not been replicated.

(8) *Tetrabenazine.* A small study by Jain et al. (2006) summarizes the clinical experience with this drug, a presynaptic dopamine depleter that does not cause tardive dyskinesia, but has possible side-effects of akathisia and depression.

(9) *Aripiprazole.* Cui et al. (2010) performed an 8-week pilot study and found a significant reduction in tics by week 8, with few extrapyramidal symptoms and no significant weight gain. Masi et al. (2012) reported success with tics in a 12-week open-label study, but all SGAs can cause weight gain (Maayan and Correll 2011).

(10) *Hyperprolactinemia.* Elevated prolactin levels occur in about 70% of patients receiving antipsychotic medications, thought to be caused by the blocking of D2 receptors that are involved in regulation of prolactin levels (Ajnal et al. 2014). The strongest effects are from haloperidol, fluphenazine, risperidone and amisulpride. Symptoms of hyperprolactinemia in men may be gynecomastia, erectile dysfunction, loss of libido, galactorrhea, osteopenia and osteoporosis; in women, symptoms may include hirsutism, acne, irregular menses, infertility, galactorrhea and fractures. Aripiprazole does not have this effect. In the presence of hyperprolactinemia that precedes medication usage, the possibility of a pituitary or hypothalamic lesion must be ruled out.

(11) *Slow onset of change.* It can be difficult to wait for improvement. There is great individual variation. One should not abandon a medication too readily without adequately exploring the dosage range and being patient while waiting for any side-effects to diminish.

How much freedom should the patient or parent have to change dosage?
Even when a satisfactory maintenance dosage has been reached, upsurges and other factors

will often cause pressure to increase dosage. Most parents are content to consult with the prescriber for advice or approval of a change, but what if access is difficult? The temptation to do it oneself will then grow, and such changes may not be reported to the clinician later, jeopardizing the relationship and accuracy of information. It is prudent to discuss this problem before such a situation arises, and to establish clear procedures and expectations. In some instances the medication may be initiated by a specialist, then continuation delegated to the primary care physician; the responsibility should be very clear to all concerned.

Neuroleptic separation anxiety syndrome
Occasionally patients who take neuroleptic drugs develop new separation anxiety symptoms that they never had before (or worsen pre-existing symptoms), either focused on separating from parents to go to school or even to leave home to go to a workplace; sometimes the 'tipping point' dosage level is very clear and the medication can be titrated to just below that level (Hanna et al. 1999).

Neuroleptic malignant syndrome (NMS)
NMS is a rare and potentially fatal complication of antipsychotic pharmacotherapy, characterized by severe muscle rigidity, fever and tachycardia (Ananth et al. 2004, Strawn et al. 2007, Neuhut et al. 2009, Gillman 2010). Drugs most frequently involved were risperidone, olanzapine and aripiprazole, and the risk is greater with the use of multiple antipsychotics. Changes in level of consciousness and mutism may also occur. Findings include elevated creatine phosphokinase from muscle damage in all cases studied. Immediate cessation of the antipsychotic drug is imperative.

Catatonia
Catatonia is not limited to schizophrenia or mood disorder; it can occur in other neurologic and psychiatric disorders, including Tourette syndrome and especially autism with SIB, in children and adults, manifesting as mutism, negativism, rigidity, echophenomena and excitement (Cavanna et al. 2008, Dhossche et al. 2010, Weiss et al. 2012, Fink 2013). First-line treatment is a high-dose benzodiazepine and/or electroconvulsive therapy. Catatonia may overlap with neuroleptic malignant syndrome.

Tardive dyskinesia
Tardive dyskinesia is fortunately very uncommon in Tourette syndrome (Müller-Vahl et al. 2011). For an excellent review, see Wain and Jankovic (2013).

Behavioral treatment
Although behavior therapy has been tried with mostly favorable reports on single cases with short follow-up, until recently most clinicians considered it useless. However, a revolution has taken place: behavior therapy has acquired a significant evidence base (O'Connor 2005; Himle et al. 2006; Piacentini et al. 2010; Woods et al. 2008a,b, 2011; Capriotti et al. 2012,

2013, 2014a,b; Wilhelm et al. 2012; Scahill et al. 2013) in the form of the Comprehensive Behavioral Intervention for Tics (CBIT), a development of Habit Reversal Therapy (HRT). However, there are still many children who are refractory to (or not ready for) HRT/CBIT and we are in a transition period when most physicians and many psychologists are not yet trained to provide this kind of therapy. Rapid progress is being made, however.

A number of criticisms or concerns have been raised about CBIT, especially since the publication of the article by Piacentini et al. (2010). These have been answered effectively by Woods et al. (2007, 2011) and Scahill et al. (2013) with a discussion of the evidence. Briefly, the criticisms are as follows: (1) doubt that tics can be suppressed by the mobilization of environmental factors, since their neurobiological causes are assumed to be beyond their reach; (2) suppression may (or will) cause rebound (contradicted by several studies such as Himle et al. 2007, Verdellen et al. 2007, Conelea and Woods 2008, Woods et al. 2008a); (3) non-targeted tics will become worse; (4) an old tic will be replaced by a new one; and (5) focusing on tics will make them worse. There is some evidence that increasing tic salience may temporarily produce an increase in tic frequency for a small subset of individuals outside of the therapeutic situation. The objections, it is argued, do not carry much weight.

The rationale for CBIT is that tics, although largely neurobiological in origin, are partially maintained by negative reinforcement, i.e. the tic performance temporarily reduces the distressing premonitory urges (Woods et al. 2011). The patient is taught to become aware of urges or premonitory sensations, and instead of then performing the tic response, to delay the tic response for an increasingly prolonged period of time and substitute an action that is incompatible with that tic. If all goes well the patient may acquire a skill that can be applied to new tics that arise, without returning for more treatment. Among unanswered questions about the applicability of this approach at the time of writing are: (1) what the earliest age is that children can be effective partners (for some children this may be as low as 6 years); (2) whether ADHD or other comorbid disorders (including intelligence level) will be a barrier to efficacy or require modifications; and (3) whether group or remote (telemedicine) approaches can be used to make treatment availability more equitable. Current research and clinical experience should clarify these questions — an intensive (several hours on four days) outpatient treatment of two boys has been reported by Blount et al. (2014), and a pilot study in our clinic of group CBIT for children aged 9–13 years is under development.

In a recent paper, Woods et al. (2010) looked at American national treatment utilization and found that most children and adults with persistent tic disorders have not received behavior therapy. Reasons include lack of information, a shortage of providers and concern about possible negative effects. The Tourette Syndrome Association through a partnership with the US Centers for Disease Control and Prevention has pioneered a series of Behavior Therapy Institutes that enable therapists to obtain behavioral training and certification. Canada has already hosted two Institutes, and other countries are showing interest. Bringing therapists together will have the additional advantage of sharing ideas for both practice and further research. The tight methodological control of behavioral studies has already led to a byproduct: the development of researchable questions about tics, premonitory urges and other sensory phenomena (Houghton et al. 2014) that augurs well for eventual improvements in our understanding (Reese et al. 2013).

The Canadian Guidelines (Pringsheim et al. 2012) give behavioral treatment a first-line recommendation, along with clonidine and guanfacine.

Parent training

Parent training has been shown to be helpful in a small randomized trial by Scahill et al. (2006b). Ideas from attachment theory, structural family systems theory, cognitive–attribution theory and others may enable therapists to help families who are stuck.

Practice point

It should be noted again that in some instances the complex interaction effects of tics and comorbid symptoms with a patient's and family members' reactivity to environmental factors and stresses over long periods of time pose challenges to the development and maintenance of a multifaceted individualized treatment program. Generic clinicians may not know how to judge the role of tics or other symptoms, and clinicians dealing with tics may not have the requisite psychosocial skills to intervene effectively. Collaboration may be necessary and approaches may require change over time.

Other treatments

Deep brain stimulation is reviewed in the European Guidelines and the conclusion is that it should be used only in adult, treatment-resistant, severely affected patients, preferably in controlled trials (Müller-Vahl et al. 2011a, Kim and Pouratian 2014).

Cannabinoids (marijuana) have been studied because of patient claims of benefit, and some studies have given support (Müller-Vahl 2003, Müller-Vahl et al. 2003), though legal and political problems in different countries, and non-standardization of marijuana complicate adequate assessment of the benefits and harms. Reports of increased vulnerability to schizophrenia in some individuals have emerged recently.

The efficacy of botulinum toxin is not yet well supported by evidence; the recommendation is for use in disabling specific tics (some vocal and motor in upper face and neck), applied only by experienced clinicians (Simpson et al. 2008). The effects persist for a few months and the treatment must be repeated.

Interventions for comorbid tic disorders

You cannot treat all comorbid disorders and their target symptoms simultaneously, or perhaps even sequentially. Time is needed to explore response and to take into account the timing of the school year, the likelihood of symptom response and side-effects. In general, one considers the severity and impact of symptoms along with the relative likelihood of response and of side-effects.

Given the high rates of ADHD, and the follow-up study showing that 41% had at least moderate OCD symptoms at one time or another, and that these tended to peak 2 years after the worst-ever tics and to persist (Bloch et al. 2006), comorbidity treatment is the key to success for most persons with Tourette syndrome. Suggestions for each disorder may be found in the relevant chapter or section. The following pertains to tics. If treatment is needed, then one has a choice of medication or a behavioral approach (or both). Comorbid disorders are more likely to need treatment than tics; often they need to be considered before behavioral treatments are undertaken (Woods et al. 2008a).

ATTENTION-DEFICIT/HYPERACTIVITY DISORDER

This is the most common additional diagnosis in those with Tourette syndrome. Sometimes a wrong diagnosis is made because the child with significant tics looks fidgety. Pharmacotherapy for ADHD in the presence of tics has been reviewed by Prince and Wilens (2009). The most important myth to understand is that stimulant drugs (methylphenidate, dextroamphetamine) should never be given to anyone with tics or even a family history of tics. This idea is still in books and some journal articles and may not be put to rest for some time to come. It derives from an important history of legal threats when the onset of tics was assumed to be due to stimulant treatment of ADHD. (At that time Tourette syndrome was thought to be rare, and an understanding of the typical age at onset of subsequent ADHD symptoms and tics was lacking.)

Research has shown that children from disadvantaged backgrounds (where psychosocial causative factors might seem predominant) may respond just as well as others to stimulant drugs. A good summary of treatment has been provided by Scahill et al. (2006a). For children under 6 years of age, however, approval for stimulant treatment in the USA is lacking, and the review by Charach et al. (2013) shows that parent behavior training is better and safer.

Treating ADHD in the presence of severe tics can be a problem. Although one may elect to persist with a stimulant even when tics are reported to become worse, one has no margin of safety when the tics are verging on the self-injurious. High doses of dextroamphetamine may increase tics in some patients (Bloch et al. 2009) and there are anecdotal reports of increase in RMBs such as skin-picking.

Case example
'Doug' was 6 years old. He was beginning to hit his trunk with his elbow and his face with his hand, but he needed treatment for his ADHD. It was thought that there was a risk that he might have a tic increase if he received a stimulant, because the tic was very close to being self-injurious.
   Comment: *In this case second-line treatments were the preferred option.*

Clonidine is a commonly used treatment for ADHD; it was originally hoped that it would simultaneously improve tics. However, this does not appear to be the case: Hedderick et al. (2009) found clonidine's efficacy in reducing tics to be of small magnitude, although the meta-analysis by Bloch et al. (2009) is more positive. Clonidine is also used off-label for insomnia (typically 0.1mg at bedtime), but the evidence base from randomized trials is still weak (MacLeod and Keen 2014).

Other available medications are atomoxetine, guanfacine (Elbe and Reddy 2014); the antidepressants imipramine, desipramine and nortriptyline; and perhaps bupropion and modafinil. Adverse events from ADHD medications in children have been comprehensively summarized by Cortese et al. (2013) on behalf of the European ADHD Guidelines Group. They accept that stimulants may worsen tics. If tics co-exist with significant ADHD, they recommend a 3-month observation of the course of the tics before deciding upon ADHD treatment; then if tics are intolerable while on stimulant medication, expert opinion leads to the recommendation of dose reduction, medication substitution (atomoxetine) and only then an antipsychotic (tiapride or sulpiride), or clonidine. Hamilton et al. (2009) have presented guidelines concerning cardiovascular safety of stimulant medication.

Although methylphenidate and its long-acting forms are more popular in North America than amphetamine-based medications, there can be an advantage in trying both, as there is a significant advantage of one over the other in a minority of patients.

Sleep problems are common in ADHD, and an excellent review of assessment and management has been provided by Cortese et al. (2013). Melatonin is frequently used for insomnia (3–5mg half an hour before bedtime) but correcting any problems with sleep hygiene first is advisable (Weiss et al. 2006).

Neurofeedback has some advocates and there is limited and mixed evidence for efficacy in ADHD (Lofthouse et al. 2012) but it has not yet been well studied in Tourette syndrome (Nagai et al. 2009). Zhuo and Li (2013) reported successful treatment of two children with Tourette syndrome who had been refractory to pharmacotherapy.

Obsessive–compulsive disorder
Medications used for OCD include the tricyclic clomipramine (the first effective drug) and the SSRIs fluvoxamine, sertraline, fluoxetine, citalopram, and to some extent paroxetine, duloxetine and venlafaxine. These medications are also used for anxiety, and for depression in adults (but the only medication with evidence in childhood depression is fluoxetine, and that has been questioned recently by Sparks and Duncan 2013). The onset may be slow, and several weeks may be necessary to ascertain the full benefit, with multiple increases often necessary to fully explore the dosage range.

Complications include *activation* especially in children with a family history of bipolarity, and the *discontinuation syndrome* (Hosenbocus and Chahal 2011). This latter reaction is not well known among child and adolescent psychiatrists, and it needs to be. The syndrome refers to a set of fairly typical reactions when the medication is withdrawn or reduced suddenly in relation to the particular drug's half-life, implying that fluoxetine is less likely to show such a reaction. (In children other factors may be involved than the half-life.) A study in adults indicated a rate of symptom appearance of 25% to 67% with paroxetine, less with fluvoxamine, 2% to 3% with sertraline and none for fluoxetine, while another study's rates were proportionately higher. The worst rates were for venlafaxine and paroxetine. Symptoms can be few or many, and include dizziness, nausea, lethargy, lightheadedness, headache, poor concentration and, in adults, paresthesias. Diagnostic criteria for adults (assumed for now to probably be applicable to children, too) include two or more symptoms occurring within 1–7 days after stopping or reducing the dosage; after at least 1 month's usage; causing significant distress or impairment; and not caused by a medical condition or mental disorder. Most reactions are mild. They usually resolve within a day or two to upwards of a week. These reactions are most likely to occur in the following situations.

- After the initial period when they have been successfully convinced that it will take a few weeks to work, but unpleasant side-effects continue beyond this time.
- When there are no regular physician follow-up visits.
- When using short half-life medications (especially paroxetine).
- Patients or parents feel empowered to make changes on their own.
- Family situations including clinic visits with an estranged or medication-averse parent, or disorganized families who fail to keep track of their pill supply or have insufficient funds.
- Teenagers who stop medication on weekends because of planned usage of alcohol or recreational drugs.

Misdiagnosis of the cause of discontinuation symptoms may lead to cycles of restarting medication and continuing longer than necessary, or undergoing unnecessary medical tests.

Behavior therapy
CBT is considered first-line and has a strong evidence base, but is expensive and not yet widely available. Efforts are under way to increase access by using a group format or a family-based online program (Storch et al. 2011).

Caution with attention-deficit/hyperactivity disorder treatment in patients with obsessive–compulsive disorder
Abramovitch et al. (2013) warn that ADHD-like symptoms in OCD may result from OCD symptomatology, and that stimulant medication for ADHD in children with OCD may exacerbate their OCD symptoms.

WEIGHT GAIN FROM ANTIDEPRESSANTS AND MOOD STABILIZERS
Relative risks of weight gain with the use of some antidepressants and mood stabilizers have been presented by Dent et al. (2012). These drugs are, in descending order of likelihood, paroxetine, amitriptyline, citalopram, nortriptyline, clomipramine, desipramine, duloxetine and escitalopram. Of those commonly used (including for anxiety) the following have minimal to no effect on weight: fluvoxamine, venlafaxine, sertraline, trazodone and fluoxetine. Bupropion may cause weight loss. Of the mood stabilizers, those causing weight gain are valproate and lithium; weight-neutral are carbamazepine, lamotrigine and topiramate.

TREATMENT FOR ANXIETY

There is a long history of medication trials for anxiety disorders, with SSRIs the most often tried. Results are less predictable in children than in adults. CBT is a first-line treatment approach, and online interventions such as computerized self-help are acquiring a positive evidence base (Christensen et al. 2014). Attention bias modification treatment is also showing good results (Eldar et al. 2012, MacLeod 2012).

TREATMENT FOR OPPOSITIONAL–DEFIANT DISORDER AND DISRUPTIVE BEHAVIOR

ODD is often treated with medication, either those used for ADHD, or risperidone. An excellent book with an individualized program of CBT for anger and aggression in children has been published by Sukhodolsky and Scahill (2012), including all the forms needed to conduct the therapy. Pharmacotherapy may be combined with CBT.

SITUATIONS OF HIGH COMORBIDITY

Some children and adults seem to have everything. They are likely to have been given diagnoses of ADHD, OCD, SLD, anxiety, mood instability, disruptive behavior, sleep problems, and often some ASD traits, as well as tics. There is typically a history of nothing working well for the combination of these disorders. The recognition of tics or the diagnosis of Tourette syndrome may create a new optimism that this will finally provide an answer. This is not reasonable to expect. One needs to explore all previous treatments, how thoroughly they were done, as well as changes in home, school or work that could have contributed to current instability.

Management of the 'everything' individual is likely to be long-term because of the often frustrating work that must be done to maintain or improve support (beyond just medication). Such supports are typically multifaceted and often cross over boundaries of government bureaucracies. In the magnificent book *Molecular Biology of the Cell* (Alberts et al. 2008), on page 67 is an all-too-believable photo of a neat, orderly room, followed by a time lapse showing the development of a mess. This is a vivid illustration of entropy. If entropy is the tendency toward increasing disorder, fragmentation and chaos without constant input of energy, then what is needed to maintain services for our patients is an anti-entropic force. Someone must take responsibility for keeping support in place through various staff and bureaucratic changes, lest progressive disorganization ensue; too often this falls to a parent rather than an experienced clinician who has 'clout' and the necessary contacts (Miller et al. 2009). The point is that otherwise sustained stability is not to be expected.

TREATMENT FOR COPROPHENOMENA

Are coprophenomena less or equally susceptible to treatment by medication or behavioral methods than other complex tics? There are no helpful studies yet to answer this question, so the working assumption is that the therapeutic response of coprophenomena will be about the same as that of other motor and vocal tics. Ben Djebara et al. (2008) treated an adult man with severe and persistent coprolalia who was oversensitive to neuroleptics with aripiprazole and obtained a continuing 75% reduction in his tic.

> **Case example**
>
> *'Earl' was 30 years old when he developed copropraxia. 'Giving the finger' was solved by his binding up that finger with the adjacent one (he did not mirror the gesture with his other hand). Later this same young man developed a transient urge to swerve while driving his car (but he never had an accident).*

TREATMENT FOR 'RAGE'

Outbursts of severe anger with or without aggression have been discussed in Chapter 10 (under ADHD). These episodes, often the reason for visits to emergency departments and hospitalization, are not typical of tic disorders without comorbidity. They are much more likely to occur when the patient has ADHD and/or OCD. They are a frequent justification for medication, but there is no drug truly specific for them. Risperidone is one of the popular drugs at present, paroxetine in the recent past, and assumptions of concurrent mood disorder may seem to justify valproic acid, lithium or other 'mood stabilizers'. This subject has been explored most thoroughly by Budman (2006) and Budman et al. (2003, 2008). In the DSM-5 these rages can be a component of the official diagnostic categories 'disruptive mood dysregulation disorder' (with onset before age 10) or 'intermittent explosive disorder'.

Alternative approaches

It is well known that many parents and patients utilize so-called alternative or 'complementary' methods, of which there are always many (including homeopathic and Chinese medicines). The internet is the modern home for many of these. We would like to believe that if a method that is outside the mainstream of medicine and psychology proves to have an evidence base for efficacy, it would become part of our armamentarium. However, in most instances such 'treatments' or 'methods' that may make sense to lay persons are suspect because of the following characteristics: (1) broad claims for improvement of diseases or symptoms that have no obvious relationship to each other, and if true, would merit a Nobel Prize; (2) dependence upon testimonials without replicated studies to support claims, although weak studies may be cited; (3) vague statements to encourage purchase, such as 'acclaimed by doctors' without saying what kind of physicians or with what qualifications; (4) use of the description 'all-natural' to imply complete safety; and (5) short times needed for results. Frequently clinicians are not told about these therapies (and may not ask), and patients are taking medications from clinicians at the same time, so that any results are impossible to sort out. It is rare that after initial hopes are disappointed, the patient or parents will admit to having been taken in; rather, the usual response is that it did help — but not enough. It is up to the clinician to decide whether embarking upon alternative therapies is in conflict with his or her approach, or one of the approaches should be delayed until the results of the other are clear. A rigid attitude is seldom helpful. The level of education seems to be an unimportant factor, since physicians, nurses, psychologists and doctorate degree holders of various sorts are all vulnerable to claims without an evidence base (Offit 2012).

One recent controlled study suggested that the popular Omega-3 fatty acid supplements can reduce tic-related impairment even though tic scores were themselves unchanged (Gabbay et al. 2012). Self-hypnosis has been described and the literature reviewed by Lazarus and Klein (2010). These approaches are not yet well accepted.

Additional considerations with medicolegal implications

The variable course of chronic tic disorders merits special consideration by physicians. The relative importance of the following points may differ by country and region, and by malpractice insurers.

- Families with limited English will need more time and perhaps the attendance of an interpreter, or by more language-competent family members or friends, not only for good understanding but more specifically to meet requirements for informed consent.
- Checking to ensure that points and directions for treatment are understood, with printed material if possible. (It would be useful if service organizations in different countries were to contribute to a list of materials that they have available in different languages (such as a Chinese brochure in Australia).
- When medication requires changing dosages or drugs, asking that medication bottles be brought to the session.
- Clarity about common side-effects and adverse effects of prescribed drugs (e.g. pimozide and some macrolide antibiotics).
- Establishment of contact procedures; if electronic, policies and expectations require clarity.
- Awareness that the names of generic and brand names of drugs are often used inconsistently, are confusing, and may sound similar (e.g. fluvoxamine and fluoxetine).
- Dosage numbers are not indications of 'strength' or 'power' as may be assumed by some patients or parents; this requires explanation.

Experience with the use of e-mail for communication with parents with limited English has shown that older children in a family are more likely than their parents to be competent with electronic devices, but depending upon them for communication requires good agreement by all concerned, and even then may fail.

National differences in medication availability

Table 15.1 shows drugs commonly used for tics by geographic region or country, as indicated in the comprehensive Martindale compendium (Royal Pharmaceutical Society 2014). To some extent this accounts for differences in recommendations made by clinicians and researchers. Note that this list does not discriminate between approved drug indications and off-label usage, nor indicate differences in recommended age ranges. (Many other drugs with a weaker evidence base have been tried.)

TABLE 15.1

Availability of medications for tics by geographic region or country[a]

Drug	Action/P450	Peak (hours)	½-life (hours)	Country/region[b]
Clonidine	A$_{2A}$-adrenergic agonist	3–5	6–24	Aus/NZ, Can, Eu, HK, In, Ind, Isr, Jp, Mal, Phil, Rs, SA, SAm, Sg, Thai, UK, US
Guanfacine	A$_{2A}$-adrenergic agonist, CYP3A4	1–4	10–30	Eu, Jp, Rs,UK, Ukr, US
Extended range guanfacine	As above	5	18	Can, US
Haloperidol	CYP2D6, 3A4	Unavail.	12–38	Aus/NZ, Can, Eu, HK, In, Ind, Isr, Mal, Mex, Phil, Rs, SA, SAm, Sg, Thai, Tu, UK, US
Pimozide	CYP2D6, 3A4	4–12	55+	Aus/NZ, Can, Eu, HK, In, Ind, Isr, Jp, SA, Sg, Thai, Tu, UK, US
Risperidone	CYP2D6	1–2	20	Aus/NZ, Can, Eu, HK, In, Ind, Isr, Jp, Mal, Mex, Phil, Rs, SA, Sg, Thai, Tu, UK, Ukr, US
Ziprasidone[c]	CYP3A4, D$_2$, 5HT$_2$	6–8	7	Aus/NZ, Can, Eu (not UK), HK, In, Isr, Mal, Mex, Phil, Rs, SA, Sg, Thai, Tu, US
Fluphenazine	CYP2D6, similar to CPZ	Unavail.	14.7	Aus/NZ, Can, Eu, HK, In, Ind, Isr, Jp, Mal, Mex, Phil, Rs, SA, SAm, Sg, Thai, Tu, UK, Ukr, US
Olanzapine	CYP1A2	5–8	30–38	Aus/NZ, Can, Eu, HK, In, Ind, Isr, Jp, Mal, Mex, Phil, Rs, SA, SAm, Thai, Tu, UK, Ukr, US
Aripiprazole	CYP3A4, 2D6	3–5	75–95	Aus/NZ, Can, Eu, HK, In, Ind, Isr, Jp, Mal, Mex, Phil, Rs, SA, Sg, Thai, Tu, UK, US
Quetiapine	CYP3A4, D$_1$, D$_2$, 5-HT$_2$	1.5	6–7	Aus/NZ, Can, Eu, HK, In, Ind, Isr, Jp, Mal, Mex, Phil, Rs, SA, SAm, Sg, Thai, Tu, UK, Ukr
Clonazepam	Similar to diazepam	1–4	20–40	Aus/NZ, Can, Eu, HK, In, Ind, Isr, Mal, Mex, SA, Sg, Thai, Tu, UK, Ukr, US
Sulpiride	D$_2$, D$_3$, D$_4$ antagonism	3–6	8–9	Eu, HK, In, Ind, Isr, Jp, Mal, Mex, Phil, Rs, SAm, Sg, Tu, UK, Ukr
Tiapride	Like sulpiride	1–2	3–4	Eu (not UK or Ireland), HK, Isr, Jp, Rs, Sg
Amisulpride	D$_2$, D$_3$	1–3	12	Aus/NZ, Eu, HK, In, Ind, Isr, Mal, Mex, Phil, Rs, SA, Sg, Tu, UK, Ukr
Tetrabenazine	Central dopamine depleter; CYP2D6	Erratic	Erratic	Aus/NZ, Can, Eu, In, Isr, UK, US

[a]Listing here should not be taken to mean that the drug has an approved indication for treatment of a tic disorder at any particular age: many usages are 'off-label'. Times to peak blood level and half-life are average figures taken from *Martindale: The Complete Drug Reference* (Royal Pharmaceutical Society 2014). Country indicators are current from early 2014 and are subject to change.

[b]Country/region codes: Aus/NZ, Australia/New Zealand; Can, Canada; Eu, Europe; HK, Hong Kong; In, India; Ind, Indonesia; Isr, Israel; Jp, Japan; Mal, Malaysia; Mex, Mexico; Phil, Philippines: Rs, Russia; SA, South Africa; SAm, South America; Sg, Singapore; Thai, Thailand; Tu, Turkey; UK, United Kingdom; Ukr, Ukraine; US, USA.

[c]The US Food and Drug Administration issued a safety announcement on December 11, 2014 for ziprasidone, warning of a rare but potentially fatal drug reaction (druginfo@fda.hhs.gov).

REFERENCES

Abramovitch A, Dar R, Mittelman A, Schweiger A (2013) Don't judge a book by its cover: ADHD-like symptoms in obsessive compulsive disorder. *J Obsess-Compuls Relat Disord* 2: 53–61. doi: 10.1016/j.jocrd. 2012.09.001.

Ajmal A, Joffe H. Nachtigall LB (2014) Psychotropic-induced hyperprolactinemia: a clinical review. *Psychosomatics* 55: 29–36.

Alberts B, Johnson A, Lewis J, et al. (2008) *Molecular Biology of the Cell, 5th edn.* New York: Garland Science/Taylor & Francis.

Ananth J, Parameswaran S, Gunatilake S, et al. (2004) Neuroleptic malignant syndrome and atypical antipsychotic drugs. *J Clin Psychiatry* 65: 464–70.

Ben Djebara M, Worbe Y, Schüpbach M, Hartmann A (2008) Aripiprazole: a treatment for severe coprolalia in 'refractory' Gilles de la Tourette syndrome. *Mov Disord* 23: 438-40. doi: 10.1002/mds.21859.

Bennett SM, Keller AE, Walkup JT (2013) The future of tic disorder treatment. *Ann NY Acad Sci* 1304: 32–9. doi: 10.1111/nyas.12296.

Bloch MH, Peterson BS, Scahill L, et al. (2006) Adulthood outcome of tic and obsessive–compulsive symptom severity in children with Tourette syndrome. *Arch Pediatr Adolesc Med* 160: 65–9. doi: 10.1001/archpedi.160.1.65.

Blount TH, Lockhart A-LT, Garcia RV, et al. (2014) Intensive outpatient comprehensive behavioral intervention for tics: a case series. *World J Clin Cases* 2: 569–77. doi 10.12998/wjcc.v2.i10.569.

Budman C (2006) Treatment of aggression in Tourette syndrome. *Adv Neurol* 99: 222–6.

Budman CL, Rockmore L, Stokes J, Sossin M (2003) Clinical phenomenology of episodic rage in children with Tourette syndrome. *J Psychosom Res* 55: 59–65. doi: 10.1016/S0022-3999(02)00584-6.

Budman C, Coffey BJ, Shechter R, et al. (2008) Aripiprazole in children and adolescents with Tourette disorder with and without explosive outbursts. *J Child Adolesc Psychopharmacol* 18: 509–15. doi: 10.1089/cap.2007.061.

Calarge CA, Nicol G, Schlechte JA, Burns TL (2014) Cardiometabolic outcomes in children and adolescents following discontinuation of long-term risperidone treatment. *J Child Adolesc Psychopharmacol* 24: 120–9. doi: 10.1089/cap.2013.0126.

Capriotti MR, Brandt BC, Ricketts EJ, et al. (2012) Comparing the effects of differential rerinforcement of other behavior and response-cost contingencies on tics in youth with Tourette syndrome. *J Appl Behav Anal* 45: 251–3. doi: 10.1901/jaba.2012.45-251.

Capriotti MR, Espil FM, Conelea CA, Woods DW (2013) Environmental factors as potential determinants of premonitory urge severity in youth with Tourette syndrome. *J Obsess-Compuls Relat Disord* 2: 37–42. doi: 10.1016/j.jocrd.2012.10.004.

Capriotti MR, Brandt BC, Turkel JE, et al. (2014a) Negative reinforcement and premonitory urges in youth with Tourette syndrome: an experimental evaluation. *Behav Modif* 38: 276–96. doi: 10.1177/0145445514531015.

Capriotti MR, Himle MB, Woods DW (2014b) Behavioral treatments for Tourette syndrome. *J Obsess-Compuls Relat Disord*, 3: 415–20. doi: 10.1016/j.jocrd.2014.03.007.

Cath DC, Hedderly T, Ludolph AG, et al. (2011) European clinical guidelines for Tourette syndrome and other tic disorders. Part I: Assessment. *Eur Child Adolesc Psychiatry* 20: 155–71. doi: 10.1007/s00787-011-0164-6.

Cavanna AE, Robertson MM, Critchley HD (2008) Catatonic signs in Gilles de la Tourette syndrome. *Cogn Behav Neurol* 21: 34–7. doi: 10.1097/WNN.0b013e318165a9cf.

Charach A, Carson P, Fox S, et al. (2013) Interventions for preschool children at high risk for ADHD: a comparative effectiveness review. *Pediatrics* 131: e1584-e1604. doi: 10.1542/peds.2012-0974.

Chen JJ, Ondo WG, Dashtipour K, Swope DM (2012) Tetrabenazine for the treatment of hyperkinetic movement disorders: a review of the literature. *Clin Ther* 34: 1487–504. doi: 10.1016/j.clinthera.2012.06.010.

Christensen H, Batterham P, Calear A (2014) Online interventions for anxiety disorders. *Curr Opin Psychiatry* 27: 7–13. doi: 10.1097/YCO.0000000000000019.

Conelea CA, Woods DW (2008) The influence of contextual factors on tic expression in Tourette's syndrome: a review. *J Psychosom Res* 65: 487–96. doi: 10.1016/j.jpsychores.2008.04.010.

Correll CU, Manu P, Olshanskiy V, et al. (2009) Cardiometabolic risk of second-generation antipsychotic medications during first-time use in children and adolescents. *JAMA* 302: 1765–73. doi: 10.1001/jama.2009.1549.

Cortese S, Holtmann M, Banaschewski T, et al. (2013) Current best practice in the management of adverse events during treatment with ADHD medications in children and adolescents. *J Child Psychol Psychiatry* 54: 227–46. doi: 10.1111/jcpp.12036.

Crume TL, Harrod CS (2013) Childhood obesity: is there effective treatment? *JAMA Pediatr* 167: 697–9 (editorial). doi: 10.1001/jamapediatrics.2013.102.

Cui Y, Zheng Y, Yang Y, et al. (2010) Effectiveness and tolerability of aripiprazole in children and adolescents with Tourette's disorder: a pilot study in China. *J Child Adolesc Psychopharmacol* 20: 291–8. doi: 10.1089/cap.2009.0125.

Dent R, Blackmore A, Peterson J, et al. (2012) Changes in body weight and psychotropic drugs: a systematic synthesis of the literature. *PLoS ONE* 7: e36889. doi: 10.1371/journal.pone.0036889.

Desmarais JE, Beauclair L, Margolese HC (2011) Switching from brand-name to generic psychotropic medications: a literature review. *CNS Neurosci Ther* 17: 750–60. doi: 10.1111/j.1755-5949.2010.00210.x.

Dhossche DM, Reti IM, Shettar SM, Wachtel LE (2010) Tics as signs of catatonia: electroconvulsive therapy response in 2 men. *J ECT* 26: 266–9. doi: 10.1097/YCT.0b013e3181cb5f60.

Eggers C, Rothenberger A, Berghaus U (1988) Clinical and neurobiological findings in children suffering from tic disease following treatment with tiapride. *Eur Arch Psychiatr Neurol Sci* 237: 223–29.

Elbe D, Reddy D (2014) Focus on guanfacine extended-release: a review of its use in child and adolescent psychiatry. *Can J Child Adolesc Psychiatry* 23: 48–60.

Eldar S, Apter A, Lotan D, et al. (2012) Attention bias modification treatment for pediatric anxiety disorders: a randomized controlled trial. *Am J Psychiatry* 169: 213–20. doi: 10.1176/appi.ajp.2011.11060886.

Fink M (2013) Rediscovering catatonia: the biography of a treatable syndrome. *Acta Psychiatr Scand* 127 (Suppl 441): 1–47.

Frank AW (2002) *At Will of the Body: Reflections on Illness.* Boston: Houghton Mifflin.

Gabbay V, Babb JS, Klein RG, et al. (2012) A double-blind, placebo-controlled trial of omega-3 fatty acids in Tourette's disorder. *Pediatrics* 129: e1493–e1500. doi: 10.1542/peds.2022-3384.

Gillman PK (2010) Neuroleptic malignant syndrome: mechanisms, interactions, and causality. *Mov Disord* 25: 1780–90. doi: 10.1002/mds.23220.

Groner JA, Joshi M, Bauer JA (2006) Pediatric precursors of adult cardiovascular disease: noninvasive assessment of early vascular changes in children and adolescents. *Pediatrics* 118: 1683–91. doi: 10.1542/peds.2005-2992.

Hamilton R, Gray C, Bélanger SA, et al. (2009) Cardiac risk assessment before the use of stimulant medications in children and youth: a joint position statement by the Canadian Paediatric Society, the Canadian Cardiovascular Society and the Canadian Academy of Child and Adolescent Psychiatry. *J Can Acad Child Adolesc Psychiatry* 18: 349–55.

Hanna GL, Fluent TE, Fischer DJ (1999) Separation anxiety in children and adolescents treated with risperidone. *J Child Adolesc Psychopharmacol* 9: 277–83. doi: 10.1089/cap.1999.9.277.

Hedderick EF, Morris CM, Singer HS (2009) Double-blind, crossover study of clonidine and levetiracetam in Tourette syndrome. *Pediatr Neurol* 40: 420–5. doi: 10.1016/j.pediatrneurol.2008.12.014.

Himle MB, Woods DW, Piacentini JC, Walkup JT (2006) Brief review of habit reversal training for Tourette syndrome. *J Child Neurology* 21: 719–25. doi: 10.1177/08830738060210080101.

Himle MB, Woods DW, Conelea CA, et al. (2007) Investigating the effects of tic suppression on premonitory urge ratings in children and adolescents with Tourette's syndrome. *Behav Res Ther* 45: 2964–76. doi: 10.1016/j.brat.2007.08.007.

Ho J, Panagiotopolous C, McCrindle B, et al. (2011) Management recommendations for metabolic complications associated with second-generation antipsychotic use in children and youth. *J Can Acad Child Adolesc Psychiatry* 20: 234–41.

Hosenbocus S, Chahal R (2011) SSRIs and SNRIs: a review of the discontinuation syndrome in children and adolescents. *J Can Acad Child Adolesc Psychiatry* 20: 60–7.

Houghton DC, Capriotti MR, Conelea CA, Woods DW (2014) Sensory phenomena in Tourette syndrome: their role in symptom formation and treatment. *Curr Dev Disord Rep* 1: 245–51. doi: 10.1007/s40474-014-0026-2.

Jacoby DL, DePasquale EC, McKenna WJ (2013) Hypertrophic cardiomyopathy: diagnosis, risk stratification and treatment. *CMAJ* 185: 127–34. doi: 10.1503/cmaj.120138.

Jain S, Greene PE, Frucht SJ (2006) Tetrabenazine therapy of pediatric hyperkinetic movement disorders. *Mov Disord* 21: 1966–72. doi: 10.1002/mds.21063.

Kenney C, Hunter C, Mejia NI, Jankovic J (2007) Tetrabenazine in the treatment of Tourette syndrome. *J Ped Neurol* 5: 9–13.

Kim W, Pouratian N (2014) Deep brain stimulation for Tourette syndrome. *Neurosurg Clin N Am* 25: 117–35. doi: 10.1016/j.nec.2013.08.009.

Kompoliti K, Stebbins GT, Goetz CG, Fan W (2010) Association between antipsychotics and body mass index when treating patients with tics. *J Child Adolesc Psychopharmacol* 20: 277–81. doi: 10.1089/cap. 2009.0091.

Lazarus JE, Klein SK (2010) Nonpharmacological treatment of tics in Tourette syndrome adding videotape training to self-hypnosis. *J Dev Behav Pediatr* 31: 498–504.

Lofthouse N, Arnold LE, Hersch S, et al. (2012) A review of neurofeedback treatment for pediatric ADHD. *J Atten Disord* 16: 351–72. doi: 10.1177/1087054711427530.

Lombroso PJ, Scahill L (2008) Tourette syndrome and obsessive–compulsive disorder. *Brain Dev* 30: 231–7. doi: 10.1016/j.braindev.2007.09.001.

Maayan L, Correll CU (2011) Weight gain and metabolic risks associated with antipsychotic medications in children and adolescents. *J Child Adolesc Psychopharmacol* 21: 517–35. doi: 10.1089/cap.2011.0015.

MacLeod C (2012) Cognitive bias modification procedures in the management of mental disorders. *Curr Opin Psychiatry* 25: 114–20. doi: 10.1097/YCO.0b013e32834fda4a.

MacLeod RL, Keen DV (2014) Innovations in practice: 'off-label' clonidine: UK paediatric and child and adolescent psychiatry prescribing practice for sleep problems. *Child Adolesc Ment Health* 19: 147–50. doi: 10.1111/camh.12032.

Masi G, Gagliano A, Siracusano R, et al. (2012) Aripirazole in children with Tourette's disorder and co-morbid attention-deficit hyperactivity disorder: a 12-week, open-label, preliminary study. *J Child Adolesc Psychopharmacol* 22: 120–5. doi: 10.1089/cap.2011.0081.

Meidinger AL, Miltenberger RG, Himle M, et al. (2005) An investigation of tic suppression and the rebound effect in Tourette's disorder. *Behav Modif* 29: 716–45. doi: 10.1177/0145445505279262.

Miller AR, Condin CJ, McKellin WH, et al. (2009) Continuity of care for children with complex chronic health conditions: parents' perspectives. *BMC Health Serv Res* 9: 242. doi: 10.1186/1472-6963-9-242.

Morrato EH, Nicol GE, Maahs D, et al. (2010) Metabolic screening in children receiving antipsychotic drug treatment. *Arch Pediatr Adolesc Med* 164: 344–51. doi: 10.1001/archpediatrics.2010.48.

Müller-Vahl KR (2003) Cannabinoids reduce symptoms of Tourette's syndrome. *Expert Opin Pharmacother* 4: 1717–25.

Müller-Vahl KR, Schneider U, Prevedel H, et al. (2003) Δ9-tetrahydrocannabinol (THC) is effective in the treatment of tics in Tourette syndrome: a 6-week randomized trial. *J Clin Psychiatry* 64: 459–65.

Müller-Vahl KR, Cath DC, Cavanna AE, et al. (2011) European clinical guidelines for Tourette syndrome and other tic disorders. Part IV: Deep brain stimulation. *Eur Child Adolesc Psychiatry* 20: 209–17. doi: 10.1007/s.00787-011-0166-4.

Murphy TK, Lewin AB, Storch EA, Stock S (2013) Practice parameter for the assessment and treatment of children and adolescents with tic disorders. American Academy of Child and Adolescent Psychiatry Committee on Quality Issues. *J Am Acad Child Adolesc Psychiatry* 52: 1341–59. doi: 10.1016/j.jaac. 2013.09.015.

Nagai Y, Cavanna A, Critchley HD (2009) Influence of sympathetic autonomic arousal on tics: implications for a therapeutic behavioral intervention for Tourette syndrome. *J Psychosom Res* 67: 599–605.

Neuhut R, Lindenmayer J-P, Silva R (2009) Neuroleptic malignant syndrome in children and adolescents on atypical antipsychotic medication: a review. *J Child Adolesc Psychopharmacol* 19: 415–22. doi: 10.1089/cap.2008.0130.

Nussey C, Pistrang N, Murphy T (2013) How does psychoeducation help? A review of the effects of providing information about Tourette syndrome and attention-deficit/hyperactivity disorder. *Child Health Care Dev* 39: 617–27. doi: 10.1111/cch.12039.

O'Connor KP (2005) *Cognitive Behavioral Management of Tic Disorders*. New York: John Wiley.

Offit PA (2012) Studying complementary and alternative therapies. *JAMA* 307: 1803–4. doi: 10.1001.jama. 2012.518.

Olufs EL, Himle MB, Bradley AR (2013) The effect of generic versus personally delivered education and self-disclosure on the social acceptability of adults with Tourette syndrome. *J Dev Phys Disabil* 25: 395–403. doi: 10.1007/s10882-012-9317-x.

Panagiotopoulos C, Ronsley R, Davidson J (2009) Increased prevalence of obesity and glucose intolerance in youth treated with second-generation antipsychotic medications. *Can J Psychiatry* 54: 743–9.

Panagiotopoulos C, Ronsley R, Elbe D, et al. (2010) First do no harm: promoting an evidence-based approach to atypical antipsychotic use in children and adolescents. *J Can Acad Child Adolesc Psychiatry* 19: 124–37.

Patten SB, Waheed W, Bresse L (2012) A review of pharmacoepidemiologic studies of antipsychotic use in children and adolescents. *Can J Psychiatry* 57: 717–21.

Piacentini J, Woods DW, Scahill L, et al. (2010) Behavior therapy for children with Tourette disorder: a randomized controlled trial. *JAMA* 303: 1929–37. doi: 10.1001/jama.2010.607.

Prince JB, Wilens TE (2009) Pharmacotherapy of ADHD and comorbidities. In: Brown, TE, ed. *ADHD Comorbidities: Handbook for ADHD Complications in Children and Adults.* Arlington, VA: American Psychiatric Publishing, pp. 339–84.

Pringsheim T, Gorman G (2012) Second-generation antipsychotics for the treatment of disruptive behaviour disorders in children: a systematic review. *Can J Psychiatry* 57: 722–7.

Pringsheim T, Panagiotopoulos C, Davidson J, Ho J (2011) Evidence-based recommendations for monitoring safety of second-generation antipsychotics in children and youth. *J Can Acad Child Adolesc Psychiatry* 20: 218–33.

Pringsheim T, Doja A, Gorman D, et al. (2012) Canadian guidelines for the evidence-based treatment of tic disorders. Pharmacotherapy. *Can J Psychiatry* 57: 133–43.

Reese HE, Scahill L, Peterson AL, et al. (2013) The premonitory urge to tic: measurement, characteristics, and correlates in older adolescents and adults. *Behav Ther* 45: 177–86. doi: 10.1016/j.beth.2013.09.002.

Rizzo R, Eddy CM, Calì P, et al. (2012) Metabolic effects of aripiprazole and pimozide in children with Tourette syndrome. *Pediatr Neurol* 47: 419–22. doi: 10.1016/j.pediatrneurol.2012.08.015.

Robertson MM, Schnieden V, Lees AJ (1990) Management of Gilles de la Tourette syndrome using sulpiride. *Clin Neuropharmacol* 13: 229–35.

Roessner V, Plessen KJ, Rothenberger A, et al. (2011a) European clinical guidelines for Tourette syndrome and other tic disorders. Part II: Pharmacological treatment. *Eur Child Adolesc Psychiatry* 20: 173–96. doi: 10.1007/s00787-011-0163-7.

Roessner V, Rothenberger A, Rickards H, Hoekstra PJ (2011b) European clinical guidelines for Tourette syndrome and other tic disorders. *Eur Child Adolesc Psychiatry* 20: 153–4 (editorial). doi: 10.1007/s00787-011-0165-5.

Ronsley R, Rayter M, Smith D, et al. (2012) Metabolic Monitoring Training Program implementation in the community setting was associated with improved monitoring in second-generation antipsychotic-treated children. *Can J Psychiatry* 57: 292–9.

Royal Pharmaceutical Society (2014) *Martindale: the Complete Drug Reference.* London: The Pharmaceutical Press.

Ryan ND, Leventhal BL (2012) What to do when it is not so clear what to do: or, what to do until the data arrive. *J Child Adolesc Psychopharmacol* 22: 385–7. doi: 10.1089/cap.2012.2262.

Sandor P, Carroll A (2012) Canadian guidelines for the evidence-based treatment of tic disorders. *Can J Psychiatry* 57: 131–2 (editorial).

Scahill L, Erenberg G, Berlin CM, et al. (2006a) Contemporary assessment and pharmacotherapy of Tourette syndrome. *NeuroRx* 3: 192–206.

Scahill L, Sukhodolsky DG, Bearss K, et al. (2006b) Randomized trial of parent management training in children with tic disorders and disruptive behavior. *J Child Neurol* 21: 650–6. doi: 10.1177/08830738060210080201.

Scahill L, Woods DW, Himle MB, et al. (2013) Current controversies on the role of behavior therapy in Tourette syndrome. *Mov Disord* 28: 1179–83. doi: 10.1002/mds.25488.

Scott S, Dadds MR (2009) When parent training doesn't work: theory-driven clinical strategies. *J Child Psychol Psychiatry* 50: 1441–50. doi: 10.1111/j.1469-7610.2009.02161.x.

Sellers EAC, Panagiotopoulos C, Lawson ML (2008) Type 2 diabetes in children and adolescents. Canadian Diabetes Association 2008 clinical practice guidelines for the prevention and management of diabetes in Canada. *Can J Diabetes* 32 (Suppl 1): S162–7.

Simpson DM, Blitzer A, Brashear A, et al. (2008) Assessment: Botulinum neurotoxin for the treatment of movement disorders (an evidence-based review): Report of the Therapeutics and Technology Assessment Subcommittee of the American Academy of Neurology. *Neurology* 70: 1699–706.

Sparks JA, Duncan BL (2013) Outside the black box: re-assessing pediatric antidepressant prescription. *J Can Acad Child Adolesc Psychiatry* 22: 240–6.

Steeves T, McKinlay BD, Gorman D, et al. (2012) Canadian guidelines for the evidence-based treatment of tic disorders: behavioural therapy, deep brain stimulation, and transcranial magnetic stimulation. *Can J Psychiatry* 57: 144–51.

Storch EA, Caporino NE, Morgan JR, et al. (2011) Preliminary investigation of web-camera delivered cognitive–behavioral therapy for youth with obsessive–compulsive disorder. *Psychiatry Res* 189: 407–12. doi: 10.1016/j.psychres.2011.05.047.

Strawn JR, Keck PE, Caroff SN (2007) Neuroleptic malignant syndrome. *Am J Psychiatry* 164: 870–6.

Sukhodolsky DG, Scahill L (2012) *Cognitive–Behavioral Therapy for Anger and Aggression in Children.* New York: Guilford Press.

Tourette Syndrome Study Group (1999) Short-term versus longer term pimozide therapy in Tourette's syndrome: a preliminary study. *Neurology* 52: 874–7.

Varda NM, Gregoric A (2009) Metabolic syndrome in the pediatric population: a short overview. *Pediatr Rep* 1: e1. doi: 10.4081/pr.2009.e1.

Varley CK, McClellan J (2009) Implications of marked weight gain associated with atypical antipsychotic medications in children and adolescents. *JAMA* 302: 1811–2. doi: 10.1001/jama.2009.1558.

Verdellen CWJ, Hoogduin CAL, Keijsers GPJ (2007) Tic suppression in the treatment of Tourette's syndrome with exposure therapy: the rebound phenomenon reconsidered. *Mov Disord* 22: 1601–6. doi: 10.1002/mds.21577.

Verdellen C, van de Griendt J, Hartmann A, Murphy T (2011) European clinical guidelines for Tourette syndrome and other tic disorders. Part III: Behavioural and psychosocial interventions. ESSTS Guidelines Group. *Eur Child Adolesc Psychiatry* 20: 197–207. doi: 10.1007/s00787-011-0167-3.

Wain O, Jankovic J (2013) An update on tardive dyskinesia: from phenomenology to treatment. *Tremor Other Hyperkinet Mov (NY)* 3: tre-03-161-4138-1. Published online Jul 12, 2013 (http://tremorjournal.org/article/view/161).

Weiss M, Allan B, Greenaway M (2012) Treatment of catatonia with electroconvulsive therapy in adolescents. *J Child Adolesc Psychopharmacol* 22: 96–100. doi: 10.1089.cap.2010.0052.

Weiss MD, Wasdell MB, Bomben M, et al. (2006) Sleep hygiene and melatonin treatment for children and adolescents with ADHD and initial insomnia. *J Am Acad Child Adolesc Psychiatry* 45: 512–9. doi: 10.1097/01.chi.0000205706.78818.ef.

Wenzel C, Kleimann A, Bokemeyer S, Müller-Vahl KR (2012) Aripiprazole for the treatment of Tourette syndrome: a case series of 100 patients. *J Clin Psychopharmacol* 32: 548–50. doi: 10.1097/JCP.0b013e31825ac2cb.

Wilhelm S, Peterson AL, Piacentini J, et al. (2012) Randomized trial of behavior therapy for adults with Tourette syndrome. *Arch Gen Psychiatry* 69: 795–803.

Wittmeier BA, Wicklow BA, Sellers EAC, et al. (2012) Success with lifestyle monotherapy in youth with new-onset type 2 diabetes. *Pediatr Child Health* 17: 129–32.

Woods DW, Conelea CA, Walther MR (2007) Barriers to dissemination: exploring the criticisms of behavior therapy for tics. *Clin Psychol Sci Prac* 14: 279–82.

Woods DW, Himle MB, Miltenberger RG, et al. (2008a) Durability, negative impact, and neuropsychological predictors of tic suppression in children with chronic tic disorder. *J Abnorm Child Psychol* 36: 237–45. doi: 10.1007/s10802-007-9173-9.

Woods DW, Piacentini JC, Chang SW, et al. (2008b) *Managing Tourette Syndrome: a Behavioral Intervention – Parent Workbook.* New York: Oxford University Press.

Woods DW, Walther MR, Bauer CC, et al. (2009) The development of stimulus control over tics: a potential explanation for contextually-based variability in the symptoms of Tourette syndrome. *Behav Res Ther* 47: 41–7. doi: 10.1016/j.brat.2008.10.013.

Woods DW, Conelea CA, Himle MB (2010) Behavior therapy for Tourette's disorder: utilization in a community sample and an emerging area of practice for psychologists. *Prof Psychol Res Prac* 4: 518–25. doi: 10.1037/A0021709.

Woods DW, Piacentini JC, Scahill LD, et al. (2011) Behavior therapy for tics in children: acute and long term effects on secondary psychiatric and psychosocial functioning. *J Child Neurol* 26: 858–65. doi: 10.1177/0883073810397046.

Zhuo C, Li L (2013) The application and efficacy of combined neurofeedback therapy and imagery training in adolescents with Tourette syndrome. *J Child Neurol* 29: 965–8. doi: 10.1177/0883073813479999.

16
WORKING WITH SCHOOLS (ADVOCACY)

Children spend much of their lives in school and doing school-related homework, and their school experiences can have a lasting impact. Tics can have important modifying effects. Teachers and other school staff are likely to have had no formal education about tics or only minimal and possibly stereotyping experiences with one or a few such children. Possibilities for misunderstanding tic-related behavior are endless, especially the belief that tics are deliberate and therefore subject to discipline, or completely and always involuntary. Medical information provided to the school may languish in files without having the desired effect and require repetition. The complexity of comorbidity may pose a serious obstacle to providing appropriate support. The development of a fear of going to school or physical symptoms only on school days merits immediate attention, as does a widening communication gap between parent and school.

A satisfactory school year is a blessing, but it may be easily disrupted, and Tourette syndrome and associated problems can do this. Unrecognized SLD or an insufficiently supportive school can create difficulties immediately. Personal sensitivities, anxiety, peer-group problems or pressures, OCD symptoms, mismatch with a teacher and new tics may trigger a crisis, even ruin a school year. For example, Brad Cohen recounts:

> One day we had a substitute teacher in one of my high school classes, and it was [on] a day that my tics were especially bad. I assumed that the sub had been told about my tics, but apparently that was not the case. It didn't help that this particular substitute had no patience with kids. She kept asking me to be quiet, even though I had told her I had Tourette's and couldn't control my outbursts. (Cohen and Wysocky 2008, p. 76)

There are many reasons why schools may misunderstand Tourette syndrome, and especially TS+, including the following.

- If they are told the diagnosis but the child has a mild case, especially without comorbidity, they may not believe it, or they may have incorrect expectations that coprolalia or aggressive behaviour will develop. Whether they should be told, when no medication is to be administered in school, is debatable.

- "It's not like on TV" (or "… not like that other child I knew"). It often isn't.
- Automatic (and maybe some voluntary) suppression is occurring in school.
- Misinterpretation of tics as something else, especially deliberate misbehavior. Coprophenomena can do this. New tics of certain kinds are likely to be interpreted this way: touching, making noises, echoing, 'talking back'. More tics in one class and not another, or more at one time of day can convince someone that the tics are just manipulative or attention-seeking.
- An experienced teacher, especially one who has known one child with the diagnosis (but not many), may be too firmly convinced about the meanings of behavior.
- Comorbidities with tics: rituals, compulsions, obsessional slowness, ADHD 'fidgeting' and disorganization combined with tics, anxieties and many other problems can cause difficulties.
- SLDs may interact with compulsions or ADHD.
- DCD and graphomotor disorders can be exacerbated by tics.
- One should never forget that a child could be faking or exaggerating symptoms.

There is a paradox: we may not want to tell teachers that a child has Tourette syndrome, rather say 'tics', yet if we don't, then their attitude that Tourette syndrome is terrible is likely to persist.

Whatever the pattern in school — and it can evolve or be different with different teachers — it must first be satisfactorily described. Parents may not be fully aware of what is happening in school; the school is often either unaware of much that goes on at home, or is influenced by gossip or bits of information without adequate context. Parents may hear about the school, a teacher or head, and believe the worst, sometimes affected by their own school experiences. Negative reports from their children may be exaggerated. Simplistic theories may be invoked. Direct contact between clinician and school is therefore often necessary. The problem is that there is no short-cut that is dependably successful, and clinician time may not be fully reimbursed. A phone call is a minimum, but may not be good enough because more staff are typically involved than the one with whom one is speaking, especially as the child progresses from elementary through to secondary classes in the school system. A formal school report often tells little. A letter from the clinician might be helpful, but may not match the need for a clarification of meanings, and could seem arrogant or presumptuous.

Case example

During an unusually severe influenza epidemic, 'Philip', who was 11 years old, encountered special difficulty: his vocal tics (throat-clearing, coughing and snorting) were interpreted as being caused by an upper respiratory infection; he was considered likely to be 'infectious' and was not allowed to be in school. The hospital posted signs that anyone coming to the Emergency Department who had upper respiratory symptoms was not to enter, so this effectively barred him from attending the neuropsychiatric clinic for his tics.

> **Comment:** *Even at times with lesser public health concern, such symptoms may make attendance problematic and may require explanation.*

Parents attempting to interpret their child's needs or behaviors to the school may find that they are not believed, even if (or sometimes especially if) the parent is a clinician. A clinician's letter or other corroboration may be necessary. There are certain helpful caveats, especially when conflict has developed between parents and the school. For the clinician, credibility may be limited if you go into a school — or even write a letter that seems to take sides with the parents — without prior contact with the school.

If a better understanding of their child by the school seems necessary, to whom do the parents address their concerns? In an elementary school this might well be the class teacher, principal or head teacher. But in a middle or secondary school where many teachers are involved with the child, it is necessary to consider who is central within the table of organization to diffuse the information to the involved staff. This is not always obvious and is likely to be less so for parents with limited skills in the local language. It may then fall to the clinician to help them with the necessary advocacy.

> **Practice point**
> Initial school contact by the clinician should be with the principal, head teacher or vice-principal, not (yet) with the child's teacher. This is both simple courtesy and an avoidance of unintentionally causing trouble or confusion within the school's organization.

A common complaint of parents is that the school does not understand the medical information that was provided, staff have not read it, or they forget what was in it. Above all, parents need to understand that after clinician information is sent to the school, it may not be enough for it to be available in a file, especially when new staff are involved. It may be necessary to repeat it in context and ensure it is read by next year's teacher.

Child abuse reporting

In places where child abuse reporting is mandatory, a child's description of acts of parental frustration or failure to provide breakfast (whether exaggerated or not) may require reporting by the school and result in an investigation. Many parents are horrified, embarrassed or fearful when this happens. I have experience of immigrant families (in whose country of origin a visit from a government official would be a serious threat) finding themselves de-skilled in applying any discipline and (in a sense) held hostage by their child who threatens to report them yet again. This kind of situation calls out for skilled and persistent intervention.

Teasing and bullying

Many children report to their parents (and sometimes to school staff) that they are being teased or bullied (Storch et al. 2007). Some schools have 'Zero Tolerance Policy' proudly and prominently displayed on the school signage. It is arguable that this impossible goal makes it less likely that actual teasing or bullying will be believed and acted upon.

Case example

'Adam' was 12 when the diagnosis of Tourette syndrome was made. He hated school. The hospital chart showed that from the age of 6 years he had been seen by multiple specialists because of frequent disruptive throat-clearing and restlessness in school. A respirologist and an otolaryngologist both mentioned tics as a possibility, but arranged for adenoidectomy and allergy testing. His teachers considered his throat-clearing to be deliberate and he was singled out for discipline, and when teased by other children his reactions resulted in him being suspended from school or from its activities. Classmates took the opportunity to make fun of him or sometimes to physically provoke him. No communication with the school had been suggested.

Comment: Adam's tics were misunderstood. Whose responsibility was it, among the physicians who saw him, to institute corrective action in school, or to even inquire further? This was unclear. Would the family physician have the experience or time? The pediatrician? Perhaps. In the event it was the psychiatrist.

Informing the school of the diagnosis

This may not be simple to decide. Who needs to know, and why? If the tics are not noticed, then maybe nothing needs to be done. If tics are noticeable and the subject of staff misunderstanding, then staff need information, though using the term 'Tourette' may be misunderstood; 'tics' may be preferable and is also correct. Comorbid disorders if present often require further explanation, the nature of which may change with a changing clinical picture. A more difficult question is what to tell the student's class, sometimes the entire school (with severe tics, especially vocal ones), and whether to use 'Tourette' or 'tics'. The child's need to be involved in the decision to inform the class with him there or absent is also a consideration. In general, it is a good idea to individualize these decisions. Tourette syndrome support groups may have a representative assigned or available to talk to a class about tics, though the child's clinician may have no way to know how accurate and relevant the information given will be to the particular class. A good way to approach this need has been established by Tourettes Action in the UK (www.tourettes-action.org.uk), which has a variety of materials designed exactly for this purpose, for primary, secondary and post-secondary settings. Other Tourette organizations may also have or develop equivalent services that take into account national legal standards, for example.

Nussey et al. (2014) studied the effects of psychoeducation directed toward school classes that have a child with Tourette syndrome as a member. Results indicated that the presentation was well received and appeared to improve self-confidence of children with Tourette syndrome.

The problem of expectations

Most physicians have little training in school consultation, and know little about school bureaucracy, policies and politics. If they go to a patient's school to observe in class or to attend a school meeting, they may feel like a fish out of water. It may be much better to emphasize that you are there to learn more about the child than to make recommendations too soon. A school visit when a child has one teacher is much simpler than at a later point when up to five or more teachers, ancillary staff and a principal are involved, each with different experiences, beliefs and opinions.

How everyday routines and rules may interact with child characteristics

Schools are complicated organizations that require rules and routines to function, but in so doing conflicts around individual problems and characteristics may result. It is not only the tics that may cause difficulty, but the comorbid disorders, symptoms and personality features as well. Children may feel a strong need to avoid displaying their weaknesses or vulnerabilities that may well be taken into account at home: for example, avoiding changing clothing in front of others, manipulating buttons when changing clothing in a limited time frame, not going on a field trip or participating in activities where their physical skill will be (or they fear may be) on display, tolerating high noise levels around their locker, writing on the chalk board in front of the class or using the school washroom. Many other examples could be given. Children may not talk about these matters to their clinician, maybe not even to their parents.

Case example

'Tammy' had many tics and some other stereotypic movements, as well as ADHD and Tourette syndrome, but what caused trouble for her in school was her DCD. She took more time to use buttons and change clothing quickly. She was intolerant of loud noises. When the class was going on a field trip that included a climbing wall she knew she would appear clumsy and had to avoid going. However, a new young teacher found a work-around: she lent Tammy her camera so she could be the activity photographer and have her photos in the school yearbook. This gave Tammy a useful role and avoided displaying her lack of physical prowess.

Rutter et al. (1982) in their important study of London schools showed that a school's atmosphere had strong independent effects on a child's mental health. Here is an example.

Case example

'Brendan' is a bright 10-year-old, burdened with Tourette syndrome, ADHD, OCD, DCD and anxiety. In school he showed perfectionistic tendencies, and he was socially both shy and competitive. Engaging him in conversation about his symptoms seemed pointless and unproductive. As school work became increasingly complex his anxiety level rose and he developed trichotillomania for the first time; his school tried to modify

---

> *the demands he felt by reducing pressures on him, to no avail, partly because he was painfully aware of what their efforts meant about his being so different. The difficult decision was reached to remove him from school and enroll him in a homebound online program.*

Children who may have learning problems will need special support and a close relationship between parent and teacher or school counselor (Packer 2005, Dornbush and Pruitt 2008, Packer et al. 2010). A special-needs designation, termed 'statementing' in the UK, must often be obtained.

Post-secondary education

Many universities and community colleges in developed countries have arrangements to take into account the needs of students with disabilities, in some places associated with legislation. When made aware of the disability and its implications, the school staff may (for example) sanction special arrangements for examinations. However, the breadth of experience required in the field of disability is so large that the understanding of tics may be absent or minimal and require clinician advocacy. Excellent information is available from Tourettes Action in the UK (see p. 287) and some other service organizations.

School refusal

Finally, it is of great importance to respond quickly to a situation in which a young child starts to refuse to go to school or complains of physical symptoms on the first school day of the week, symptoms which quickly abate when he or she remains at home. This may be due to self-consciousness based upon poorly written output or inability to perform as expected in front of others, social anxiety, or perceived criticism or humiliation from the teacher or classmates.

REFERENCES

Cohen B, Wysocky L (2008) *Front of the Class: How Tourette Syndrome Made me the Teacher I Never Had.* New York: VanderWyk & Burnham.

Dornbush MP, Pruitt SK (2008) *Tigers, Too: Executive Functions/Speed of Processing/Memory.* Atlanta, GA: Parkaire Press.

Nussey C, Pistrang N, Murphy T (2014) Does it help to talk about tics? An evaluation of a classroom presentation about Tourette syndrome. *Child Adolesc Ment Health* 19: 31–8. doi: 10.1111/camh.12000.

Packer LE (2005) Tic-related school problems: impact on functioning, accommodations, and interventions. *Behav Modif* 29: 876–99.

Packer LE, Pruitt SK (2010) *Challenging Kids, Challenged Teachers: Teaching Students with Tourette's, Bipolar Disorder, Executive Dysfunction, OCD, ADHD, and More.* Bethesda, MD: Woodbine House.

Rutter M, Maughan B, Mortimore P, Ouston J (1982) *Fifteen Thousand Hours: Secondary Schools and Their Effects on Children.* Cambridge, MA: Harvard University Press.

Storch EA, Lack CW, Simons LE, et al. (2007) A measure of functional impairment in youth with Tourette's syndrome. *J Pediatr Psychol* 32: 950–9. doi: 10.1093/jpepsy/jsm034.

17
WORKING WITH FAMILIES

Working with families — which in some cases includes grandparents or other relatives acting as caregivers — is essential. Disagreements over the extent and variety of symptoms and the meanings attached to these are common and should not be assumed to indicate pathology in relationships. Some of the information that is important to live well with tic disorders is not easy to impart in one initial meeting, so that some repetition over time is often necessary, particularly when cultural differences are active. Genetic information is difficult to grasp and absorb. Theories of causation and triggering factors held by patients and parents may clash with those of the clinician. The feelings and roles of siblings need to be considered, and strong efforts should be made to overcome language limitations by using proper interpreting services, not another relative with a smattering of English.

With limited time, what can one expect to be accomplished? If family issues are an important component of the child's problems, parents often do not bring them up, and discovering them takes time, a supply of which is often short. Recommendations for medication may be the only action available. Paradoxically, although parents want help quickly, they often are negative about medication, and more so the younger the child and the less the time the clinician spends with them. That may be one of the reasons they ask about diet. There seems to be no easy remedy for this situation.

An unpleasant experience is to see your child 'ticcing up a storm' while you are making dinner — or worse, in a school play while you sit helplessly in the audience and hear whispered comments from other parents like "That child should never have been allowed to perform" or "What's the matter with him?" (Similar embarrassing situations can occur with adults who have obvious tics.)

Predicaments
Some parents may have special problems with Tourette syndrome because of the irregular unpredictable nature and comorbidity, and — as already mentioned — the feeling during an upsurge that their child has a progressive neurological disease. It may be helpful to contrast Tourette syndrome with other common childhood conditions that usually have a good prognosis, but whose exacerbations are of severity, not of kind (e.g. asthma, eczema). This helps to partly account for their anxiety with upsurges. Of course each story is different. If adaptation does not occur after a few upsurges, further exploration may be required.

> **Practice point**
> Get a good description of the meanings associated with tics before giving advice. That includes premature reassurance!

Hunter (1991) has provided a very helpful understanding of the incommensurability of patients' and doctors' stories of an illness or disorder, and the possibilities of reconciliation.

Counseling as a process has rather vague meanings. It can be informative and educational, and/or psychotherapeutic (Freeman and Pearson 1978).

Genetic information in relation to tics is especially confusing because of the lack of a mendelian pattern (which is usually the only aspect educated parents know) and the possibility of genetic heterogeneity with multiple factors involved. Even in mendelian conditions genetic risks tend to be misunderstood (Klitzman 2010), and the confusing boundaries of the tic disorder categories may add to the difficulty.

Issues in working with families

Each family member may see/feel the child and the child's symptoms differently, and specifically differently than you do. This can cause problems that may never be made explicit, even if there were time and opportunity to talk about it. Parents do not expect physicians to take such an interest. For example, a fairly hopeful attitude toward the child's Tourette syndrome for the future may not accord with the pain the parent is suffering, the basis for which may not be what they know now but rather past expectations of a normal child that have now been demolished, and fear of social ostracism in the future. It is important to recognize that there are at least three contributory factors: (1) the waxing–waning course with sometimes major upsurges (that will top out when?) that make it feel like a progressive disease; (2) extreme cases on the internet and information in many home medical encyclopedias that do not apply accurately to most children; (3) the counseling that describes that the variation may increase into puberty (which may be years away), and the assumption that everything will be worse in adolescence. Furthermore, cultural beliefs and values are always important, whether explored or not. Even when clinicians and familes are members of the same ethno-cultural group, beliefs about health and illness very likely differ, because medical systems of understanding constitute a different culture.

> **Case study**
> *'Janice' was first seen at age 13. She presented with worsening predominantly right-sided tics, first noticed at age 11, which were severe enough for her to be briefly hospitalized. (Her brother also had tics and was seen later.) Her tics included her right arm, shoulder and face, along with humming, blowing, shouting and echolalia. There had been some mild obsessive–compulsive symptoms: lining her stuffed animals up, having to walk a specific route through the house, and tapping objects. Family dynamics were problematic. Despite education about it, her mother believed that because the tics were worse at the end of the day at home, Janice was doing it deliberately. She*

resisted believing that some of Janice's behaviors were due to her increasing OCD. At age 17 Janice was using up all the toilet paper and causing problems with their septic tank because of her uncertainty about how much was enough, and all the hot water because of prolonged showers (unsure at what point she was clean enough). Cabinet doors had to be slammed just right, leading to breakage. These symptoms added stress to an already fragile marriage. Clomipramine initially had a beneficial effect but later caused sleepiness. She was then lost to follow-up.

Comment: *Janice had remarkable ability to describe her inner states and was appreciated by all clinicians who saw her as a person with a fine spirit and many positive attributes. Unfortunately her parents were unable at the time to share in this appraisal and thus her symptoms aggravated an already precarious relationship. This can happen despite proper education about Tourette syndrome and OCD; perhaps the limited clinical contact due to the family living a long way from the hospital imposed intractable limits.*

This comment was written based entirely upon old records. Her mother was located and phoned decades later, and was pleased to provide an update. The parents had separated. Janice was working successfully as a married pharmacist. She still had tics but they were stable and not a problem. Her brother's tics had worsened, then gradually subsided and in adulthood were rarely seen. The mother reported that in retrospect she had been unable to believe that there was not something seriously and specifically wrong with Janice's brain, such as a brain tumor. She still saw high fevers the children had had as a causative factor in their Tourette syndrome.

Note that at the time Janice was first seen, patterns we now understand could not be explained: the worsening of tics toward the end of the day at home — misinterpreted as deliberate because controllable at school — and the typical improvements in adulthood.

When one parent seeks to minimize stress (because it is assumed to exacerbate tics, possibly permanently), the other may not feel that need. It is a common clinical situation for the father (who often has less time with the child) to minimize the symptoms and to attribute the mother's concern to her oversensitivity. Since fathers are more likely to have had tics than mothers, they may also see themselves in their child. What to do? It may be helpful as an initial entry into an exploration of this pattern to acknowledge that it is common for parents to have disagreements over the importance of symptoms, and that each may actually encounter different tics or severity of tics. It is then important to ensure that both parents participate in meetings with you, or as a minimum to make a phone call to the absent parent to equalize the information.

Practice point

Always seek to meet with both parents for psychoeducation, if at all possible, or to talk with the absent parent separately or by phone. It is not sufficient to talk to one parent (usually the mother) who then must try to adequately answer questions by the other parent who was not there.

Caregiver strain

This has been studied and shown to be important (Cooper et al. 2003, Wilkinson et al. 2008). Mothers were seen to carry a disproportionate burden as compared with fathers. It is the presence of comorbid disorders (and especially disruptive externalizing behavior disorders) that seems most important, more than tic severity alone. School-based interventions did not seem to diminish strain, but more comprehensive interventions did. In designing interventions for Tourette syndrome, family-based help (including respite and support groups) is important to include in order to reduce stress (Wrigley et al. 2000).

Threat statements

Parents may, after severe or chronic frustration, issue a threat that they would never have imagined themselves making, like: "If this continues, you may have to live somewhere else!" or "Maybe you'd prefer another family…" You may not be told about this, or in a better mood they may not think that their child took it seriously, or how seriously. The boundary of the child's zone of tolerance of tics may have been changed thereby. The idea of a parental 'zone of tolerance' is complex: including reactions when out in public with the child, when at home, or when mommy has a headache.

Increased interparental conflict

Parents may hate the tics and the effect they have on them and their child, and their reaction to the child; and they may hate their powerlessness to stop the tics or their reactions to the tics. It is important to be aware of complex interactions within the family between the child's tics and other factors.

Results of parental suffering

A 10-year-old boy had longstanding encopresis, averaging five days a week. While his mother was out of the office briefly, his father responded to a question by reporting that episodes had decreased to an average of two days a week. The clinician was pleased. When mom returned, she was asked about her reaction. She said (with disgust) that only a decrease to zero would please her after all the messes she'd had to deal with.

Practice point

It is important to recognize that parents who have become very negative about their child's behavior may not spontaneously report improvement that is less than complete or almost complete. Another factor may be an underlying bias toward negative thinking.

Theories about tics

Theories about tics can have important consequences. These theories may have several different sources: (1) observations of variations in tic severity; (2) cultural attitudes; (3) the internet; (4) personal experience; (5) clinician's statements; and (6) read or overheard statements in the media, from friends, or from persons with tics. Intake information can sometimes give an early indication of a problematic theory.

Case examples

'Ruth', age 9, had developed noticeable tics that upset both parents. The father, who had suffered from inflammatory bowel disease aggravated (he felt) by emotional stress, had observed fluctuations in Ruth's tics and decided that they could probably be controlled if her stress could be minimized. Attempts to accomplish this, unsupported fully by her mother and sometimes defied by Ruth, led to potentially destructive conflict that required family intervention.

'Allyson', age 7, had some obvious tics that were causing no problems in school or for her mother. Her tic exacerbations were typical and not unusual. Her father, however, had an anxiety disorder, and with each upsurge of Allyson's tics he was the one who seemed to suffer the most, with powerful images of a negative future. Reassurance by the mother (a health professional) was ineffective and led to serious marital strain. The father had a longstanding tendency to catastrophize, so that increases in tics were particularly threatening to him. Looking for information from persons he knew with tics or the internet failed to assuage his suffering. These crises required the clinician to repeatedly engage in counseling by telephone for the first year after diagnosis.

*   **Comment:** How this would eventuate in the years to come was initially unclear, but with a later tic exacerbation and more extensive counseling the father's over-responsivity diminished; the need for frequent reassurance abated and has continued at only a low level.*

Siblings

These are the lost souls in many families. It is often worth talking with them, to get their view of the situation, to provide information, and to understand their feelings about the inevitable changes in their family wrought by a tic disorder. Sometimes they have unrecognized mild tics or non-tic repetitive motor behaviors that scare them or their families, recognition and clarification of which can be very helpful. Others feel overly responsible for their sibling, or that they will be caretakers forever, and suppress any negative feelings. Others feel that the sibling with tics is treated better and receives more attention, and that the entire situation is unfair.

Practice point

In a family where the child has a disability or significant disorder, unaffected siblings often criticize the parents for their differing expectations, potentially aggravating family stress. This is probably normal and to be expected.

Relatives

Both parents may be working outside the home. Child-minding may be by relatives (frequently grandparents). They may disagree about the child's problem and its management, and have strong ideas about what should be done. This can cause significant problems with (or between) parents. When genetic factors are brought up, grandparents may react in varied ways that are typically not brought into the clinical situation (Lehmann et al. 2011). With parental agreement, it may be good for the clinician to see them, or at least to offer to do so.

Parental thinking about education

Clinician advice, especially when given piecemeal and without integration with advice from others, can be overwhelming, and the parent may not be able to judge the relative importance or the certainty of that advice. Often explanations must be offered more than once over the years.

The following frequently reveal gaps in parental thinking and education.
* Probability/risk (e.g. risk of a treatment compared with risk of no treatment)
* *Post hoc ergo propter hoc* fallacy (after this, because of this) concerning 'causes' of tics
* The difference between correlation and causation
* The difference between high-quality evidence and testimonials
* Multiple factors in causality, association and triggers
* Limitations and uses of categorization
* Comorbidity overlaps
* Overrides (e.g. reaction by emotion rather than logical thinking)
* 'Binary trap' thinking (that a phenomenon must be either/or).

Families from different cultures

In many parts of the world immigration and an influx of refugees have increased and pose new challenges to health and related services. For example, in the major cities of Canada at the time of the 2006 national census, Asian and African immigrants and refugees represented one-third or more of the population.

Specifically with regard to tics, in many if not most parts of the world, and in many poorly educated segments of a society, there may be no concept of a tic as distinct from any other 'twitch'. This is itself a barrier to explanation and counseling. Time may need to be taken to distinguish common tics from benign ocular or other myokymia, sleep starts, stereotypies, some habits, and other repetitive motor behaviors.

Case example
'Kevin', an 11-year-old boy, had had longstanding nose-picking, occasionally causing nose-bleeds. When he developed Tourette syndrome, the nose-picking was reclassified by the parents as a tic. His teacher apparently was sensitive about germs and made him wash his hands each time he was observed to pick his nose.

Comment: In such a situation it was unclear what to do about the teacher. Should he or she be contacted and the issue explored? Questions were raised about possible

---

triggers such as dryness of his mucous membranes, allergies (which he had) and the possibility of an otolaryngology referral. His parents were told that nose-picking is common with or without tics and that the main problem seemed to be his teacher's reaction.

It is often hard work to deal with the many issues and myths when a family uses a different language through an interpreter. Immigrants from some countries are suspicious of interpreters who may come from a subgroup, tribe, or different social class or religion of their country of origin (which may be in conflict with theirs), or who represent a regime they have fled, or may even be an informer who can affect family members still in their country of origin. The clinician is unlikely to be aware of this. However, success can often be achieved by repeated visits, and respect for fears and ideas.

To be realistic, it can be impracticable to work out periodic two-sided interpreter services to monitor progress, appointment arrangements and medication; in such instances it may be necessary to invoke a very imperfect solution: using a sibling's e-mail (who is often more competent in English than the parents) or even that of a relative or neighbor.

Case study

'Ralph' was just 7 years old when referred because of uncooperative behavior, blurting out words in class, reported by his school as "repetitive, disruptive verbal vocalizations; uncontrolled facial grimaces and eye-twitching, sucking on clothing, difficulty focusing, at times anxious and inability to self-regulate", starting about 6 months previously. The referring physician indicated the urgent need for further assessment of ADHD, ODD, probable cognitive delay, and some tics. His family did not speak English, so an interpreter was arranged. When the mother and Ralph arrived they asked that the interpreter be sent away because they had a family friend with them who could serve in that capacity. They explained through her that they were not comfortable coming to a mental health facility with an interpreter from their ethnic group. After confidence was established the recent history slowly unfolded. Ralph was usually a caring, dependable boy, helpful with his baby sister, but had started to swear frequently for no apparent reason. This was only in English, not their native language, and the mother imitated: "Fuh!" His sleep became more difficult and his behavior in school deteriorated. His mother was unable to describe any previous symptoms including tics. In the interview obvious eye-blinking and facial grimacing were observed, but his behavior was exemplary, without any indication of impulsivity, distractibility or cognitive delay. A phone call with his teacher revealed the same description as his mother had given and that his current behavior was not a problem. Furthermore, when she had told him to stop his swearing he had said that he was unable to, but tried and was fairly successful in replacing it with a shrieking noise.

Comment: *Two points are worth consideration. The parental reluctance to accept a qualified interpreter should be understood in light of the reality that there are factions* *in the ethnic community and in the native country that can make private behavior and even opinions hazardous. Second, it appears likely that this was the onset of multiple tics including coprolalia, with the latter limited to one language and transient. The most probable course will be another upsurge with or without coprolalia.*

In some countries or social classes a visit to a physician almost always means receiving a prescription for whatever symptoms one has; without one the encounter is judged incomplete. This may be true for tics. We have seen overmedicated children and adolescents who had no tics because they appeared zombie-like from high dosages of neuroleptic drugs. The concept of 'no medication unless compellingly necessary' may be incomprehensible to these families without diligent education, but it can often be successfully imparted.

Case study of 'Joshua' [continued from Chapter 7, p. 49]
It took eight sessions to obtain what seemed to be a realistic view of what had developed in his family because of the violent neck tic. After many visits it became clear that the uncertainty of the danger was playing a central role for everyone concerned, including the physicians. (No one could say what was safe to do and what was not.) Joshua claimed that playing computer games was his sole source of pleasure, and refused to accept the argument that he could play computer games freely "when you grow up". He stated that "I love my childhood; I hate growing up." This was not all. He was threatening to do the dangerous tic if he did not get his way, no matter what the result. This emotional blackmail put his tic literally in charge of every contentious decision in the family, and it was difficult initially for them to confess that they had lost control.

> *Comment: Again, this was not all. In this family's country of origin a child with a disability was often treated as deserving compensatory attention and to be sheltered from any frustration. He had been indulged since the diagnosis was made. Furthermore, the parents and relatives disagreed about the approach to his destructive omnipotence. He had no concept of his duty to his family, nor any experience with frustration tolerance. Re-training proceeded slowly, but with some success using a family approach.*

Case example
A 10-year-old boy with obvious tics was from a family that had immigrated recently from China. The relatives' importance was revealed only after a few visits to the clinician. Every night the parents displayed the boy's tics, via Skype, to the grandparents in China, who then gave advice.

> *Comment: This not only indicates a degree of involvement rare among most Westernized parents, but is also a commentary on how technology can affect family patterns.*

Marriageability of a child and the need for parents to present their child as normal or better can be demolished by Tourette syndrome. Concepts of disease causation that clash with modern Western thinking may not be evident. Many immigrant families are living with — or in close communication with — relatives whose ideas about the problem and its treatment may be important but not volunteered to the clinician.

Case example

'Liam' is an 8-year-old boy with significant tics and ADHD. The parents separated and his father was not initially seen. When specifically invited, he came in. It was immediately obvious that he had significant tics of his own. He saw his son as just like himself (although he had had no understanding as a child/adolescent of his tics or other patterns). The parents disagreed over management, but rather than the father opposing the mother, he felt that despite his and his son's tics, a sense of consequences and responsibility had to be inculcated and that the tics were not completely involuntary, whereas the mother seemed to feel that Liam's tics and behavior patterns were completely involuntary and the school had to be told that he was not responsible in any way.

*   **Comment:** *These types of disagreements are common between parents, even those with a good relationship. Each may feel in the face of their helplessness that "if only my spouse would consistently do what I think is best, the symptoms would improve" (but neither has an opportunity to prove it).*

Families' understanding of a 'familial' disorder

Although specific genes have not been identified, family members learn (if they did not know already), that heredity is involved in some way, not only with tics but with comorbidity. Just as the limitation has previously been pointed out that Tourette syndrome *as such* is not inherited, family members need a nuanced understanding that 'familiality' is not totally deterministic with regard to the kind of life their child or relative will lead. Environmental factors and personal decisions are also involved (Kendler 2013).

REFERENCES

Cooper C, Robertson M, Livingston G (2003) Psychological morbidity and caregiver burden in parents of children with Tourette's disorder and psychiatric comorbidity. *J Am Acad Child Adolesc Psychiatry* 42: 1370–5. doi: 10.1097/01.CHI.0000085751.71002.48.

Freeman RD, Pearson PH (1978) Counselling with parents. In: Apley J, ed. *Care of the Handicapped Child. A Festschrift for Ronald Mac Keith. Clinics in Developmental Medicine no. 67.* London: Mac Keith Press, pp. 35–47.

Hunter KM (1991) *Doctors' Stories: The Narrative Structure of Medical Knowlege.* Princeton, NJ: Princeton University Press.

Kendler KS (2013) What psychiatric genetics has taught us about the nature of psychiatric illness and what is left to learn. *Mol Psychiatry* 18: 1058–66. doi: 10.1038/mp.2013.50.

Klitzman RL (2010) Misunderstandings concerning genetics among patients confronting genetic disease. *J Genet Counsel* 19: 430–46.

Lehmann A, Speight BS, Kerzin-Storrar L (2011) Extended family impact of genetic testing: the experiences of X-linked carrier grandmothers. *J Genet Counsel* 20: 365–73.

Wilkinson BJ, Marshall RM, Curtwright B (2008) Impact of Tourette's disorder on parent reported stress. *J Child Fam Stud* 17: 582–98. doi: 10.1007/s10826-007-9176-8.

Wrigley K, Mason A, Lambert S, et al. (2000) A specialist service for children and adolescents with Tourette syndrome: problems and attempted solutions. *Clin Child Psychol Psychiatry* 5: 247–57.

18
PEER RELATIONSHIPS AND TEASING/BULLYING

> Bullying is a worldwide problem. Teasing is virtually a universal experience and persons with obviously unusual behavior (such as many with tics), comorbidities like ADHD, and sometimes weak social skills or social anxiety are more likely targets than others. Having friends is a protective factor that often is a major concern of parents and teachers. Finding ways to support or intervene early is advisable, but knowing how is often lacking, and therapeutic services targeting peer problems may be unavailable. Cyberbullying has recently become a serious problem that may have devastating consequences for some children and adolescents.

Having friends is a moderating influence on children's behavior and developmental problems. Much recent research, however, shows that children (and presumably adults) with noticeable tics have a reduced quality of life and more difficulty with peer relationships when compared with persons with typical development (Stokes et al. 1991; Bawden et al. 1998; Boudjouk et al. 2000; Elstner et al. 2001; Storch et al. 2007a,b,c; Conelea et al. 2011; Cavanna et al. 2013; Wadman et al. 2013). In some studies the role of comorbidity, and specifically ADHD, was the major predictor of behavioral and social problems (Hoekstra et al. 2004). One-third of children reported some teasing (Storch et al. 2007a). The definition of teasing and bullying (when combined constituting 'victimization') varies within different studies, cited statistics, and as reported by children of different ages.

Bullying and teasing
Bullying is reported to be a problem worldwide. Although few examples of serious bullying specifically on account of tics have come to our attention, the presence of tics provides another focus for a bully, and children with Tourette syndrome are more likely than children with typical development to be victimized (Storch et al. 2007c). Several problems exist in making a general statement about it, though.

• Children who are more anxious or sensitive are more likely to report teasing, and perhaps to promote the naming of their experiences of teasing into 'bullying'. Nowakowski et al. (2013) found that persons with social anxiety tend to interpret ambiguous interactions negatively, and teasing as malicious.

- Schoolmates' imitation of tics may be interpreted or reported as teasing, especially by young children.
- Children who are prime targets for teasing may attribute it solely to tics; tics may be easier to conceptualize or to admit to than other characteristics that are targeted, such as personality characteristics or weak social skills.
- Reasons for becoming and staying a target are often mixed.
- Parents who expect tic severity at school to equate to tic severity at home may be anticipating teasing and then may assume their child's reports of teasing and reasons for it are fully accurate and valid.

A recent paper (Zinner et al. 2012) reported a survey of children with Tourette syndrome, of whom 26% reported being victimized; this is a substantial rate that must be taken seriously. School-based surveys of reports of being bullied were examined in a study by Smith and Madsen (1999). They analyzed the age decline (between 8 and 16 years) in reports, and examined four hypotheses: (1) that younger children have many older children above them who are in a position to bully them; (2) that younger children haven't yet come to understand that you should not bully others; (3) that younger children have yet to acquire social and assertiveness skills to cope effectively with bullying; and (4) that definitions of what bullying consists of change with increasing age. The last-named may account for high reports by younger children. The authors concluded that there is support for hypotheses (1) and (3). Public and professional concern about bullying has increased with worldwide distribution of video-related cases of teenage bullying, including cyberbullying, sometimes leading to death.

Childhood gross motor clumsiness was found to be strongly associated with peer victimization in a study of 277 patients by Bejerot and Humble (2013). Karlsson et al. (2013) studied urban American students and found that internalizing symptoms were predictive of peer victimization. Both parental warmth and teacher support were protective factors. Being overweight is a predictor of bullying (Jansen et al. 2014), and one should not forget the possibility of teasing and bullying by a sibling (Bowes et al. 2014).

A few caveats are important to note. Some schools have adopted a 'zero-tolerance' policy that is prominently posted on and inside the school. Although this is an important indicator of official policy, its appropriateness is sometimes questioned because school staff cannot supervise and become aware of all teasing and bullying, since there are unsupervised times such as recess. Might some incidents not be taken seriously because they go against the school policy, which *should* be successful? Victimization may also be an overly broad category, and rather than concentrate only on bullies, a more sophisticated approach might be to also examine factors that signal the victim's vulnerability (but this may come too close to 'blaming the victim').

Most children report being teased at some time, occurring either in school or the community, or sometimes with siblings in the family — see further discussion in Twemlow and Sacco (2012), who have presented programs for preventing bullying, and Christoffersen (2010) who directed a large Danish national study that showed that social support moderated the effect of early adversity (poor parenting and abuse) and reduced the risk of suicide. Children in care were three times more likely to be bullied than those living with their parents. One problem is that once a child acts the bully, he or she may be gaining a new and negative identity that will have consequences. There are thus problems on the part of the victim as well as the bully.

Cyberbullying has increased the impact, spread and permanence of bullying; it has affected about 1 in 10 secondary school students in Canada (Stanbrook 2014) and an even higher proportion in other countries (Kiriakidis and Kavoura (2010). The onset of new behavioral problems, unexplained medical symptoms, or a decline in school performance should be an occasion for inquiry about possible bullying.

A recent publication of the TSA-USA, *A Family's Guide to Tourette Syndrome* (Walkup et al. 2012), has much helpful information. It is an up-to-date guide available at a very reasonable price through the organization's online store at http://store.tsa-usa.org. Much other useful material is available on the www.tsa-usa.org website. This includes 'Bullying 101: What Children, Parents, and Teachers Need to Know' (2010) and 'Bullying Prevention: Positive Strategies' (2011). Although these publications include American-oriented legal provisions, they make many useful suggestions both for parents, children and adolescents, and for clinicians throughout the world, and further updates can be expected.

REFERENCES

Bawden HN, Stokes A, Camfield CS, et al. (1998) Peer relationship problems in children with Tourette's disorder or diabetes mellitus. *J Child Psychol Psychiatry* 39: 663–8.

Bejerot S, Humble MB (2013) Childhood clumsiness and peer victimization: a case–control study of psychiatric patients. *BMC Psychiatry* 13: 68. doi: 10.1186/1471-244X-13-68.

Boudjouk PI, Woods DW, Miltenberger RG, Long ES (2000) Negative peer evaluations in adolescents: effects of tic disorders and trichotillomania. *Child Fam Behav Ther* 22: 17–28.

Bowes L, Wolke D, Joinson C, et al. (2014) Sibling bullying and risk of depression, anxiety, and self-harm: a prospective cohort study. *Pediatrics* 134: e1032–e1039. doi: 10.1542/peds.2014-0832.

Cavanna AE, Luoni C, Selvini C, et al. (2013) Disease-specific quality of life in young patients with Tourette syndrome. *Ped Neurol* 48: 111–4. doi: 10.1016/j.pediatrneurol.2012.10.006.

Christoffersen MN (2010) *Child Maltreatment, Bullying in School and Social Support: a Social Psychological Study of Self-Esteem and Suicidal Behaviour Based on a National Sample of Young People.* Copenhagen: Danish National Centre for Social Research.

Conelea CA, Woods DW, Zinner SH, et al. (2011) Exploring the impact of chronic tic disorders on youth: results from the Tourette Syndrome Impact Survey. *Child Psychiatry Hum Dev* 42: 219–42. doi: 10.1007/s10578-010-0211-4.

Elstner K, Selai CE, Trimble MR, Robertson MM (2001) Quality of life (QOL) of patients with Gilles de la Tourette's syndrome. *Acta Psychiatr Scand* 103: 52–9. doi: 10.1111/j.1600-0447.2001.00147.x.

Hoekstra PJ, Steenhuis M-P, Troost PW, et al. (2004) Relative contribution of attention-deficit hyperactivity disorder, obsessive–compulsive disorder, and tic severity to social and behavioral problems in tic disorders. *J Dev Behav Pediatr* 25: 275–9.

Jansen PW, Verlinden M, Dommisse-van Berkel A, et al. (2014) Teacher and peer reports of overweight and bullying among young primary school children. *Pediatrics* 134: 473–80. doi: 10.1542/peds.2013-3274.

Karlsson E, Stickley A, Lindblad F, et al. (2013) Risk and protective factors for peer victimization: a 1-year follow-up study of urban American students. *Eur Child Adolesc Psychiatry* 23: 773–81. doi: 10.1007/s00787-013-0507-6.

Kiriakidis SP, Kavoura A (2010) Cyberbullying: a review of the literature on harassment through the internet and other electronic means. *Fam Commun Health* 33: 82–93.

Nowakowski ME, Antony MM (2013) Reactions to teasing in social anxiety. *Cogn Ther Res* 37: 1091–100.

doi: 10.1007/s10608-013-9551-2.

Smith PK, Madsen KC (1999) What causes the age decline in reports of being bullied at school? Towards a developmental analysis of risks of being bullied. *Educ Res* 41: 267–85.

Stanbrook MB (2014) Stopping cyberbullying requires a combined societal effort. *CMAJ* 186: 483 (editorial). doi: 10.1503/cmaj.140299.

Stokes A, Bawden HN, Camfield PR, et al. (1991) Peer problems in Tourette's disorder. *Pediatrics* 87: 936–42.

Storch EA, Lack CW, Simons LE, et al. GR (2007a) A measure of functional impairment in youth with Tourette's syndrome. *J Pediatr Psychol* 32: 950–9. doi: 10.1093/jpepsy/jsm034.

Storch EA, Merlo LJ, Lack C, et al. (2007b) Quality of life in youth with Tourette's syndrome and chronic tic disorder. *J Clin Child Adolesc Psychol* 36: 217–27. doi: 10.1080/15374410701279545.

Storch EA, Murphy TK, Chase RM, et al. (2007c) Peer victimization in youth with Tourette's syndrome and chronic tic disorder: relations with tic severity and internalizing symptoms. *J Psychopathol Behav Assess* 29: 211–9. doi: 10.1007/s10862-007-9050-4.

Twemlow SW, Sacco FC (2012) *Preventing Bullying and School Violence.* Washington, DC: American Psychiatric Publishing.

Wadman R, Tischler V, Jackson GM (2013) 'Everybody just thinks I'm weird': a qualitative exploration of the psychosocial experiences of adolescents with Tourette syndrome. *Child Care Health Dev* 39: 880–6. doi: 10.1111/cch.12033.

Walkup JT, Mink JW, McNaught KStP, eds (2012) *A Family's Guide to Tourette Syndrome.* Bloomington, IN: iUniverse/Bayside; NY: Tourette Syndrome Association.

Zinner SH, Conelea CA, Glew GM, et al. (2012) Peer victimization in youth with Tourette syndrome and other chronic tic disorders. *Child Psychiatry Hum Dev* 43: 124–36. doi: 10.1007/s10578-011-0249-y.

19
CONTROVERSIES

PANDAS

From the parents' point of view, if a shockingly abrupt onset of tics and/or OCD occurs, previous infection may understandably be linked as a plausible cause. Visiting PANDAS (*p*ediatric *a*utoimmune *n*europsychiatric *d*isorders *a*ssociated with *s*treptococcal infections) websites may convert the plausibility into a certainty. The experience of a sudden onset of tics and/or OCD can be quite traumatic for the parents, as if their child had been replaced by another, a 'changeling' (Gabbay et al. 2008).

The PANDAS hypothesis has now been around for almost 20 years, and in an era where molecular aspects of neuroimmunology have come to the fore, it has seemed a possible explanation of 'molecular mimicry' (in which an antigen in the coat of the streptococcus bacterium is similar enough to part of the nervous system of the patient that it can elicit an antibody reaction to it; thus the body's immune system is attacking the part of itself that mimics part of the streptococcus). Yet despite much research and the application of rather invasive treatments, the concept remains unclear and fraught with technical problems. Some researchers and clinicians have portrayed it as settled, others remain sceptical. Since treatments advocated by some are potentially hazardous, the subject is certainly important, so a brief outline of the problems with the hypothesis is provided here, based upon the excellent summary by Singer et al. (2012).

In considering the PANDAS hypothesis, the following points should be considered.
- The abruptness criterion is not operationalized.
- The temporal association between infection and symptom exacerbation could lag for many months, making significant determination unclear.
- The pattern of response is not limited to the effects of Group A beta-hemolytic streptococcus (GABHS).
- Carrier status in children is common, and not eliminated by a throat culture determination; carriers can have protracted elevated titers.
- A single antistreptococcal titer (as in some studies) is insufficient.
- Tics occur in 20% to 30% of school-age children.
- Claimed quick or immediate benefit from antibiotics is not consistent with an immunological process; antibody levels do not correlate with exacerbations (Morris-Berry et al. 2013).
- Improvements with standard treatment occur, as in non-PANDAS cases.

One reasonable conclusion at this point is that the concept is still unproven and inappropriate to apply to community cases, given that children with this pattern have a clinical course indistinguishable from non-PANDAS cases and that the specific treatments recommended (long-term antibiotics, steroids, intravenous immunoglobulins, plasmapheresis) are not without risk.

A nonspecific role for GABHS and other triggers is likely, with genetic vulnerability involved, but GABHS is not the only trigger and the PANDAS criteria are not specific enough (Kurlan et al. 2008, Shulman 2009, Murphy et al. 2010, Brilot et al. 2011, Murphy 2013).

Finally, one of the latest summaries in this contentious area is by Singer et al. (2012) who proposed abandoning the connection with GABHS in favor of a new acronym with broader scope: CANS, *c*hildhood *a*cute *n*europsychiatric *s*ymptoms (later renamed as *p*ediatric *a*cute-onset *n*europsychiatric *s*yndrome or PANS). As proposed, this syndrome requires acute dramatic onset of neuropsychiatric symptoms (not only tics or OCD), a comprehensive history and examination, consideration of differential diagnoses, an active search for a specific etiology, and treatment with the most appropriate therapy. A consensus conference on PANS was held in 2013 (Chang et al. 2014). The paper has an elaborate history of the concept and a helpful review of acute-onset severe symptoms in children with autoimmune and autoinflammatory disorders as well as those meeting the proposed criteria for PANS and PANDAS. Negative critiques of the concepts are omitted. Murphy et al. (2014) have characterized what they feel is the PANS phenotype and state that it represents a subtype of OCD marked by an abrupt onset or exacerbation of neuropsychiatric symptoms.

Among both clinicians and parents there is a group of firm believers on both sides of the argument, so that the validity of the diagnosis and treatment of PANDAS is unlikely to be fully resolved at the time of writing.

The US National Institute of Mental Health (NIMH), where the concept arose, has the following statement on their website regarding the use of long-term prophylactic antibiotics.

Can penicillin be used to treat PANDAS or prevent future PANDAS symptom exacerbations?
Penicillin and other antibiotics kill streptococcus and other types of bacteria. The antibiotics treat the sore throat or pharyngitis caused by the strep by getting rid of the bacteria. However, in PANDAS, it appears that antibodies produced by the body in response to the strep infection are the cause of the problem, not the bacteria themselves. Therefore one could not expect antibiotics such as penicillin to treat the symptoms of PANDAS. Researchers at the NIMH have been investigating the use of antibiotics as a form of prophylaxis or prevention of future problems. At this time, however, there isn't enough evidence to recommend the long-term use of antibiotics.

An additional question is posed:

What about treating PANDAS with plasma exchange or immunoglobulin (IVIG)?
The results of a controlled trial of plasma exchange (also known as plasmapheresis) and immunoglobulin (IVIG) for the treatment of children in the PANDAS subgroup was [sic] published in "The Lancet", Vol. 354, October 2, 1999. All of the children participating in the study had clear evidence of a strep infection as the trigger of their OCD and tics, and all were severely ill at the time of treatment. The study showed that plasma exchange and IVIG were both effective for the treatment of severe, strep triggered OCD and tics, and that there were persistent benefits of the interventions. However, there were a number of side-effects associated with the treatments, including nausea, vomiting, headaches and dizziness. In addition, there is a risk of infection with any invasive procedure, such as these. Thus, the treatments should be reserved for severely ill patients, and administered by a qualified team of health care professionals.

(These and other helpful statements can be found on the NIMH website: http://www.nimh. nih.gov/health/publications/pandas/index.shtml.)

Of note, a separate study was conducted to evaluate the effectiveness of plasma exchange in the treatment of chronic OCD (Nicolson et al. 2000). None of the children benefited, suggesting that plasma exchange or intravenous immunoglobulin (IVIG) is not helpful for children who do not have strep-triggered OCD or tics.

Prodrome before tic onset

In some young children with unclear psychopathology (especially if someone in the family has tics) a question may be raised as to whether the symptoms or problems could be 'early Tourette syndrome' before any tics appear. This poses a conceptual problem, yet occasionally one encounters this idea: Tourette syndrome lurking as a malign but as yet unrevealed potential in the child's development. No evidence-based support has been forthcoming.

Personal responsibility?

Suppose a child's tics are neither exclusively voluntary or involuntary (so-called 'unvoluntary'), but when he gets into trouble in school he is not held responsible for his behavior because it's believed to be involuntary, and as he matures he knows this blanket excuse isn't valid. What then? Can and do patients sometimes fake their tics? Yes, it is possible. Also, what if a child or adolescent's symptoms are an alternative expression of negative emotions, as can happen in a 'conversion disorder' (Chapter 9)?

Premonitory sensations as a dependable distinguishing feature of tics

Do premonitory sensations that characterize most tics really distinguish them from other movement disorders as many textbooks and articles say (e.g. stereotypies)? Where is the evidence? Research to clarify this point is needed. Clinical examples to challenge this supposed dependability may be found in Chapter 11 and in Ricketts et al. (2013).

REFERENCES

Brilot F, Merheb V, Ding A, et al. (2011) Antibody binding to neuronal surface in Sydenham chorea, but not in PANDAS or Tourette syndrome. *Neurology* 76: 1508–13. doi: 10.1212/WNL.0b013e3182181090.

Chang K, Frankovich J, Cooperstock M, et al. (2014) Clinical evaluation of youth with pediatric acute onset neuropsychiatric syndrome (PANS): recommendations from the 2013 PANS Consensus Conference. *J Child Adolesc Psychopharm* (epub ahead of print). doi: 10.1089/cap.2014.0084.

Gabbay V, Coffey BJ, Babb JS, et al. (2008) Pediatric autoimmune neuropsychiatric disorders associated with streptococcus: comparison of diagnosis and treatment in the community and at a specialty clinic. *Pediatrics* 122: 273–8. doi: 10.1542/peds.2007-1307.

Kurlan R, Johnson D, Kaplan EL, Tourette Syndrome Study Group (2008) Streptococcal infection and exacerbations of childhood tics and obsessive–compulsive symptoms: a prospective blinded cohort study. *Pediatrics* 121: 1188–97. doi: 10.1542/peds.2007-2657.

Morris-Berry CM, Pollard M, Gao S, et al. (2013) Anti-streptococcal, tubulin, and dopamine receptor 2 antibodies in children with PANDAS and Tourette syndrome: single-point and longitudinal assessments. *J Immunol* 264: 106–13. doi: 10.1016/j.jneuroim.2013.09.010.

Murphy TK (2013) Infections and tic disorders. In: Martino D, Leckman JF, eds. *Tourette Syndrome.* New York: Oxford University Press, p. 168.

Murphy TK, Kurlan R, Leckman J (2010) The immunobiology of Tourette's disorder, pediatric autoimmune neuropsychiatric disorders associated with streptococcus, and related disorders: a way forward. *J Child Adolesc Psychopharmacol* 20: 317–31. doi: 10.1089.cap.2010.0043.

Murphy TK, Patel PD, McGuire JF, et al. (2014) Characterization of the pediatric acute-onset neuropsychiatric syndrome phenotype. *J Child Adolesc Psychopharmacol* (epub ahead of print). doi: 10.1089/cap. 2014-0062.

Nicolson R, Swedo SE, Lenane M, et al. (2000) An open trial of plasma exchange in childhood-onset obsessive–compulsive disorder without poststreptococcal exacerbations. *J Am Acad Child Adolesc Psychiatry* 39: 1313–5.

Ricketts EJ, Bauer CC, Van der Fluit F, et al. (2013) Behavior therapy for stereotypic movement disorder in typically developing children: a clinical case series. *Cog Behav Pract* 20: 544–55. doi: 10.1016/j.cbprac. 2013.03.002.

Shulman ST (2009) Pediatric autoimmune neuropsychiatric disorders associated with streptococci (PANDAS): update. *Curr Opin Pediatr* 21: 127–30.

Singer HS, Gilbert DL, Wolf DS, et al. (2012) Moving from PANDAS to CANS. *J Pediatr* 160: 725–31. doi: 10.1016/j.peds.2011.11.040.

20
REFRACTORY CASES

> There are sensible patient and medication factors to review if treatments continue to fail, as well as some form of consultation with those who are more expert or just have a different perspective. Sometimes a life change (of job or residence) may make a significant difference, or reduction in a source of psychological or social stress. More extreme cases may require deep brain stimulation or transcranial magnetic stimulation.

In any condition, treatment can fail. There are some general principles that apply to approaching this problem constructively.

- Review previous medications: how they were given, for how long, with what targets, how monitored, at what dosages, and with what side-effects.
- If the treatment was behavioral, was the therapist adequately trained for the appropriate approach, and was the relationship cordial and supportive?
- Has something been missed? Is there some stress that has not been identified?
- Obtain a consultation, even if only by phone or e-mail.
- From the behavioral standpoint, an excellent discussion focused upon 'complex and refractory cases' is available in McKay and Storch (2009).

In extremely serious cases with major impairment where everything has been given a good chance to succeed, more 'last resort' measures may be needed. These include electroconvulsive therapy (in the rare case where tics may be signs of catatonia: Dhossche et al. 2010), transcranial magnetic stimulation (Edwards et al. 2008, Steeves et al. 2012) and deep brain stimulation (Müller-Vahl et al. 2011, Steeves et al. 2012, Kim and Pouratian 2014). All of these require assessment and second opinions at an experienced tertiary center and are beyond the scope of this book.

Some serious and long-term problematic cases may do better with a change of occupational situation or residence, as in the following example.

> **Case example**
> *A 35-year-old man suffered from severe treatment-refractory tics, OCD, ADHD, anxiety disorder with panic attacks, and several medical problems as a result of a motor vehicle accident, after which his tics worsened. He became unable to work and subsisted on a small disability pension and his wife's employment. The reactions of others to his*

obvious tics added considerably to his sense of isolation. Follow-up after a move from the large city to a small town showed that he was much happier because he knew everyone and "They've become used to my tics. There aren't those surprises any more."

Comment: *Facing strangers had been a factor in maintaining a high stress level.*

REFERENCES

Dhossche DM, Reti IM, Shettar SM, Wachtel LE (2010) Tics as signs of catatonia: electroconvulsive therapy response in 2 men. *J ECT* 26: 266–9. doi: 10.1097/YCT.0b013e3181cb5f60.

Edwards MJ, Talelli P, Rothwell JC (2008) Clinical applications of transcranial magnetic stimulation in movement disorders. *Lancet Neurol* 7: 827–40. doi: 10.1016/S1474-4422(08)70190-X.

Kim W, Pouratian N (2014) Deep brain stimulation for Tourette syndrome. *Neurosurg Clin N Am* 25: 117–35. doi: 10.1016/j.nec.2013.08.009.

McKay D, Storch EA, eds (2009) *Cognitive Behavior Therapy for Children: Treating Complex and Refractory Cases*. New York: Springer.

Müller-Vahl KR, Cath DC, Cavanna AE, et al. (2011) European clinical guidelines for Tourette syndrome and other tic disorders. Part IV: Deep brain stimulation. *Eur Child Adolesc Psychiatry* 20: 209–17.

Steeves T, McKinlay BD, Gorman D, et al. (2012) Canadian guidelines for the evidence-based treatment of tic disorders: behavioural therapy, deep brain stimulation, and transcranial magnetic stimulation. *Can J Psychiatry* 57: 144–51.

21
SERVICE PROVISION: A FEW CONSIDERATIONS

The heterogeneous and dynamically varying aspects of tic disorders, especially in child-hood, make service provision challenging and conventional arrangements inadequate. The question of how to match services to the inherently variable course and content of tic upsurges and comorbidities has been mentioned before, but needs further exploration.

• The expertise of the clinician is likely to be very variable and probably limited because relatively few have concentrated their learning and experience in developmental disorders.

• Some access to a higher level of expertise may be or become necessary, but this may not be readily available, if at all. Reading material will be available, but sorting through it to find information directly applicable to your patient is onerous and can be frustrating.

• Treatment guidelines may have limited utility in unique predicaments.

• Community services may reject patients with significant tics outright, stating that they do not have the requisite expertise, or may fail to appreciate the variable role of tics in the patient's problems. A collaborative relationship between knowledgeable developmental disability experts and community services may offer the most practical solution.

• Encourage professional and service organizations dedicated to developmental disabilities or disorders to include (or increase) programs and in-service training that develops expertise in tic disorders. Participate in your national or regional Tourette syndrome organization.

• Finally, you should not despair. Take a broad view of the situation and try out some simple, straightforward and available interventions.

22
SUPPORT GROUPS

> Support groups are a valuable resource and are growing in importance. They offer patients and family members new ideas to improve their quality of life and reduce the sense of isolation that may follow the diagnosis. There may also be problems that one should be aware of.

Support groups are a common function of Tourette syndrome organizations, or may be independent. Like other service components they have potential benefits and harms.

Benefits include reducing a sense of isolation, that the child is a rare and freaky creature, and learning that one's struggles and occasional triumphs can be shared and appreciated. New ways of coping can be learned and suffering expressed. Many new child patients say that they know of no one else who has tics, though you may know that with the size of their school there must be some there, even with mild tics. Would it bring some relief from isolation to help them (in a planned way) meet someone with tics?

A downside can be that, in a mixed group of those recently diagnosed and those who have been attending for years, the newcomers may see and hear worse symptoms than their child has and fear that that is the future, or what is presented as typical by someone may be the result of complex comorbidity or special circumstances. Those who have had their symptoms for a considerable time and are doing well are less likely to attend than those dissatisfied with their progress and with more severe or complex symptoms.

One way to cope with the uncertainty is for parents to attend first, without their child, to assess the factors mentioned here. (Some larger organizations run support groups for parents without children, for children separately, or for adults only.)

Practice point

Encourage parents and adults who are interested in learning more about tics to join their national and local Tourette syndrome groups. For US residents, if they are competent in English they can profit from joining the Tourette Syndrome Association (USA) because of its highly developed newsletter and publications and can visit other Tourette syndrome group websites (see Appendix 3).

23
TIC DISORDERS AND THE LAW

> Persons with chronic tic disorders are not more likely to commit breaches of the law, but their unusual behavior may be subject to misunderstandings that can have serious consequences. The issue of the degree of voluntariness (voluntary, involuntary or semi-voluntary) may well arise and also be complicated by comorbidity and medication effects. A well-informed defense attorney with access to expert testimony may be crucial so that justice can be done.

If Tourette syndrome were an impulse control disorder (in the general sense, not just for tics), one would expect a significant increase in the rate of criminal acts and other breaches of the law. Insofar as is known, this is not the case. Such a finding would be complicated by the likelihood of proper identification as a person with the diagnosis of Tourette syndrome or other tic disorder, uncertainty as to comorbid disorders, and misunderstandings of the symptoms as purely voluntary or deliberate. The high rate of co-occurrence of ADHD and OCD would make a valid general statement about tic disorders highly problematic. Experience with hundreds of patients, many followed into adult life, does not suggest that persons with tic disorders are likely to be law-breakers. A more significant factor is the chance that a person with a tic disorder who is charged with an offense will be misunderstood and "at risk of potential mistreatment by the courts of justice" (Wright et al. 2012, p. 25). Justice demands the availability of a well-informed defense with access to expert information (Jankovic et al. 2006).

> **Case example**
> *'Tara' was 20 years old when she was charged with refusing to take a breathalyzer test by the police. Although she was driving, her boyfriend had been drinking and the officer smelled alcohol when they were stopped at a checkpoint during the night. When she failed to breathe out adequately, as directed, she was deemed uncooperative and she was not allowed to try again. She had had respiratory tics for years as part of her Tourette symptomatology, although not recently when her tics had mostly subsided. Under the stress of the situation her forced expiration was not smooth and sustained enough to complete the test satisfactorily. Provided with a full explanation, the court dismissed the charge, which could otherwise have had serious consequences.*

If a person with a tic disorder who is on maintenance medication for tics is initially incarcerated, his or her medication may not be immediately continued and the diagnosis may not be believed. The discontinuation and the new situational stress may result in a serious regression in symptom control and possibly mistreatment by other inmates or staff. The consequences of not correcting the problem may be serious but only the prescribing physician may be able to intervene to bring the regression under control.

Under stress, tics may temporarily increase. For instance, one may be questioned at an international border or when arriving at an airport in another country, and officers may profile (for further examination) people who are 'acting nervous'. A recent reality TV program centered on border security showed an example of two such persons asked "Why are you so nervous?"   one had tics, and the other was perspiring profusely (the officers did not consider tics or hyperhidrosis as health-related reasons). A person with a moderately severe tic disorder, aware of his or her tendency to have more tics in such situations, may find it useful to carry a physician's note to help ease such a situation.

There is a potential (and controversial) problem that is not usually discussed. That is the tendency of service organizations for tics and Tourette syndrome, the internet, many clinicians and parents to assert, in defining tics, that they are involuntary. This raises the always difficult issue of the degree of personal responsibility. How much of a 'free pass' does this give to a person with a tic disorder whose behavior interferes with others, and may violate their personal space by touching, poking, spitting and so forth? Are we to expect that after successful public education everyone will accept this, because they understand the person cannot help it? This subject has been discussed in Chapter 19. It should not be ignored.

REFERENCES

Jankovic J, Kwak C, Frankoff R (2006) Tourette's syndrome and the law. *J Neuropsychiatry Clin Neurosci* 18: 86–95.

Wright A, Rickards H, Cavanna AE (2012) Impulse-control disorders in Gilles de la Tourette syndrome. *J Neuropsychiatry Clin Neurosci* 24: 16–27. doi: 10.1176/appi.neuropsych.10010013.

24
TOURETTE SYNDROME, EMPLOYMENT AND INSURANCE

> Future employment opportunities and maintenance of employment in the face of significant or changing symptoms is a complex issue. Applications for insurance will often require signing a statement to the effect that all past health information has been provided. In childhood you cannot foresee whether honest replies about previous health on an application form will cause later problems for your child, nor can you assume that later explanations will remove or modify actuarial or employment policies.

Questions sometimes arise around a new tic disorder diagnosis: will it hurt one's employment chances or make it more difficult to obtain insurance later in life? This is especially commonly asked by parents about their child. It arises because of parental awareness about the public's misunderstandings about tics and Tourette syndrome, and especially because of the typically improving life course, which should be considered by anyone judging the patient later (but often isn't). In other words, if Tourette syndrome isn't likely to be limiting to the person as an adult, should one tell 'the whole truth' on an application? Advice on this question is not straightforward. In some places, like the USA, insurance eligibility or rates may depend upon 'telling the whole truth', because if you don't, a meticulous investigation of every medical/surgical event will unearth it and you may be denied coverage or be uprated. Such conditions vary by country and type of situation as well as by the standards required for some specific types of employment. Helpful publications are available through some service organizations such as Tourettes Action in the UK (www.tourettes-action.org.uk) that contain very useful ideas for employers and employees, and include country-specific legal provisions (Shady et al. 1995).

Although it may be true that some progress is being made in public and clinician education, this is slow and uneven, and cannot be expected to solve the problem by the time the child is at an age when a job application may be made; even then, the complexity and variability within the diagnosis will remain an issue.

Explaining to parents that one needn't tell "the whole truth" because by that time the condition will likely be minimal in its impact and those requiring the information "aren't really referring to something like that" is unwise because one cannot safely make such an assumption.

In other different situations tics may cause difficulty on a job because of misunderstanding of tics or of tic severity that is causing disturbance to co-workers or the public.

Three case examples

The first adult, a firefighter, had significant tics remaining (as well as some ADHD) that in themselves were not affecting his job, but he still required medication which appeared to be causing tremor. This became more obvious when he was under stress, and lately it had been noticed by others when he was working in a major accident situation. He did better when switched from pimozide to aripiprazole.

The second adult wanted to join a police force. In order to accomplish this he had to fill out a form and also submit to a polygraph test; he was worried that he would fail the test if he did not tell 'the whole truth' about his childhood diagnosis of Tourette syndrome. In his case having the diagnosis would not exclude him from joining the force, provided he could provide a medical opinion to the effect that his tics would not render him unsuitable for the job. This was provided; he was accepted for training and completed it successfully, becoming a fully fledged officer.

The third adult had applied for, and been accepted for, employment as a teacher. Before starting his new position there was a very widely publicized case of murder by a person diagnosed with Tourette syndrome, OCD and ADHD. The diagnostic categories were invoked by lawyers on both sides to bolster their case. The job offer to the patient was withdrawn during the period when the murder case was in the public eye, a clear case of prejudice.

Finally, it should be said that adults with obvious residual tics have been successfully employed as police, firefighters, border guards, prison guards, physicians, teachers and lawyers. Whether they had difficulty in obtaining and maintaining their job is not always known, nor the status of their tics at the time of application.

REFERENCE

Shady G, Broder R, Staley D, et al. (1995) Tourette syndrome and employment: descriptors, predictors, and problems. *Psychiatr Rehab J* 19: 35–42.

25

AND NOW FOR SOMETHING COMPLETELY DIFFERENT

> Tics represent deviation from the norm and therefore pathology, even when they may not be very noticeable or cause impairment. So it is a change of assumption to realize that sometimes tics — or their result — can be positive or appreciated for highly individual reasons. At least their potentially manipulative function should be appreciated as a possibility. It can be enlightening to ask your patient whether he or she would actually like to have *all* tics gone for good.

We have already seen in the chapter on stereotypic movement disorder (Chapter 11) that one of its common features is that its practitioners like it and may feel they need it or are more creative when doing it (regardless of what others think about it), and furthermore that its form has been developed out of early experimentation with the creation of an altered mental state. Is it possible that this could apply to some other repetitive patterns, at least some of the time? Yes, it has been shown in the quotation in Chapter 12 from Rohinton Mistry (p. 166) that this can be true of an RMB. In Chapters 7 and 17 we saw that for 'Joshua' his dangerous SIB-causing tic was used partly to control his parents. So we may entertain the possibility (virtually never mentioned) that tics might sometimes come to be valued for their effect. Here is another example.

> **Case example**
> *A boy of 10 with Tourette syndrome, OCD and anxiety developed a marked fear of intruders in his home when his parents were away. He modified one of his vocal tics to be more like a loud honking of a goose and explained that he then felt safer because an intruder would realize that there was someone in the house and go away. However, a few days later he noted that he was making this new tic outside of his home at other times. That awareness re-awakened his specific fear and horrific images, so he no longer felt that the tic was a successful defense.*
>
> ***Comment:*** *This is one example of the functional complexity of a tic involving interaction between environmental and emotional factors.*

Tics have a potential manipulative power and the capability to confuse others as to one's motives. This bears further exploration, particularly because it is traditionally believed that if there is an effect of tics it is negative and the attitude toward tics is always negative. It seems that there has been no study of this factor, but such should be simple to design and perform.

26
SOME PROBLEMS TICS CAN CAUSE FOR OTHERS

Specialists have several obstacles in dealing with persons with Tourette syndrome. First is the lack of time; second, the unfortunate fact that training usually includes little about tics. Third, specialists may not ask about symptoms in any part of the body outside of their area of expertise. To not miss a possibly important role of one or more tics, questions must be asked. Lastly, examination may require the patient (or a part of the patient's body) to remain still during the examination or procedure. Failure to do this may be interpreted as willful behaviour and may lead to injury or to future patient anxiety because of being (or feeling) blamed for involuntary movements.

Otolaryngology

In 1989 Fred Kozak, I and our co-workers published the first article on Tourette syndrome in the English ear, nose and throat literature (Kozak et al. 1989). Since then our experience has broadened. 'Cough' clinics have been established in recent years. Only some of them recognize that a 'cough' can be a respiratory tic. Uncontrollable movements during examination or procedures, especially if not anticipated, can cause injury and a negative interaction between surgeon and patient. Vocal tics can be caused by — or confused with — gastroesophageal reflux, which is itself not always easy to diagnose and treat (Richter 2004). In some instances it may be appropriate to institute a trial of treatment for gastroesophageal reflux disorder before assuming that a symptom is a tic. Quite odd sounds and symptoms that may seem to fall into an otolaryngologist's area may occur.

Ophthalmology/optometry

Eye-related tics are common, but contrariwise, eye 'twitches', which almost everyone has sometimes, are usually not tics. These are termed 'benign ocular myokymia' and sometimes 'fasciculations', though sometimes a distinction is made between these two.

Brief blepharospasm was the most frequent eye manifestation in an ophthalmologic study of 16 children (Tatlipinar et al. 2001), but 'involuntary gaze deviation' was also found. Typically the urge to move the eyes includes the felt need to reach the maximum deviation in each direction, causing muscle soreness in some patients, especially when the tic's onset is recent. The brief relief from the unpleasant urge is not sufficient when the eye is deviated less than fully.

Eye infections from rubbing or touching the eyelids are sometimes seen.

Sudden unanticipated movements of patients with Tourette syndrome can pose a risk of injury during eye examination. Margo (2002) described two such instances in adults and recommended 'mental preparedness' for such situations.

The possibility that an eye condition or behavior is caused by tics can often be clarified by asking about tics or 'repetitive twitches' of muscles in other parts of the body.

Allergy

Allergic symptoms can trigger or exacerbate tics. Some specific distinctions are hard to make. Sniffing, for instance, could be caused by allergies, or by a tic. If a tic, it is likely to be associated with others or to occur in a specific or unusual pattern. One child, for example, had a regular 'cough–sniff' sequence.

Respirology

A 'cough' can be a respiratory tic. Sometimes this has been termed a 'habit cough' and not realized to be a tic (Irwin et al. 2006). At other times 'atypical asthma' may be diagnosed, itself a controversial subject, and treated unnecessarily. Various interruptions in the pattern of inspiration and expiration may be encountered. Respiratory tics might interfere with tests of pulmonary function.

Orthopedic surgery

Pain can be the result of pushing joints to extreme positions. New tics can produce soreness. In rare cases fractures of the clavicle (Yamada et al. 2004), ribs or spine (Isaacs et al. 2010) have been reported. Further references may be found in Chapter 12 in the section on SIBs. Conservative measures are indicated, at least initially.

Dermatology

Excoriations, bruising, and variations of skin-picking may be seen (Jankovic and Sekula 1998). This is not unique to Tourette syndrome, and can occur in OCD. Lip-licking, already discussed in Chapter 12, can be quite troublesome. There is an association with trichotillomania.

Many drugs used in neuropsychiatry may have dermatologic side-effects (Mitkov et al. 2014), the result of which may be a need to change medications. For antipsychotics used in treating tics, skin rash was reported in 0.3%, as well as pigmentary and photosensitivity effects (Mitkov et al. 2014). This paper has a list of drug-related cutaneous reactions.

Education

It is very important to not attribute every problem to Tourette syndrome, such as anger, learning and behavior problems. Another pitfall is to interpret tics as deliberate, as if they must be one or the other (involuntary or 'behavioral'). This seems especially likely with noise-making or touching.

Teachers without in-depth understanding of tics may be vulnerable to misunderstanding because the information provided by child, parents or printed materials may be in error.

In complex situations, schools may have to ask for permission to contact the clinician, and recognizing the importance of the school experience, clinicians should be willing to act in this capacity, bearing in mind that communications between clinician and school should always include parents.

New or apparently new tics may seem to 'appear' in school because former active suppression has become less effective or a comorbid disorder's symptoms have entered the picture.

In rare instances deaf children with Tourette syndrome may manifest coprolalia in sign language (Morris et al. 2000, Rickards 2001). Special education teachers should be aware of this possibility that may require the assistance of a native signer to determine.

Dentistry and dental hygiene
'Keeping still' can be a problem, and since many patients have head-shaking or mouth-opening as part of their repertoire of tics, they may be blamed for their involuntary movements, contributing to their fear of dentists and dental hygienists. It needs to be recognized by dentists that the patient's very awareness that he or she should not move may paradoxically aggravate the problem. Also, sensitivity may be more marked (Stein et al. 2011) and be conducive to SIB (Friedlander and Cummings 1992, Leksell and Edvardson 2005). The latter authors were the first specialists to suspect Tourette syndrome in a 4-year-old girl with self-extraction of teeth and resulting dental pain as a consequence of her tics.

Dentists need to be aware that a patient's unwanted sudden movements may be due to a tic disorder, and this can include biting of a dentist's finger. It is highly desirable for medical clinicians whose patients have tic disorders to communicate with dentists and orthodontists about unwanted movements but also about effects of medication, SIB, speech peculiarities and bruxism.

Practice point
Medical clinicians should communicate with dentists and orthodontists about tic patients whose tics or associated disorders or symptoms may affect dental care. Communication in the other direction can also be helpful, as when dental work changes intraoral perceptions and may trigger new tics, or there are interactions between local anesthetics and medications the patient is taking.

Another concern is that vasoconstrictors in local anesthetics may interact with medications the patient is taking, the latter medications causing hypotension in some instances. Preoperative consideration needs to be given to this point (Yoshikawa et al. 2002).

Bruxism is a complex and confusing area (Lobbezoo et al. 2013); temporomandibular joint syndrome may result and produce pain (Huynh et al. 2013). Abnormal tooth wear and jaw muscle tenderness may occur; bed partner sleep may be impaired by the noise. Certain drugs have been reported to be conducive to the development of sleep bruxism, including antipsychotics, amphetamines and SSRIs (Huynh et al. 2013). Masseter muscle hypertrophy may be seen. Jaw-cracking can be like a tic and can produce secondary symptoms.

Orthodontic appliances, adjustments and temporary fillings are examples of situations in which the patient may detect (at least initially) a change in the way his or her mouth feels, and this can be a trigger for a new tic or SIB.

In 2013 Dr John Walkup, Former Chair of the TSA Medical Advisory Board, was awarded a research grant by the TSA to perform a randomized controlled trial of an oral orthotic device claimed to be effective in ameliorating the effects of Tourette syndrome and being offered by some dentists in Canada and the USA.

Speech and language pathology

Given that vocalizations are a necessary criterion for the diagnosis of Tourette syndrome, one would think that there should be many studies and publications reflecting research on this topic. But no, there are only a handful. There are several on stuttering and dysfluency (Abwender et al. 1998, Van Borsel and Vanryckeghem 2000, Van Borsel et al. 2004, De Nil et al. 2005; see also Chapter 12).

Special situations

The unpredictable nature of many tics provides challenges, of which only a few can be mentioned here. Unusual stress leading to temporarily increased tics may be a factor.

Airline travel presents several possibilities: personnel in charge have the power to make instant decisions as to who can board a flight when there is a question as to problem behavior and safety; and delayed flights, long flights with little opportunity for sleep, and changed seating due to aircraft substitutions can all increase tics in some persons. If this is a possibility, carrying a letter from a doctor may be of help when a decision needs to be made by the flight crew. This also applies to children with unusual behavior likely to be misunderstood. Prearranged seating to avoid bothering the passenger sitting in front of the child may be arranged by the physician involved.

Case example

An adult with Tourette syndrome was going on a very long flight to take a temporary job in another country. He had the opportunity to carry a medical letter with him, but declined to do so. His flight encountered a considerable departure delay. The associated stress led to an increase in his vocal tics that led to airline personnel questioning him; the added stress resulted in a resurgence of a spitting tic which was perceived as an attack upon airline personnel. He was refused boarding and became increasingly agitated, with a final result of being denied subsequent travel.

Comment: It is possible that carrying a doctor's letter could have prevented this unfortunate escalation.

There are situations where a person's ability to sit still may pose trouble; one aspect, injury, has already been mentioned. Others that have occurred because the tics were misunderstood have involved barbers, hairdressers and podiatrists. Although no case has come to light, one can also imagine a problem with tattooing. Standing in line waiting patiently for service may expose a person with tics to the ire of others waiting who take the tics as impatience and an effort to gain unfair attention.

When a person has loud vocal tics, attendance at a concert or cinema or at a quiet restaurant may cause trouble, and considerations of 'rights' may arise. Attempts to explain the interruptions to strangers en masse cannot generally succeed. In considering staying away, rather than becoming angry that Tourette syndrome is being specifically targeted, one can point out that it is not only vocal tics that cause such discrimination: a person with a bad cold or bronchitis will have the same difficulty in having the noises tolerated by others, for the same reasons.

REFERENCES

Abwender DA, Trinidad KS, Jones KR, et al. (1998) Features resembling Tourette's syndrome in developmental stutterers. *Brain Lang* 62: 455–64. doi: 10.1006/brln.1998.1948.

De Nil LF, Sasisekaran J, Van Lieshout PHHM, Sandor P (2005) Speech disfluencies in individuals with Tourette syndrome. *J Psychosom Res* 58: 97–102. doi: 10.1016/j.jpsychores.2004.06.002.

Friedlander AH, Cummings JL (1992) Dental treatment of patients with Gilles de la Tourette's syndrome. *Oral Surg Oral Med Oral Pathol* 73: 299–303.

Huynh MT, Emami E, HelmanJI, Chervin RD (2013) Interaction between sleep disorders and oral diseases. *Oral Dis* 20: 236–45. doi: 10.1111/odi.12152.

Irwin RS, Glomb WB, Chang AB (2006) Habit cough, tic cough, and psychogenic cough in adult and pediatric populations: ACCP evidence-based clinical practice guidelines. *Chest* 129: 174S–179S.

Isaacs JD, Adams M, Lees AJ (2010) Noncompressive myelopathy associated with violent axial tics of Tourette syndrome. *Neurology* 74: 697–8.

Jankovic J, Sekula S (1998) Dermatological manifestations of Tourette syndrome and obsessive–compulsive disorder. *Arch Dermatol* 134: 113–4.

Kozak F, Freeman RD, Connolly JE, Riding KH (1989) Tourette syndrome and otolaryngology. *J Otolaryngol* 18: 279–82.

Leksell E, Edvardson S (2005) A case of Tourette syndrome presenting with oral self-injurious behaviour. *Int J Paediatr Dentistry* 15: 370–4. doi: 10.1111/j.1365-263X.2005.00652.x.

Lobbezoo F, Ahlberg J, Glaros AG, et al. (2013) Bruxism defined and graded: an international consensus. *J Oral Rehabil* 40: 2–4. doi: 10.1111/joor.12011.

Margo CE (2002) Tourette syndrome and iatrogenic eye injury. *Am J Ophthalmol* 134: 784–5.

Mitkov MV, Trowbridge RM, Lockshin BN, Caplan JP (2014) Dermatologic side-effects of psychotropic medications. *Psychosomatics* 55: 1–20. doi: 10.1016/j.psym.2013.07.003.

Morris HR, Thacker AJ, Newman PK, Lees AJ (2000) Sign language tics in a prelingually deaf man. *Mov Disord* 15: 318–20. doi: 10.1002/1531-8257(200003).

Richter JE (2004) Ear, nose and throat and respiratory manifestations of gastro-esophageal reflux disease: an increasing conundrum. *Eur J Gastroenterol Hepatol* 16: 837–45.

Rickards H (2001) Signing coprolalia and attempts to disguise in a man with prelingual deafness. *Mov Disord* 16: 790–1. doi: 10.1002/mds.1158.

Stein LI, Polido JC, Mailloux Z, et al. (2011) Oral care and sensory sensitivities in children with autism spectrum disorders. *Spec Care Dentist* 31: 102–10.

Tatlipinar S, Iener EC, Ilhan B, Semerci B (2001) Ophthalmic manifestations of Gilles de la Tourette syndrome. *Eur J Ophthalmol* 11: 223–6.

Van Borsel J, Vanryckeghem M (2000) Dysfluency and phonic tics in Tourette syndrome: a case report. *J Commun Disord* 33: 227–39. doi: 10.1016/S0021-9924(00)00020-4.

Van Borsel J, Goethals L, Vanryckeghem M (2004) Dysfluency in Tourette syndrome: observational study in three cases. *Folia Phoniatr Logop* 56: 358–66. doi: 10.1159/000081083.

Yamada K, Sugiura H, Suzuki Y (2004) Stress fracture of the medial clavicle secondary to nervous tic. *Skeletal Radiol* 33: 534–6. doi: 10.1007/s00256-004-0766-x.

Yoshikawa F, Takagi T, Fukayama H, et al. (2002) Intravenous sedation and general anesthesia for a patient with Gilles de la Tourette's syndrome undergoing dental treatment. *Acta Anaesthesiol Scand* 46: 1279–80. doi: 10.1034/j.1399-6576.2002.461018.x.

27
CODA

It is time for some final thoughts.

Tics are a challenge to our clinical and research skills because their essence seems unknowable owing to the very high frequency of associated symptoms and disorders, and the mixture of observable and unobservable phenomena that they entail. Their relationship to other repetitive and stereotypic behaviors is complex and may be too often neglected in clinical thinking. Grasping the role that tics and other features play in a person's life is rarely straightforward and often requires experience, engagement, time and an openness to revise one's conclusions.

Two important cautions must not be forgotten: (1) Tourette syndrome is unusual in that no impairment is necessary for the diagnosis; and (2) some movements seen, heard or reported may not be tics. The implications are that impairment or distress may not result directly from the tics themselves; other factors such as tic tolerance must be considered; and the presence of non-tic repetitive behaviors may bring the diagnosis into doubt or cause confusion.

It seems that many of our patients are not well enough attuned to their sensations and experiences to describe them. With encouragement, more may be formulated and shared. A proverbial 'goldmine' of clinical nuggets then awaits the prepared mind.

The changing nature of childhood tics and the accompanying problems make the school situation crucial for the quality of life of many children. At the same time, the complexity of schools poses a challenge to clinicians who should give schooling a high priority in their thinking but rarely have time to understand the setting and the interactions that take place there.

The comorbidity of most patients entails a very large number of symptoms and some overlapping category boundaries. Once you assign the categories, circular reasoning can then 'explain' any symptom by referring back to the category definitions and descriptions. This is loose thinking of which one should beware.

While research continues to find causal factors in neurodevelopmental disorders, treatment effects remain generally modest. This situation has a corollary that needs to be appreciated: small improvements can be made that have small effect sizes, but in the aggregate can with high probability tip the developmental balance and make a difference.

Finally, for many clinicians and their patients, time is the enemy. The case for flexible support (and sometimes treatment) in consonance with the often dramatic and irregular symptoms in chronic tic disorders — especially in children and adolescents — has been made. Yes, most of their tics will improve by the time they are adults, but what will their childhood and adolescence have been like? When lack of sufficient time (for whatever reason) prevents these needs being met, health care falls far short of its ideals. The recent revolution in carefully planned behavioral research and intervention bodes well for the future, but has barely begun, and can be expected to inform — and be informed by — neuro-biological, genetic, phenomenological and narrative discoveries.

If you have interest, curiosity and of course time, there is more to learn from persons with Tourette syndrome (and those with lesser versions of it) than meets the eye or ear. Although motor and vocal tics are the most obvious elements, and have received most atten-tion, the associated urges (and their awareness or lack thereof) and the lived experiences are relatively neglected or totally ignored. Only some clinicians will take an opportunity to pursue this aspect wherever it may lead, but all should be aware that there is much more involved than what we call tics.

The goals advocated in this book have been developed and are supported by a logical and coherent view of the usual natural course of tic disorders and how they are experienced by those who encounter them as patients, significant others, and society at large. It is fur-thermore argued that these goals rightly belong to medicine as a whole and to our under-standing of the nature of human suffering. Rather than utopian, the unspoken moral stance taken is to reflect the famous old saying attributed to Hippocrates, "to cure sometimes, to harm never, to comfort always", which, while apparently simple, requires repeated contem-plation. Although 'cure' is still beyond our reach, there has been substantial improvement in understanding and care for persons with tics over the past 45 years, well illustrated by the 'Then and Now' cases in Appendix 2.

This book began with a confession, and will close with another. For some 10 years I have been collecting information and experience to complete this book. In that time I have felt myself become better attuned to what I am told and observe, yet, in a clinic waiting room where my patients and their parents are exposed to the jerking, hooting and other tics of other patients, never — *not once* — have I thought to ask them when they accompany me to my office: "What is that like for you?" I have no idea why this has eluded me when now it seems so obvious, but perhaps it is an indication of how much is happening of which I, and perhaps you, dear reader, can be unaware.

There is much to be done, but while awaiting those benefits, however great they turn out to be, much that has already been learned can be better applied and even more awaits our careful attention. In the words of TS Eliot, "We shall not cease from exploration, and the end of all our exploring will be to arrive where we started and know the place for the first time" (*Little Gidding*, Four Quartets).

Appendix 1
How Accurate is Information on the Internet?

Since most parents cannot resist the temptation to 'educate' themselves about tics, it's usually safe to assume that they have availed themselves of information on the internet. Reichow et al. (2013) evaluated the characteristics and quality of websites providing information about developmental disabilities. Those sites were best that were not sponsored by a for-profit company, did not contain advertisements, and had a top-level domain of *.gov* or *.org*. However, parents and patients need to be vigilant. Table A1.1 shows a list of the inaccuracies (by category) found in a survey of the first 35 websites accessed.

It is easy for clinicians to be critical of information that has such uneven value, but it is only fair to appreciate that presenting balanced, comprehensive information about tics that also includes the often-related comorbidities is a daunting task.

TABLE A1.1
Websites showing errors in describing Tourette syndrome (n=35)

Item	n	Comments
Genetic/familial disorder	8	
Vocal or phonic or verbal?	7	
Frequency of coprolalia	6	
Stimulant drugs for ADHD	5	
Ignore tics (or else…)	5	
Prognosis; worst-ever time	4	
Diagnostic categories, criteria	4	
Prevalence of tics	3	
Comorbidity; relation to symptoms	2	
Tics continue in sleep?	2	Confidently asserted: no
Symptoms included as vocal tics	2	Sniffing, whistling
Medications for tics, OCD, ADHD	2	
Coprolalia always shouting, loud	2	No site said that coprolalia could be a minor symptom
Causes of tics	1	
PANDAS	1	
Rages	1	No indication that comorbidity, especially ADHD, is typical
Cures via CAM	1	

ADHD, attention-deficit/hyperactivity disorder; OCD, obsessive–compulsive disorder; PANDAS, pediatric autoimmune neuropsychiatric disorders associated with streptococcal infections; CAM, complementary/alternative medicine.

REFERENCE

Reichow B, Shefcyk A, Bruder MB (2013) Quality comparison of websites related to developmental disabilities. *Res Dev Disabil* 34: 3077–83. doi: 10.1016/j.ridd.2013.06.013.

Appendix 2
Then and Now

It isn't often that a clinician has the opportunity to review his files from 45–50 years ago, but in my case (perhaps due to a touch of hoarding?) retention of some old case records has enabled a partial analysis of changes in how some children with Tourette syndrome and their parents were understood and treated, insofar as these were reflected in the reports.

Example 1

'Alan' was 13 and was receiving psychotherapy weekly with a community child psychiatrist for his multiple tics. He was referred and admitted to hospital 'to rule out organic factors'. The therapist wanted him to be separated from his parents because his tics worsened when he returned to them from a trip. The boy described his tics as always worse at night, and that they hurt. Tics were most obvious in the interview when he started talking about entering high school in the near future. The tics were interpreted as the result of psychological conflict involving family and other factors.

*   ***Treatment recommendation:*** *No organic factors identified; referred back to his therapist for further psychotherapy.*

Example 2

'Anton', a 12-year-old boy with tics of fluctuating severity, had been seen previously in both clinic and private psychiatric practice. He was described as sensitive, overly affectionate with his parents, and had a parting ritual at bedtime. He was quite indecisive in the interview. Impression: "nothing to indicate a true Gilles de la Tourette syndrome"; "a mixed compulsive-tic picture."

*   ***Treatment recommendation:*** *A more intensive course of psychotherapy "although even that would not guarantee any benefit." Because of the severity of his tics, haloperidol, 1mg/d, was started and in a few days this was increased to 2mg/d. Anton developed an acute dystonic reaction (about which the parents had been warned), requiring intravenous diphenhydramine.*

Example 3

'Blaine', age 11, was referred with constipation, enuresis and possible Tourette syndrome. Many kinds of tics had begun at age 5; medications tried were unhelpful, and he was diagnosed elsewhere as having "chorea of unknown etiology". During some runs of tics he was described as "out of contact" and therefore was also diagnosed with "petit mal epilepsy". Again no medication was helpful. He showed difficulty focusing, was slow to give answers, and had reading difficulty. He described tension building up before the tics, which was worse with any kind of excitement. He had throat-clearing "but no vocalization". Several EEGs were done, one of which showed nonspecific abnormalities. His father reported that he himself had had worse tics; he was observed in the interview to have a "nervous tic". The parents were confused by the diagnosis of chorea and epilepsy. John said he hated school. The school's impression was of intellectual disability, but psychological testing showed average intelligence with "no organic signs".

*   ***Treatment recommendation:*** *Psychotherapy. After receiving psychotherapy he was better for 4 months; the tics then returned, psychotherapy was resumed, and then the tics recurred. The neurologist included in his impressions that "there are many suspicious psychogenic factors and a history of improvement with psychiatric care". Note that throat-clearing was not considered a vocal tic.*

Example 4

'Blake', age 8, was first seen at age 5 at another hospital, and after an admission of 11 days there was diagnosed with "St Vitus' Dance" secondary to acute rheumatic fever (he had had numerous throat infections). Complex tics followed an infection and there was a past history of febrile seizures. He showed whole-body jerking, foot stamping, mouth opening, loud screaming and "barking like a dog". He was then diagnosed at a second hospital with "Sydenham chorea, emotional disturbance and multiple tics". Admitted to our hospital, he had an electroencephalogram and skull radiograph, then was referred for psychiatric help. While watching TV he'd repeat the last word said. His mother seemed overprotective. His father had tics, and played down Blake's tics, which were said to be "much worse when the parents argue". His tested IQ was 92, classified as "borderline retarded". His father felt that his admission to several hospitals with several diagnoses had affected Blake. Psychotherapy had been recommended but it seemed that this had not been pursued. His father "appeared to be hostile and bitter". Blake showed tangential thinking in interviews. He was felt to fit Gilles de la Tourette's description: "borderline psychotic with organic factors in the past"

Treatment recommendation: *"...urgent psychotherapy to avoid a full-blown psychosis, and casework help for the parents to reduce factors obviously stimulating him towards further disintegration of his personality."*

Comment: *There is an acceptance here of Tourette's original conclusion that tics progress into psychosis. The confusion about his intellectual level and how the hospitalizations had affected him were not explored according to the report.*

Example 5

'Bruce', an only child who was born preterm, was 8 years old when admitted to our hospital after being excluded from school for defiance, making noises and acting restless. The referring clinic wanted evaluation of his "neurologic cerebral damage in association with behavioral problems". Tics were not mentioned as such, rather "bizarre movements of the hands, head and feet". He repeated first grade and developed "vulgar language" at age 7, which was very distressing to the family and resulted in corporal punishment. This was apparently followed by a number of different tics including coughing, grunting, kissing sounds, sucking, spitting, eye-blinking, eyebrow-raising, facial grimacing, poking his mouth, and stabbing, punching and licking movements that never actually connected. He appeared distractible and fidgety. In play he had marked aggressive fantasies. His mother was anxious about his preterm birth and was perfectionistic, like her family. It was felt that she had infantilized him. There was conflict in the family about how to manage his symptoms. Bruce's tics were interpreted (by me) as growing out of aggressive impulses and defenses against them, "as he is able to stop just short of hitting or kicking." I made the diagnosis of Tourette syndrome, "a rather unusual condition". Sydenham chorea was ruled out by cardiology consultation. Psychological testing revealed average intelligence and immature emotional control with "a suspicion of organicity" and a strong recommendation for psychotherapy and a comment that "the pathognomonic coprolalia has not been observed here."

Comment: *The movements that just missed their apparent goal made a plausible case for conflict over unacceptable aggressive impulses; this common feature of Tourette syndrome was not generally known at the time, nor was the association of tics with 'perfectionism'. The concept of 'organicity' was extremely vague as was the role and efficacy of psychotherapy.*

Impressive is the focus on psychological or psychogenic factors. Characteristics that we would see today as typical of most cases (waxing/waning symptoms, tics worse at the end of the day, positive family history especially in males, echolalia, multiple factors) played no role in understanding. There was no knowledge about the natural history of Tourette syndrome, so parents were not given any positive or reassuring information. Tourette's original criteria, including impending psychosis, were still lurking in the background. What parents did receive, when symptoms were prominent (whether mixed with other disorders or symptoms or not), were

- Varying diagnoses of the tics, often with sometimes prolonged hospitalizations
- Tic upsurges were attributed to psychological factors, by the neurologist as well

- Parental frustrations were not understood as possibly a reaction to prolonged iatrogenic confusion; any anger on their part was thought to reflect a causative psychogenic factor of the tics; little or nothing was said about the unique family situation or medical encounters in which the tics were occurring
- Treatment was always to be individual and family psychotherapy, but no actual case formulation was presented that would justify this approach
- No mention was made of the importance of school understanding or support
- Only one medication was available at the time, and the dosage was increased too aggressively (by current practice), causing a dystonic reaction in one case.

It is interesting that at a meeting, Prof. René Cruchet, a French neurologist, advocated that: "In general, one must remove tiqueurs, especially if children, from their environment. I always advise parents to allow me to admit the child into my hospital service for nervous and abnormal children at Bouscat, near Bordeaux for a month or two" (Wilson 1927, p. 107).

In a book by two highly respected pediatricians, *The Child and His Symptoms* (1968), Apley and Mac Keith included a section on tics. Tics were seen as psychosomatic and an indicator of deep-seated psychological problems based in the family. "Underlying tension nearly always exists, though in some cases it is deeply hidden" (p. 123). The diagnosis required the presence of emotional disturbance, and they even went so far as to say that "in a happy, secure child tics are never serious and do not persist... The tic acts as a motor release for emotional tension" (p. 123).

Our situation now seems to have significantly advanced: children are rarely hospitalized for tics, the diagnosis is often made quickly once the specialist is seen; although the etiology isn't known in detail, biological and genetic factors are invoked with psychological stresses understood as secondary modifiers; the typical course and characteristics of Tourette syndrome are used to make a formulation and are interpreted to the family, and if treatment of tics is needed, psychodynamic psychotherapy is not invoked as a directly curative approach. The school's understanding is considered important, and modified if necessary. The usual prognosis is for improvement in the tics during and after adolescence. This radically alters parent counseling.

Having said this, can we predict with any confidence what a future clinician will see as advances from our current position? I think not.

REFERENCES

Apley J, Mac Keith R (1968) *The Child and His Symptoms: a Comprehensive Approach, 2nd edn.* Oxford: Blackwell Scientific.

Wilson SAK (1927) The tics and allied conditions. *J Neurol Psychopathol* 8: 93–108.

APPENDIX 3
Web Resources

If you don't explore the innovative and useful projects and services being developed around the world by Tourette syndrome organizations, you're really missing the action! These organizations and groups are now starting to use social media as well.

USA

Tourette Syndrome Association (TSA): www.tsa-usa.org
• Through its partnership with the US Centers for Disease Control and Prevention, the TSA has developed a number of important initiatives including the CBIT treatment concept and evidence base. The TSA's Behavioral Science Consortium provides the Tourette syndrome Behavior Therapy Institute (TS-BTI) that is filling gaps in the availability of clinicians trained in this new and important approach.
• The TSA's Medical Advisory Board and Scientific Advisory Board have traditionally had Canadian members in addition to Americans, but have recently added Dr Andrea Cavanna (Birmingham, UK), so now have a European reach as well.
• Consortium for Genetics, grants.
• Medication trials.
• Youth Ambassador Program, bringing young people aged 13–17 years to Washington, DC, to advocate for Tourette syndrome with their representatives.
• Deep brain stimulation, international database of around 70 researchers (see website).
• National neuroimaging group.
• Newsletter, videos, books; brochures on advocacy, airline travel, aging, bullying, employment, college and university entrance, dating, housing, military service, ticcing in public, and sports.

NIH re PANDAS: www.nimh.nih.gov/health/publications/pandas/index.shtml

Leslie Packer (US psychologist specializing in TS+): www.tourettesyndrome.net
• An excellent and informative website.

Canada

Tourette Canada (formerly Tourette Syndrome Foundation of Canada): www.tourette.ca
• Online videos, DVDs, books, brochures, *Green Leaflet* (a triannual news magazine produced in French and English), annual conference, discussion forum, social media, regional and provincial chapters and support.

Europe

European Society for the Study of Tourette Syndrome: www.tourette-eu.org

Austria

Gilles de la Tourette Syndrom Österreich: www.tourette.at

Belgium

Vlaamse Vereniging Gilles de la Tourette: www.tourette.be (Flemish)

Denmark

Dansk Tourette Forening: www.tourette.dk

France

Association Française du Syndrome de Gilles de la Tourette (AFSGT): www.france-tourette.org

Germany

Tourette Gesellschaft Deutschland: www.tourette-gesellschaft.de
• Has excellent materials, several comprehensive books for clinicians and books for parents and persons with Tourette syndrome, and a newsletter.

Iceland

Tourette-samtökin á Íslandi: www.tourette.is

Ireland

http://www.tsireland.ie

Italy

Associazone Sindrome di Tourette Siamo in Tanti: www.sindromeditourette.it

Netherlands

www.tourette.nl

Norway

Norsk Tourette Forening: www.touretteforeningen.no

Spain

Asociación Española para Pacientes con Tics y Síndrome de Tourette: www.astourette.com

Switzerland

Tourette Gesellschaft Schweiz: www.tourette.ch

UK

Tourettes Action–UK: www.tourettes-action.org.uk
• Informative website with description of their help line, camps, job assistance, research blog, publications, video talks, an online forum, presentation materials for adults, primary and secondary schools, and much more. Covers England, Wales and Northern Ireland; for Scotland, see:

Tourette Scotland: www.tourettescotland.org

Touretteshero: www.touretteshero.com
• Website co-founded by Jessica Thom, a woman with Tourette syndrome, aiming to provide "a place to celebrate the humour and creativity of Tourettes … reclaiming the most frequently misunderstood syndrome on the planet and … changing the world one tic at a time".

Australia

TSA of Australia: www.tourette.org.au

Other disorders (selected examples)

OCD: International OCD Foundation: www.ocfoundation.org
• Has a distinguished Scientific Advisory Board with excellent material and a very informative newsletter.

ADHD: CHADD (Children and Adults with Attention-Deficit/Hyperactivity Disorder): www.chadd.org
• *Caveat:* their website allows advertising of a wide variety of 'natural' remedies (herbal, homeopathic) and video/computer games, with 'proven' results supported by testimonials, and simultaneously is supported by pharmaceutical donations or advertising.

Anxiety: www.anxietybc.com
• Has an excellent free set of videos, an app, and newsletters and more. One of the best!

Mood disorders:
• There are research and support groups in many countries including the National Institute of Mental Health

287

in the USA (www.nimh.nih.gov/health/topics/depression) and the Mood Disorders Association of Canada (www.mooddisorderscanada.ca).

SLD: Learning Disability Association of America: www.ldanatl.org, www.ldonline.org

Trichotillomania: www.trich.org

NICE clinical guidelines for the UK (www.nice.org.uk) include bipolar disorder (CG185, 2014), depression in children and young people (CG28, 2005), and depression in adults (CG90, 2009).

APPENDIX 4
Publications of the *TIC* Consortium

Fiala O, Růžička (2002) International database of Tourette syndrome: pilot study of the project in Czech Republic. *Homeostasis* 41: 146–51.

Freeman RD, Fast DK, Burd L, et al. (2000) An international perspective on Tourette syndrome: selected findings from 3500 individuals in 22 countries. *Dev Med Child Neurol* 42: 436–47.

Freeman RD, Fast DK, Burd L, et al. (2001) An international perspective on Tourette syndrome: reply. *Dev Med Child Neurol* 43: 428–9 (letter).

Burd L, Freeman RD, Klug MG, Kerbeshian J (2005) Tourette syndrome and learning disabilities. *BMC Pediatr* 5: 34.

Burd L, Freeman RD, Klug MG, Kerbeshian J (2006) Variables associated with increased tic severity in 5,500 participants with Tourette syndrome. *J Dev Phys Disabil* 128: 13–24.

Pringsheim T, Freeman R, Lang A (2007) Tourette syndrome and dystonia. *J Neurol Neurosurg Psychiatry* 78: 544.

Freeman RD (2007) Tic disorders and ADHD: answers from a world-wide clinical dataset on Tourette syndrome. Tourette Syndrome International Database Consortium. *Eur Child Adolesc Psychiatry* 16 (Suppl 1): 15–23.

Roessner V, Becker A, Banaschewski T, et al. (2007) Developmental psychopathology of children and adolescents with Tourette syndrome – impact of ADHD. Tourette Syndrome International Database Consortium. *Eur Child Adolesc Psychiatry* 16 (Suppl 1): 24–35.

Freeman RD, Zinner S, Müller-Vahl K, et al. (2008) Coprophenomena in Tourette syndrome. *Dev Med Child Neurol* 51: 218–27.

Burd L, Li Q, Kerbeshian J, et al. (2009) Tourette syndrome and comorbid pervasive developmental disorders. *J Child Neurol* 24: 170–5.

Freeman RD, Soltanifar A, Baer S (2010) Stereotypic movement disorder: easily missed. *Dev Med Child Neurol* 52: 733–8.

Wanderer S, Roessner V, Freeman RD, et al. (2012) Relationship of obsessive–compulsive disorder to age-related comorbidity in children and adolescents with Tourette disorder. *J Dev Behav Pediatr* 33: 124–33.

APPENDIX 5
Stereotypy Severity Scale

Name _____ Date _____ 201 ___

Number	0	None
	1	Single stereotypy
	2	2–5 discrete stereotypies
	3	>5 discrete stereotypies

Frequency	0	Never	
	1	Rare	Not daily
	2	Occasional	Daily, but infrequent
	3	Frequent	Daily, multiple times per day
	4	Very frequent	Virtually every hour
	5	Always	Few if any, stereotypy-free intervals

Intensity	0	Absent	
	1	Minimal	Minimally forceful compared to voluntary actions and not visible
	2	Mild	Not more forceful than comparable voluntary actions and not usually noticed
	3	Moderate	More forceful than comparable voluntary actions and call attention to individual
	4	Marked	More forceful than comparable voluntary actions, exaggerated, and call attention
	5	Severe	Extremely forceful and exaggerated, call attention, may cause physical injury

Interference	0	None	
	1	Minimal	Stereotypies do not interrupt flow of behavior
	2	Mild	Stereotypies occasionally interrupt flow of behavior
	3	Moderate	Stereotypies frequently interrupt flow of behavior
	4	Marked	Frequently interrupt flow of behavior and occasionally disrupt intended action
	5	Severe	Stereotypies frequently disrupt intended action

Global Impairment Rating	0	None	
	10	Minimal	Associated with subtle difficulties in self-esteem, family, school, or social acceptance
	20	Mild	Associated with minor problems in self-esteem, family, school, or social acceptance
	30	Moderate	Associated with clear problems in self-esteem, family, school, or social acceptance
	40	Marked	Associated with major difficulties in self-esteem, family, school, or social acceptance
	50	Severe	Associated with extreme difficulties in self-esteem, family, and severely restricted life because of social stigma and school avoidance

Score = _____

(Total score maximum = 68)

From Miller et al. (2006), modified from Yale Global Tic Severity Scale (reprinted with permission of Harvey Singer, MD, and Sage Publications).

REFERENCE

Miller JM, Singer HS, Bridges DD, Waranch HR (2006) Behavioral therapy for treatment of stereotypic movements in nonautistic children. *J Child Neurol* 21: 119–25. doi: 10.1177/08830738060210020701.

APPENDIX 6
Stereotypic Movement Disorder — a Primer for Teachers

What is stereotypic movement disorder?

You may have a child in your class you're concerned about because he or she engages in unusual repetitive behavior such as arm-flapping, pacing, jumping, bouncing, finger or hand manipulations, or whole-body tensing, for no obvious reason. This can look odd, be quite intense, and the child typically cannot satisfactorily explain it. Furthermore, the activity may interfere with joining in the transition from one activity to another. The child can be brought out of the pattern by calling his or her name or perhaps a touch. Soon, however, the pattern will be repeated. The child probably is doing reasonably well academically, in spite of the pattern, but other children are noticing or asking about it, and you or other staff are wondering whether the child should have an assessment, specifically for an autism spectrum disorder, where early intervention is said to be very important, or for other conditions such as Tourette syndrome or epilepsy.

When brought to the attention of a parent, they will typically be well aware of it, and the child may have already been assessed (or such is planned). The parent is likely to express concern about future social teasing or ostracism. (Sometimes they may assert that the behavior is not important or is improving.)

Such motor patterns are common in very young children but in the cases discussed here it does not subside. It may even increase in frequency and intensity when the child first enters school. The child is not distressed and the parent may even say that it is pleasurable for the child, appearing especially with excitement.

You probably know little or nothing about stereotypic patterns because there is little education about it, and what there is, is confusing. Repetitive motor patterns (often with some vocalization accompanying it) can link with, and enhance, fantasy and imagination. (From the child's perspective, then, the pattern is positive, unlike the reaction of parents or teachers.) Young children do not yet have good inhibitory powers to enable them to limit such behavior to socially desirable situations or privacy. SMD is not by itself diagnostic of anything, though; it can be seen in children with typical development, in blind children, or in children with autism, intellectual disability, obsessive–compulsive disorder, Tourette syndrome, and some forms of genetic disorder or brain damage. In some instances it may be self-injurious (e.g. self-hitting or -biting). Thus, stereotypic behavior can be a symptom of some disorder or exist on its own, then known as stereotypic movement disorder if it causes some interference. Many of the children are highly imaginative and bright. (To complicate matters further, SMD can co-exist with tics.)

The usual course

SMD usually becomes more private as the child's social awareness and self-regulation improve, but it may be continued in private, where it typically causes no problems. Such behavior tends to run in families, though a parent who engaged in it may not mention their own pattern. The problem posed by SMD is that privatization requires years of socialization and development of self-control, so that it can't be expected to subside quickly. In a minority of individuals who engage in the pattern it may take up too much time and cause concern, but we do not yet know how common this is. In such situations a form of behavior therapy may be useful, but it will be important to specify what the level of impairment actually is. Evidence-based information on therapy is still sparse and there are few experienced therapists. However, interest is increasing and more helpful information is expected to be available in the future.

Explaining to a class

Unless the SMD is causing direct interference with activities or with other children physically (as from swinging their arms around when close to others), the issue becomes: do I need to explain anything to other children or school staff? Do I need permission to do so from the parents? Sooner or later your class may need an explanation in simple terms, with parental permission, because the pattern has been noticed, causes questions, enters others' personal space, or sometimes interferes with classroom routines. There is no agreed-upon explanation. One could say that everyone is different, and when this child is excited or imagining things, he or she flaps their arms (or whatever movement pattern they exhibit). If in fact the child in question swings their arms around and by accident sometimes hits a classmate, you could suggest giving the child some extra space and assure them that the hitting is not on purpose. (If you don't exert some control over that, other parents may complain.)

APPENDIX 7
Comments on the American Practice Parameters on Tic Disorders (Murphy et al. 2013)

Publication of these parameters is a significant advance. Because of their importance, a few points should be noted.

Vocal/phonic. These descriptors are confused, sometimes used interchangeably, at other times separately. 'Simple vocal/phonic tics' include grunting, sniffing, snorting, throat-clearing, humming, coughing, barking or screaming. 'Complex vocal/phonic tics' can be words out of context, a good point, but some individuals without tics also use repetitive phrases that are meaningless and thus 'out of context' such as "you know".

Stereotypies are given more discussion in this article than almost anywhere else, the frequent difficulty differentiating them from tics is stressed, and accompanying facial grimacing is noted, but vocalization or phonic noises occur in stereotypies as well as in tics; only repetitive speech is noted. No mention is made of stereotypies in blindness. Lack of premonitory urges is asserted without evidence and is debatable, but privatization over time is omitted.

Tics in neurologic diseases or conditions. A good point that is made is that it is rare for tics to be the only manifestation of a neurologic disease.

Clinical course. The authors omit one aspect of this: adult reduction or remission is characterized by increased *stability*, not just reduction in number, frequency or force of tics.

Aggravating factors. Although heat is mentioned as exacerbating tics and referenced by one publication, this is doubtful and is not commonly seen in patients.

Rage/anger control problems. The prevalence cited in our study (37%) (Freeman et al. 2000) is unfortunately misrepresented. The point missed is that such problems are common in TS+ but not in TS-only (anger control problem history in 10%, at registration only 5%), and that of all behavior patterns studied these problems have the strongest positive correlation with comorbidity score.

REFERENCES

Freeman RD, Fast DK, Burd L, et al. (2000) An international perspective on Tourette syndrome: selected findings from 3500 individuals in 22 countries. *Dev Med Child Neurol* 42: 436–7. doi: 10.1111/j.1469-8749.2000.tb00346.x.

Murphy TK, Lewin AB, Storch EA, et al. (2013) Practice parameter for the assessment and treatment of children and adolescents with tic disorders. *J Am Acad Child Adolesc Psychiatry* 52: 1341–59. doi: 10.1016/j.jaac.2013.09.015.

INDEX

Page numbers in *italics* refer to material in case examples/studies; page numbers in **bold** refer to material in tables. Abbreviations used: ADHD, attention-deficit/hyperactivity disorder; CBIT, Comprehensive Behavioral Intervention for Tics; CHADD, Children and Adults with Attention-Deficit/Hyperactivity Disorder; DAMP, disorders of attention, motor control and perception; DSM, *Diagnostic and Statistical Manual of Mental Disorders*; DSM-III-R, *DSM, Version 3, Revised*; DSM-IV-TR, *DSM Version 4, Text Revision*; ESSENCE, early symptomatic syndromes eliciting neurodevelopmental clinical examinations; OCD, obsessive–compulsive disorder; ODD, oppositional–defiant disorder; PANDAS, pediatric autoimmune neuropsychiatric disorders associated with streptococcal infections; SSRIs, selective serotonin reuptake inhibitors.

New titles from Mac Keith Press www.mackeith.co.uk

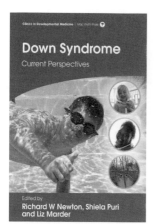

Down Syndrome: Current Perspectives
Richard W Newton, Shiela Puri, and Liz Marder (Editors)

Clinics in Developmental Medicine
2015 ▪ 320pp ▪ hardback ▪ 978-1-909962-38-5
£95.00 / €118.00 / $150.00

Down syndrome remains the most common recognisable form of intellectual disability. The challenge for doctors today is how to capture the rapidly expanding body of scientific knowledge and devise models of care to meet the needs of individuals and their families. *Down syndrome; Clinical Perspectives* provides doctors and other health professionals with the information they need to address the challenges that can present in the management of syndrome.

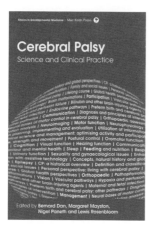

Cerebral Palsy: Science and Clinical Practice
Bernard Dan, Margaret Mayston, Nigel Paneth and Lewis Rosenbloom (Editors)

Clinics in Developmental Medicine
2014 ▪ 712pp ▪ hardback ▪ 978-1-909962-38-5
£190.00 / €235.80 / $299.95

The only complete, scientifically rigorous, fully integrated reference giving a wide ranging and in-depth perspective on cerebral palsy and related neurodevelopment disabilities. It considers all aspects of cerebral palsy from the causes to clinical problems and their implications for individuals. Leading scientists present the evidence on the role of pre-term birth, inflammation, hypoxia, endocrinological and other pathways. They explore opportunities for neuroprotection leading to clinical applications.

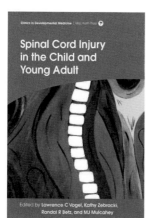

Spinal Cord Injury in the Child and Young Adult
Lawrence C Vogel, Kathy Zebracki, Randall R Betz and MJ Mulcahey (Editors)

Clinics in Developmental Medicine
2014 ▪ 460pp ▪ hardback ▪ 978-1-909962-34-7
£125.00 / €155.10 / $206.50

Compared to adult-onset spinal cord injury (SCI), individuals with childhood-onset SCI are unique in several ways. First, as a result of their younger age at injury and longer lifespan, individuals with pediatric-onset SCI are particularly susceptible to long-term complications related to a sedentary lifestyle. This book is intended for clinicians of all disciplines who may only occasionally care for young people with SCI to those who specialize in SCI as well as clinical and basic researchers in the SCI field.
.